C0-AWE-482

NORM DIFFUSION AND HIV/AIDS GOVERNANCE IN
PUTIN'S RUSSIA AND MBEKI'S SOUTH AFRICA

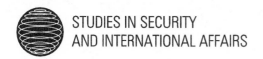

STUDIES IN SECURITY AND INTERNATIONAL AFFAIRS

SERIES EDITORS

William W. Keller
Professor of International Affairs, Center for International Trade and Security, University of Georgia

Scott A. Jones
Director of Export Control Programs, Center for International Trade and Security, University of Georgia

SERIES ADVISORY BOARD

Pauline H. Baker
The Fund for Peace

Eliot Cohen
Paul H. Nitze School of Advanced International Studies, Johns Hopkins University

Eric Einhorn
Center for Public Policy and Administration, University of Massachusetts, Amherst

John J. Hamre
The Center for Strategic and International Studies

Josef Joffe
Hoover Institution, Institute for International Studies, Stanford University

Lawrence J. Korb
Center for American Progress

William J. Long
Sam Nunn School of International Affairs, Georgia Institute of Technology

Jessica Tuchman Mathews
Carnegie Endowment for International Peace

Scott D. Sagan
Center for International Security and Cooperation, Stanford University

Lawrence Scheinman
Monterey Institute of International Studies, CNS-WDC

David Shambaugh
The Elliott School of International Affairs, George Washington University

Jessica Stern
FXB *Center, Harvard School of Public Health*

Norm Diffusion and HIV/AIDS Governance in Putin's Russia and Mbeki's South Africa

Vlad Kravtsov

The University of Georgia Press
Athens and London

RA
643.86
.R8
K73
2015

© 2015 by the University of Georgia Press
Athens, Georgia 30602
www.ugapress.org
All rights reserved
Set in 10/14 Minion Pro by Graphic Composition, Inc., Bogart, Georgia
Printed and bound by Sheridan Books
The paper in this book meets the guidelines for
permanence and durability of the Committee on
Production Guidelines for Book Longevity of the
Council on Library Resources.

Most University of Georgia Press titles are
available from popular e-book vendors.

Printed in the United States of America
19 18 17 16 15 C 5 4 3 2 1

Library of Congress Cataloging-in-Publication Data

Kravtsov, Vlad, author.
 Norm diffusion and HIV/AIDS governance in Putin's Russia and Mbeki's South Africa /
Vlad Kravtsov.
        p. ; cm. — (Studies in security and international affairs)
    Includes bibliographical references and index.
    ISBN 978-0-8203-4799-8 (hardcover : alk. paper) — ISBN 978-0-8203-4833-9 (e-book)
    I. Title. II. Series: Studies in security and international affairs.
    [DNLM: 1. Acquired Immunodeficiency Syndrome—Russia (Federation) 2. Acquired
Immunodeficiency Syndrome—South Africa. 3. HIV Infections—Russia (Federation) 4. HIV
Infections—South Africa. 5. Health Policy—Russia (Federation) 6. Health Policy—South Africa.
7. Health Services Accessibility—organization & administration—Russia (Federation) 8. Health
Services Accessibility—organization & administration—South Africa. WC 503]
    RA643.86.R8
    362.19697'9200947—dc23

                                                                            2014038948

British Library Cataloging-in-Publication Data available

CONTENTS

University Libraries
Carnegie Mellon University
Pittsburgh, PA 15213-3890

PREFACE

The porosity of current political borders does not always promote normative congruence across political spaces. Paradoxically, in the age of increased global connectivity, domestic anxieties over normative intrusions from abroad do not disappear. On the contrary, all too many politicians sense that norm diffusion threatens the ideas and sensibilities on which these politicians' authority is premised. They try to push back against external influences and defend the methods of governance they are comfortable with. This book analyzes two interesting instances of these anxieties and explores their consequences for norm diffusion and for the performance of domestic governance systems. I reach deep into the constructivist toolshed to develop an adequate analytic framework and use HIV/AIDS as an issue area to investigate systems of governance empirically.

This book is the result of a long journey, both academic and personal. I wish to express my immense gratitude for the unwavering support and friendship of my mentors Audie Klotz, Brian Taylor, and Roger Coate. I am very grateful for the advice, comments, questions, suggestions, reminders, corrections, and criticisms given by Hongying Wang, Mark Rupert, Michael Bosia, Andrew London, Linda Cook, Oxana Shavel, Tim Shaw, and Elena Dmitrieva. I thank Chris Jones, Marion Orr, and Dmitry Gorenbug for the opportunity to test some of my ideas in front of graduate students at Northern Illinois University, during a speaker series at Brown University, and during a post-Communism seminar at Harvard University, respectively. Matt Hoffman, Mark Miller, Marian Palley, and Dan Green were helpful for sustaining my early interest in the topic in particular and in political science in general. Without Jim Rosenau and Roger Coate my intellectual journey would not have even started. My friends and colleagues—Asli Ilgit, Deepa Prakash, Eric Rittenger, Chan Woong Shin, Jooyoun Lee, and Matt Walton—wherever your careers bring you, thank you for stimulating me to push my inquiry further. Without Irina Chechel's and Aleksandr Shatilov's insights, my understanding of current Russia would have been incomplete. All of you challenged me intellectually. Here is my ninety-thousand-word response to that challenge. I also greatly benefited from the thoroughgoing analysis of my text by two anonymous reviewers.

I thank Julia Ruman for the support and distraction she has been offering so generously.

A necessary note is on transliteration of Russian names into the Latin script. I chose to use the United States Board on Geographic Names and the Permanent Committee on Geographical Names for British Official Use (BGN/PCGN 1947 System). This system provides a simple way for romanization of the Russian alphabet. It has no special letters to represent distinct Russian sounds; it is intuitive to read and pronounce. I follow this system thoroughly, although I also use simplified transliterations of Russian names and surnames when doing so is conventionally accepted. All translations are mine unless indicated otherwise.

ABBREVIATIONS

AIDS	acquired immunodeficiency syndrome
ANC	African National Congress
ARVS	antiretrovirals
ATM	African traditional medicines
AZT	azidothymidine (zidovudine)
COSATU	Congress of South African Trade Unions
DST	Department of Science and Technology (South Africa)
FSKN	Federal Drug Control Service of the Russian Federation
GAK	State Antinarcotics Committee
GAP	Global AIDS Programme (WHO)
GBC	Global Business Coalition on HIV/AIDS, Tuberculosis and Malaria
GFATM	Global Fund to Fight AIDS, Tuberculosis and Malaria
GMP	good manufacturing practices
HAART	highly active antiretroviral therapy
HIV	human immunodeficiency virus
IKS	indigenous knowledge system
ITPC	International Treatment Preparedness Coalition
KFF	Kaiser Family Foundation
MCC	Medicines Control Council (South Africa)
Minekonomrazvitiya	Ministry of Economic Development of the Russian Federation
Minpromtorg	Ministry of Industry and Trade of the Russian Federation
MRC	Medical Research Council (South Africa)
NAPWA	National Association of People Living with AIDS (South Africa)
NEC	National Executive Council (South Africa)
NEDLAC	National Economic Development and Labour Council
NEPAD	New Economic Partnership for African Development
NGO	Nongovernmental Organization
NIH	National Institute of Health

NPPS	National Priority Projects
OHI	Open Health Institute (Russia)
OST	opioid substitution therapy
PEPFAR	President's Emergency Plan for AIDS Relief
PhRMA	Pharmaceutical Researchers and Manufacturers of America
PLWA	People Living with AIDS
Rosminzdrav	The Ministry of Health of the Russian Federation
Rosnano	Russian Corporation of Nanotechnologies
Rospotrebnadzor	Russian Federal Service for Surveillance on Consumer Rights Protection and Human Well-Being
Rostekhnologii	Russian Technologies State Corporation
Roszdravnadzor	Federal Service on Surveillance in Health Care
RSPP	Russian Union of Industrialists and Entrepreneurs
SANAC	South African National AIDS Council
SANCO	South African National Civil Organization
SCMS	Supply Chain Managements System
SEP	syringe exchange programs
TAC	Treatment Action Campaign
THO	Traditional Healers Organisation of South Africa
TPAA	Transatlantic Partners against AIDS
UNAIDS	Joint United Nations Programme on HIV and AIDS
UNGASS	United Nations General Assembly Special Session
USAID	The United States Agency for International Development
WHO	World Health Organization
WIPO	World Intellectual Property Organization
WTO	World Trade Organization

Introduction

The experience of the nineties demonstrates that the successful renewal of our country . . . cannot be achieved by moving abstract models and schemes drawn from foreign textbooks to Russian soil. Mechanical copying of other states' experience does not lead to success. Every country, including Russia, must find its own way to renewal.
— Vladimir Putin, "Rossiya na rubezhe tysyacheletiy" (Russia at the turn of the millennium), *Nezavisimaya Gazeta*, December 30, 1999

It is obvious that whatever lessons we have to and may draw from the West about the grave issue of HIV-AIDS, a simple superimposition of Western experience on African reality would be absurd and illogical. Such proceeding would constitute a criminal betrayal of our responsibility to our own people.
— Thabo Mbeki, "Letter to the World Leaders," a handwritten letter leaked to the *Washington Post*, April 3, 2000

VLADIMIR PUTIN AND THABO MBEKI regarded many global norms with suspicion. At the very least, as indicated in the two epigraphs that open this chapter, the two presidents shied away from any external norms, policies, or ideas that did not fit the essential (or essentialized, to be precise) features of their polities. Few, if any, foreign ideas met Russian needs, claimed Putin. Spreading without control, observed Mbeki, Western norms portended social misfortunes. Not surprisingly, resistance to international influences went hand in hand with a steadily growing devotion to localized principles of governance that Russians and South Africans applied to a variety of social practices, including public health. As it turned out, apprehension of external norms impelled these two leaders to undermine good health governance.

Although in the past Putin had been careful not to endorse any reactionary ideas, he made it explicitly clear that no changes in domestic affairs should arrive from abroad. He nourished domestic insecurities about the harmful influences of nonterritorial and foreign actors on domestic affairs. He endorsed conservative values that justified Russia's normative self-sufficiency. The more one ransacks the entire corpus of domestic political discourse, the clearer it becomes that similar hidebound sensibilities had come to be preponderant among the country's top politicians, opinion leaders, and the public. As a result, while not any external norm is now likely to carom off the Kremlin, the possibilities of what might be up for adoption are reduced considerably. How do we best conceptualize and explain Russian concerns about external recommendations and the newly acquired preference for alternative, localized policy solutions?

Contrary to conventional wisdom, Russia's diminishing willingness to recognize the validity of external norms is perplexing. Following Mikhail Gorbachev's ill-fated perestroika, post-Communist reformers had been looking outside the country in earnest hopes of finding practical governance models. External ideas, whether misunderstood or not, gained some purchase in Russia during the 1990s. A decade later, external norms, principles, and ideas would stand trial. That incompetent bureaucrats and inept politicians did not use the available external advice appropriately is apparent. But the participants in the intensifying political debates exonerated those individuals whose poor record of governance was not associated with a fondness for external assistance. Acceptance of external norms, on the contrary, became widely viewed as a social offense. Why is that so?

Conventional arguments that underscore the immutability of Russian statism and its evergreen mistrust of the outside world are insufficient and unsatisfying. They are also misleading, because they uncritically reify the isolationism inherent in Russian culture and decouple normative predispositions from the ongoing processes of social and transborder communications. Thinking afresh, therefore, requires a scholar to ponder both the current reasons of positing the state as the ultimate locus of authority and the evolving communicative structures that sustain intersubjective consensus about the nature of political authority at home. It is reasonable to postulate that the interpretation of the nature of external normative challenges depends on domestic ideational commitments. Changes in the global order often encourage previously disempowered social groups and constrain the obdurate defenders of statism. They also summon governments to reinvent the normative foundations of the state authority. Thus, it is worthwhile to explore the proposition that Russian anxiety about normative intrusions from abroad may very well stem from intersubjective commitments to achieve the state's consciously designed goals. In this, Russia is hardly unique.

The story in South Africa equally defies an easy explanation as to what the state wanted from internationally accepted norms and best practices. The current South African elite came to power aided by external coercive and normative influences.[1] Thabo Mbeki's seemingly Westernized identity, projected by his pipe, scotch, impeccable attire, and penchant for Victorian poetry, was superficial. More telling was his distaste for the "false knowledge" that he believed emanated from the colonizing West and jeopardized the country's healthy beginnings.[2] Reflecting on his central preoccupations near the end of his presidency, Mbeki proudly acknowledged that he had striven to "defend, uphold and promote our culture in the face of strong encroachments of alien cultures some of which seek deliberately to destroy our indigenous cultures."[3] These arresting words were more than an isolated outburst that simply vented his own insecurities; they captured confluent sentiments of rectitude and anxiety that had taken hold of a significant portion of the South African elite, if not of the whole country.

These sentiments are hardly intuitive. They are a definitive reversal of the earlier orientations, such as human rights and democracy promotion, that characterized Nelson Mandela's presidency. Mbeki is no Mandela; that much is clear. As the "globalist" generation wanes, South Africa has gradually relieved itself from a devotion to taxing external norms and has replaced them with locally crafted standards of appropriateness.[4] But even within the same generation, various normative orientations overlap and evolve, and thus similar experiences might not culminate in identical conventional wisdoms. Mbeki, for instance, displayed outlooks that belonged to different generations. He espoused the globalist value of market-centered society, commercialism, and technological determinism, and yet he resuscitated the Africanist stress on heritage and precolonial values as the instruments of transformation.[5] Thus, to understand the origins and implications of South African conventional wisdom, it is necessary to offer an innovative explanatory strategy.

In the two countries under investigation here, politicians aroused fears that the external world intruded in the domestic spheres of authority at the very moment when norm diffusion and policy transfer became pervasive and ordinary features of transboundary exchanges and international interactions. Contrary to Russians and South Africans, many politicians across the globe became accustomed to the idea that external decisions, practices, and recommendations could benefit them. Indeed, there are many successful examples of adopting norms that resulted in small-scale policy fixes. Moreover, many states found it useful to adopt a variety of external approaches not just to solve some narrow policy problems at home but also to alter the underlying features of doing policy business as usual. We know a lot about how prominent leaders and norm entrepreneurs import ideas and policies from elsewhere, but the question persists: How do we investigate clashes between international practices and domestic normative structures when we have strong reasons to expect conflicts of this kind to happen? Because we cannot simply infer norms from behavior, it is sensible to begin an inquiry by studying underlying normative orders and legitimate social purposes separately from policy-making behavior.

From the theoretical vantage point, the social purpose of the state is essential because it is, together with coercive material power, an indispensable component of a full political authority.[6] For the purposes of clarity, I will stick to the definition of coercive power as an elite's capability to enforce compliance, commit resources, and limit the discretion of other domestic groups to act on their own. Critical scholars who preoccupy themselves with the everything-is-power argument might insist that the distinction between material and ideational powers is bogus, but conflating coercive powers and intellectual commitments is not a good way to conceptualize the structure of political authority.

Social purposes become observable when state rulers and opinion leaders decide to rethink the nature of political authority. Decisions to do so are rather common in emergent states that have to cope with transitional crises. Russia's Putin and South Africa's Mbeki are prime examples of posttransitional leaders who envisioned and upheld a constellation of original ideas that in due course defined the nature of political authority at home. As political leaders settled on a set of specific ideational commitments, domestic opinion leaders led conceptual debates about the essential goals of the state, and their audiences eventually internalized these goals as normal and self-evident. Domestic discussions matter a great deal, because these debates may lift a promulgated set of ideas to the status of reasons for actions and, conversely, destroy the social appeal of other ideas. Depending upon their substance, social purposes can provoke interest in the indiscriminate adoption of external norms, trigger hostility to them, or adopt some of them on a selective basis. To pursue these insights further requires a thorough inquiry that probes the analytical potency of the concept of social purpose. This is the main theoretical task of this book.

OUTLINING THE ARGUMENT

Substantively, the book explores systems of AIDS governance in Russia and South Africa. To discern and analyze a coherent system of governance is to find answers to three interrelated sets of questions.[7] The first set of questions should inquire how governments understand a matter of public concern. Accordingly, chapter 4 reveals how the state frames the nature of the epidemic (is the contagion a public health crisis, a security issue, or something entirely different?) and then chooses the available biomedical tools to address such a challenge. The second set of questions should examine the core set of activities that governments undertake in order to solve the issue. Chapter 5, therefore, focuses on governmental action to remove obstacles to evidence-based prevention services and ensure universal access to proven life-saving medicines. The third set of questions should probe how states interact with the other participants in social practice. Chapter 6 discusses how governments choose health policy partners among the plethora of domestic stakeholders and what kind of limits the state imposes—or seeks to impose—on these actors' behavior and their objectives. In addition, it investigates how the state chooses to interact with the existing international health architecture or, conversely, decides to influence and change it. Structured, focused comparisons of these core aspects of health governance in the two countries organize the flow of the story. By tackling these questions, this book explains how, why, and to what extent the two transitional countries under investigation groped for alternative approaches to AIDS governance and justified their value and utility.

The short version of my central line of argument is as follows. The outbreak of HIV/AIDS (human immunodeficiency virus / acquired immunodeficiency syndrome) has forced governments to play an aggressive role in the control of the disease. Much as the spread of HIV/AIDS does not stop at the political borders we see on the map, ideas about how to respond to the virus transcend governmental purviews. International actors spread functional standards for health practices, but deeply embedded into these standards are particular conventions and organizing principles of governance that go beyond technical information of a nonethical, practical origin. Although there is a considerable diversity in the principles and norms that exist in the global realm, the ones that currently underlie standardized practices of health governance are Western in origin and liberal in nature. Put differently, they are expressions of global liberal governmentality.[8] When these organizing principles impinge on the normative dimension of domestic political authority, politicians are likely to revolt against external recommendations.

After all, when domestic actors become confident that only their (local) standards for behavior are just and right, which is certainly the case with Putin's Russia and Mbeki's South Africa, those actors shrink back from external principles of governance. Hence, in Russia and South Africa, while leaders recognized the validity of some health-related recommendations and best practices, they often failed to appreciate the underpinnings of those recommendations. Many factors could have contributed to this outcome, but ideas about the core goals of the state—the normative foundation of domestic authority—along with pledges to uphold them were most consequential. These ideas became reasons for action; they determined both leaders' point of reference concerning the appropriate social practices and their orientation toward the external organizing principles of AIDS governance. The content of these domestic ideas was not random. It materialized as a response to Russia's and South Africa's ontological need to renovate the nature of political authority at home, a task that was more than necessary after the decline of power and legitimacy that buried preceding political regimes in both countries. In summary, social purposes encompassed specific ideas that shaped the process of adopting external norms.

Next, I provide a more explicit definition of the international standards for health governance and offer a concise outline of the HIV policies that leaders of both countries under investigation implemented. Internationally, there are three main standards that describe good AIDS governance. First, although curbing HIV/AIDS requires a variety of health interventions (such as educational campaigns, prevention, etc.), governments should approach the contagion as a public health crisis and use conventional antiretroviral medicines invented to suppress the virus replication. Failure to address the spread of HIV as a matter of public health is a sign that a government is trying to fulfill objectives that might be at odds with internationally agreed-upon principles of health governance. Second, governments should ensure extensive access to the medicines and remove legal barriers to prevention services. Although the truly universal coverage of all those who qualify for antiretrovirals from the medical standpoint is not yet possible, governments should scale up treatment and underwrite HIV-related programs. That treatment is a matter of the public good and that prevention strategies should not violate human rights are now broadly understood as two interrelated principles that buttress the second dimension of AIDS governance.

Third, the state—undeniably the primary actor in health governance—should involve all key stakeholders, both international and domestic, in policy formulation and implementation. Undergirding the third guideline is the organizing principle of nonhierarchical and nonstate governance. Simply put, tight governmental control over all policy participants should be abolished so that the plurality of various societal actors can meaningfully participate in health governance.

The outline that follows gives a brief description of HIV-related policies in Russia and South Africa. The intention is to emphasize the internal coherence of policy-making behavior and the interdependence of various parts of either country's AIDS governance strategies. Further empirical observations are presented in the relevant chapters where they belong.

The Russian government framed the outbreak of AIDS as a health problem linked to dwindling demographic security, an issue that was ominous for the state. Law enforcement agents (known as *siloviki*), joined by the conservative functionaries of the Russian Orthodox Church, captured the policy debate on HIV/AIDS and influenced that debate to fit their skewed ideas. Importantly, they deemed the outbreak of the epidemic of HIV as secondary to the scourge of heroin consumption. The heavy emphasis on the war against drugs, led by the *siloviki* and conservative opinion leaders, undermined the urgency of addressing HIV as a pressing public health issue. At the same time, Russian officials resisted the idea that prevention services such as needle exchanges and opioid substitute treatments commonly referred to as harm reduction were normal and effective. Instead, because harm reduction rested on the principles of human rights, which the Kremlin came to view as subversive and inappropriate, the state intentionally erected barriers to providing prevention services for drug addicts. Since injecting drug users drove the spread of the epidemic, dismissing an effective method of mitigating HIV did more harm than good.

The official rhetoric lionized the state and downplayed the needs of vulnerable individuals. Insofar as Moscow embraced the ideas of the developmental state and its social responsibility to provide for its populace, the government increased public spending for HIV-related programs and strived to implement a working system of purchasing and distributing antiretroviral medications. But the limited administrative capacity of the state machinery exacerbated the negative externalities that emerged out of the state's overextended obligations. Not surprisingly, although state officials accepted the validity of the evidence-based medications, recurring failures to sustain the standardized protocol across the country's many regions were unstoppable.

The Kremlin's lessening tolerance for the civil society's activity, inherently antithetical to the values of statism, went hand in hand with the government's diminishing respect for international health organizations and transnational health actors that seemingly encroached on the external sovereignty of Putin's state. The officialdom was no longer interested in sustaining either internal or transboundary partnerships in response to AIDS. To weave domestic stakeholders into the state-dominated hierarchy of social relations, Russian politicians used both the carrot of generous state funding and the stick of punitive laws, thereby reducing the autonomy of the fledgling civil society. That funding promise was fulfilled, but most of the money was directed to nourish predominantly those conservative nonstate actors that had no record of external funding and no ambition to challenge Moscow's ways of governing.

Finally, to cultivate the idea of Russia as a great power and to exercise tight control over nonstate actors, the government chose to refuse international health assistance. This move allowed the Kremlin not only to shore up its identity as a transformative global leader but also to cut domestic civil society from important sources of external support. As Moscow obsessively chased the status of a global power in the international system, Russian leaders nurtured unrealistic ambitions to develop a number of evidence-based innovative drugs. But, given the numerous debilitating shortcomings that plague the health-care sector and industrial prerequisites that do not match the manufacturing standards and capacities of major global pharmaceutical firms, neither ambition—global health leadership or competitive drug manufacturing—is likely to come to fruition.

On the other side of the globe, instead of addressing the contagion as a public health crisis, Pretoria reframed HIV/AIDS as an issue that supported an emphasis on fostering local knowledge and enhancing local development. The president and his ministers supported alternative medicines and indigenous healing practices and questioned the utility of the standard evidence-based medications. As Pretoria's commitment to indigenous knowledge systems solidified, the Cabinet empowered, sometimes tacitly and sometimes explicitly, AIDS dissidents, traditional healers, peddlers of fake cures, and a variety of nutritionists. To secure their newly found predilection for medical pluralism, key officials sought to undermine the competencies of the mainstream domestic AIDS bureaucracy and paralyze its abilities to act independently.

In order to avoid undesirable expenditures, Pretoria flatly resisted the universal and free rollout of essential HIV drugs. As South African politicians

stressed market-centered empowerment and expressed their aversion to redistribution, they challenged the need to ensure extensive access to antiretrovirals in
the public health sector. Pretoria sought to protect the private sector from sharing the burden of health governance. Investments in HIV-related programs remained low. At the same time, insofar as prevention involved human rights principles, the orientation to remove legal barriers to prevention bore some fruit.
Simply put, the Cabinet was not ready to recognize treatment as a public good
but was well prepared to excoriate the advocates of treatment as the leading "detractors" of South African transformation.

Finally, Pretoria's commitment to exercise moral leadership on the continent prompted the country's leaders to challenge the authority of international
organizations, welcome the counterepistemic community of AIDS dissidents,
and tout the transformative role of traditional medicines. Pretoria picked a
rhetorical fight against the predatory pharmaceutical industry, which was seen
as yet another transmitter of global neocolonialism. But that self-righteous
obsession paralyzed the Cabinet's interest in using the available mechanisms
of international trade to secure the supply of high-quality generics. Adopting
generic drugs, the cheaper versions of brand-name pharmaceutical products
with expired or waived patents, was not a priority for Mbeki and his acolytes
anyway.

When dealing with international AIDS-related norms, both countries exhibited a peculiar combination of behaviors that cannot be easily explained, even
though, for any keen observer of Russian and South African domestic politics,
these behaviors might seem vaguely in line with the overall political orientations. On the pages that ensue, I argue that the Kremlin's responses to the international recommendations regarding AIDS control emerged from a conceptual
conflict between a rapidly maturing illiberal statism as a main component of
Russia's social purpose and those organizing principles of health governance that
were gaining momentum internationally. Pretoria's responses to international
AIDS norms were consistent with the predominant ideas regarding the indigenous and inward-looking renewal of the state circulating in South Africa. Although, from an empirical standpoint, there are multiple significant differences
between the two cases, they both illustrate the larger argument about the outcomes of norm diffusion when localized ideas about the core tasks of the state
crystallize at home. The section that follows unpacks the concept of the social
purpose as the main explanatory variable.

DEFINING THE SOCIAL PURPOSE OF THE STATE

Scholars remain all too comfortable using the notion of social purposes in its intuitive sense. Any state goal not reducible to private gains, such as the redistribution of wealth, a large public sector, and governmental intervention, can loosely typify the social purpose of the state. Sometimes this intuitive grasp of social purposes supports an empirical analysis of the unfolding processes of governance. Surely there are many legitimate and actionable ideas that float freely in a given political space, but ideas turn into social purposes only when these ideas are treated as justifications for the existence of the state. Because ideas are handled here as social phenomena, social purposes are best conceptualized as elites' commitments to a range of specific ideas on the cardinal goals of the state and the convergence of public expectations around those ideas.

To discern the rise of social purposes, it is reasonable to start by exploring ideas that domestic political and cultural elites articulate in their rhetorical pleas and put in public circulation. The emphasis on elites is not arbitrary. An elite is a small group of people with a high position in a political system. During the initial stages of social communication, such a group enjoys a tremendous opportunity to promulgate the ideas it considers just and right. Members of the elite spell out politically meaningful conceptions of the state; they also commit resources to bring this conception to life and spread it among wider audiences. Ruling groups can often exercise brute power and force compliance with their designs. At the very least, exploring an elite's commitments gives us preliminary clues about a set of ideas that underpins domestic systems of governance. Furthermore, the study of statements and arguments made by renowned opinion leaders helps us evaluate whether the elite-generated ideas have gained a strong social footing and thus became intersubjectively shared among wider audiences.[9] Two types of outcomes are worth mentioning at this point. On the one hand, various high-powered groups might fail to develop compelling justifications for the state's existence, which precludes the emergence of a consequential discourse on the core goals of the state and in the end implies the absence of any relevant social purpose. On the other hand, in favorable circumstances political groups might converge on fundamentally similar justifications for the state's existence and thus are able to promote one predominant set of ideas about the core goals of the state, which implies that the single social purpose becomes legitimate. In the former case, implications for norm diffusion will be negligible, while in the latter they might be quite profound.

While the content of ideas (understood as systems of representations and sets of meanings) is unique and contingent on an elite's subjective appraisals, the reasons why new social purposes emerge and old ones vanish are far from random. Instead of thinking about the current international system as a number of fundamentally similar territorial nation-states with analogous and immutable *raisons d'état*, it is more rewarding to imagine such a system as an assemblage that brings together individualized political spaces, each with its own distinctive identity and evolving *raison d'être*.[10] Political transitions, redistribution of power capabilities, social transformations, external shocks, sweeping financial crises, and changes in the nature of the international system summon political leaders to ponder both the meaning of their power and the nature of the authoritative structure within which they operate (i.e., the state). Further, the interaction of integrative and fragmenting forces that challenge the state as an authoritative and long-established institution is a prevalent process that shapes contemporary world affairs.[11]

In the second half of the twentieth century, the retreat of colonial powers, the demise of apartheid, and the collapse of the Second (Communist) World profoundly transformed the international system. Those changes and challenges were quite shocking both for those who experienced them firsthand and for those who observed them academically from a distance. The end of the Cold War did not signal a dawn of the unipolar moment in history, as some staunch realists would have us believe, but rather ushered in a postinternational condition that challenged the sovereign state as the only natural locus of political authority. It also challenged the prevalent reasons why a body politic had to be sustained in the form of a centralized and autonomous political unit. The state was no longer taken for granted. Newly independent Russia could not remain committed to what had been its main raison d'être: spreading Communism and counterbalancing the United States' hegemony. Similarly, for the newly democratic South Africa, the policy of separate development could not have served as a mission of the state.

Although in the early twenty-first century we have not witnessed revolutionary transformations of a magnitude comparable to the systemic shifts of the late 1980s and early 1990s, many critical events and powerful processes have continued to motivate leaders to either renegotiate the meaning and extent of their authority or search for new meanings and identities. The global force of the liberal governmentalization of international politics will continue to test domestic systems of representation regarding the state.

In these circumstances, governments either adjust their conceptions of authority to match new global realities or reinvigorate the ensemble of their earlier normative predilections. Creative constructions of authority occur when elites employ innovative ideas, including those from the outside world. Although charting a new normative terrain might be daunting, it also holds a genuine promise of social renewal. And on the contrary, when elites cling to comfortable and historically dominant notions engrained in local intellectual cultures, they resuscitate inevitably outdated normative arrangements. There is no doubt that resorting to habitual notions and long-established discourses is the path of least resistance to the hearts and minds of the populace. Inasmuch as this strategy is relatively undemanding, it is likely to be attractive to politicians and opinion leaders. But for the same reason, it is likely to be both ill suited to meet external challenges and deficient for a successful adaptation to a rapidly changing world.

Vladimir Putin's post-Communist Russia and Thabo Mbeki's postapartheid South Africa are cases in point. In both countries, political elites settled on unique understandings of the nature of each state. The Kremlin's "sovereign democracy" and Pretoria's "African Renaissance" describe these unique understandings. While these concepts surely were the thinly concealed implements of the elites' propaganda efforts, they also captured some genuine normative orientations. Lionizing "internal" and "external" sovereignty in Russia and touting indigenous revival in South Africa are the key discursive processes that convey the desired nature of domestic political authority. Russian elites decided to construct their authority based on the value of a centralized state independent from society and insulated from external influences. To be sure, these values have always floated in Russia, but Mikhail Gorbachev's perestroika and its turbulent aftermath seriously compromised the validity of statism. In the 1990s, transnational actors, the fledgling civil society, and the emergent private sector encroached on the centralized structures of authority, challenged the territorial conceptions of political power, and undermined previously incontestable statist values.

South African elites envisioned political authority being predicated on some inherent African values that the apartheid rule had threatened and nearly destroyed. It was not by accident that Mbeki echoed many other African leaders of the second half of the twentieth century who had asserted their sense of rectitude, self-efficacy, and self-esteem by crafting various innovative postcolonial concepts. Consider the following examples. *Ujamaa* (oneness) became the foundational notion for Tanzanian authority under Julius Nyerere's rule, paralleled by roughly similar constitutive ideas of *harambee* (pulling together) in Jomo Ken-

yatta's Kenya and Pan-Africanism in Kwame Nkrumah's Ghana. All these notions intended to express renovated styles of political authority in newly independent political places. The idea of the African Renaissance rightly fits this list.

Initially, in both countries under investigation wider audiences embraced the
proposed social purposes with much optimism. As the second decade of the
twenty-first century approached, it became almost impossible to imagine and
talk about the nature of the Russian political community without glorifying statism. For many Russians, the sensibilities encompassed by the discourse of sovereign democracy provided a psychological relief after the decade of political
instability and ideological uncertainty that characterized Boris Yeltsin's rule. Instead of sticking to the elusive ideals of political liberty and human rights, Russians fell prey to the elite's promise to restore the state, take care of the people,
and secure external recognition and respect. In South Africa, the originators
of the African Renaissance promised that only genuine Africanist sensibilities
would define postapartheid rule. The discourse of the African Renaissance re-
assured citizens of the authenticity of the new methods of governance and resonated with intellectuals' revolt against the supremacy of Western science. These
sensibilities also powerfully reverberate in international postcolonial theorizing.

It is worth stressing that the concept of social purpose is distinct from that
of ideology. While ideology molds actors into universalized identities and pre-
scribes standardized roles, social purposes depend on actors' identities and do
not operate outside the battlefield of clashing discourses on the nature of the
state and the common good. That is why scholars and political observers who
tried to force Putin's stated obligations and Mbeki's public commitments into the
Procrustean iron bed of any commonly recognized ideology soon realized the
futility of the task. Contrary to ideology, a robust consensus on what constitutes
the common good might not last long after its supporters fall from the commanding heights. Quite the opposite—this consensus is situational and depends
on the outcomes of domestic discursive contestation and intellectual debates.

The social purpose of the state, however, is not coterminous with the administration of a given leader. In some cases, social purposes serve longer than
their originators could have hoped. Social purposes endure when identity arguments impair alternative normative visions for the country, foreclose the debate
on suitable methods of governance, and paralyze an elite's political opponents,
thus securing the convergence of public expectations around elite-driven ideas
on the core goals of the state. Further, once widely accepted, these ideas cannot be simply discarded or rescinded. Having generated strong societal expec-

tations, elites have to oblige them, even if at some point those elites might want to change the course of policy and break free from methods of governance they set themselves.

RESEARCH APPROACH

Although it seems fruitful to focus on obvious country-specific variables shaping health governance in Russia and South Africa, finding the deep-seated and generalizable determinants of health governance is also a rewarding research strategy. In both countries, seemingly unique national responses to the looming HIV/AIDS crisis materialized concurrently with the social progression toward full-fledged social purposes. That simultaneity tentatively suggests a causal link between the enacted systems of AIDS governance and social purposes. This book is designed to probe the potency of social purposes as a concept and thus to demonstrate how local normative orders filter external organizing principles of governance. The finding that committed elites evaluate external norms and organizing principles of AIDS governance on the grounds of elites' commitment to the ideas that they perceive as crucial to fulfill the goals of the state has made me confident that social purposes are indeed a valuable explanatory variable.

In general, I follow a constructivist explanatory strategy that focuses on exploring causal mechanisms within cases, that is, processes within cases that link causes and conditions to outcomes. Such an emphasis does not negate the significance of finding and explaining an across-case general pattern as a part of the broader research strategy. That is why, although I concentrate on explaining evidence within cases, I have provided a structured, focused comparison of the systems of AIDS governance in Russia and South Africa in order to give an additional proof that the causal mechanism revealed here is not unique to one unit of analysis. The necessary caveat is that transitional powers (including Russia and South Africa, but not limited to them), as opposed to nontransitional countries, are more likely to reconceptualize the cardinal goals of the state. Both Russia and South Africa provide enough empirical material to trace the process of how some incipient ideas about the state can evolve and mature into indispensable political constructions.

In addition, comparing Russia and South Africa is fruitful because these two countries are different and do not share a common history, regional features, related sensibilities, or similar cultures. Controlling for potential independent variables becomes difficult in the context of globalization, as it ties together previously isolated political spaces. The absence of any explicit links between these two cases helps a researcher to postulate the autonomy of causal processes from any overarching influences. Although the availability of cases that lend themselves to a fruitful comparison is relatively limited, there are somewhat similar cases that naturally come to mind. The renovation of political authority in Brazil after the collapse of its autocratic military regime affected the espoused principles of health governance.[12] The Chinese state's role as a moral patron that promotes positive mores and proscribes social vices has slowed down the diffusion of some preventive measures.[13]

Another feature of constructivist theorizing is that scholars operating in this paradigm have been primarily interested in examining the impact of social purposes on international organization, ranging from the emergence of multilateral institutions to a state's exit from the economic orbit of the decaying imperial core. The pull of globalism is easy to observe. However, the opposite research strategy suggests the intriguing proposition that individualized political spaces with unique social purposes might be profoundly challenged by an intensifying transnational flow of ideas, innovations, technologies, norms, and practices. A practical task is to design a structured, focused comparison of the domestic modes of HIV/AIDS governance and demonstrate that governments in both states created political environments sanctioning a highly selective approach to international policy guidelines and best practices. The main difficulty here is to overcome the undesirable but widespread research tendency to explain governance choices simply by cherry-picking some ideational elements from a plethora of coexisting ideas whose independent causal impact could be equally plausible. Luckily, for an observer, in both countries social purposes have emerged separately from international standards for HIV/AIDS governance and for the most part prior to the moment when external standards entered the domestic policy arenas. This initial observation helps construct a research design that is safeguarded from the underhanded tautologies that often plague ideational explanations. For that reason, examining the adoption of the external best practices in HIV/AIDS governance has a considerable advantage over just looking at the internal state of affairs in policy making.

In addition, a comparison of the two countries overcomes glaring asymmetries in the broader awareness about various cases and explanatory strategies designed to illuminate them. Describing Russian health policies outside eastern European and post-Soviet epidemiological and political contexts gives us a fresher look at the country's health governance strategies. This method also helps draw attention to those elements of health governance that are either not sensationalist enough or seemingly self-explanatory for regional experts. Pro-treatment activists who wanted to expose Mbeki's erratic health policy drove global attention to the South African situation but left Russian health gover-nance unexamined. As a result, while the study of AIDS in South Africa spawned numerous commentaries and academic articles, Russian AIDS politics, with few exceptions, remained on the margins of scholarly interest and media exposure. However, the counterintuitive comparison proposed here provides us with an inroad to a better understanding of HIV/AIDS politics and the global dynam-ics behind norm diffusion, as well as the relationship between the structures of global governance and the state.

Examining Russian politics, I start with the period of the second Putin presi-dency of 2004–8. The year 2008 marked the advent of the short-lived "tande-mocracy" of Putin in his deceptively humble role as prime minister and Dmi-triy Medvedev as the presidential seat-warmer. The continuity of Russia's regime warranted an examination of what happened in the following years. In South Af-rica, however, the new president, Jacob Zuma, distanced himself from his ousted predecessor, and thus the years 2008–10 have received only brief consideration.

ORGANIZATION OF THE BOOK

This book tells a nuanced empirical story of AIDS governance and norm diffu-sion in Russia and South Africa. The plan of the book reflects the evolving logic of the questions asked. Chapter 1 first justifies the advantage of the construc-tivist framework for examining the links between the state and public health, contrasting that framework to realist, liberal, and Foucauldian approaches. The chapter then uses the concept of social purpose to sharpen the available models of norm diffusion, offers a skeletal argument, and discusses alternative explana-tions that shed additional light on domestic responses to the AIDS crisis. Chapter 2 explores social purposes in the two countries separately from each country's HIV/AIDS policy. The chapter concludes with a concise section that conceptual-izes the social purpose of the state as a variable.

Chapters 3, 4, and 5 examine the systems of AIDS governance as they so-lidified in Russia under Putin's rule and in South Africa during Mbeki's presi-dency. Chapter 3 inquires primarily how each government framed the issue of HIV/AIDS and how each one approached the medicines that suppress the virus's replication. Chapter 4 examines both access and obstacles to prevention and treatment in both countries. Chapter 5 probes the relationship between the state and other relevant stakeholders in AIDS governance. The introductory sections of all these empirical chapters examine the principles of HIV/AIDS governance in the international arena in order to set the stage for the subsequent examination of the empirical cases. I document how the international medical community, intergovernmental organizations, financial institutions, specialized health agencies, and AIDS advocacy and service organizations came to a shared understanding about the best measures to fight HIV/AIDS.

In the conclusion, I summarize my contribution to three relevant debates and offer some lessons for practitioners. In a nutshell, the book makes three contributions. First, by investigating how domestic consensus about the nature of political authority influences the adoption of external norms, it improves the standard models of global diffusion and sharpens their heuristic power. Second, the book thinks afresh about the conditions under which ideational elements play an independent causal role in governance. Third, by probing previously overlooked political determinants of health, it helps overcome a sense of disarray in health governance literature.

CHAPTER 1

Purposeful Choices

Goals of the State, Norm Diffusion, and Fighting HIV/AIDS

IN ORDER TO CONTROL the spread of AIDS, the state confronts a variety of practical problems that require domestic policy makers to make many deliberate decisions. Most importantly, governments have to frame the nature of the epidemic, select among the available biomedical tools to address the challenge, sponsor treatment programs, remove obstacles to proven prevention services, and consider which actors to invite into the health governance process and on what terms. Core concepts of security, interests, and governmentality can clarify a lot about the goals of the state and its subsequent behavior in health governance. Constructivism helps stipulate the set of goals any state tries to achieve without making strong universalized propositions about agents' objectives and thus without imposing some exogenous logic on a particular political process of goals formation.

If domestic systems of health governance are indeed suffused with ideas about the core goals of a state, as argued here, then social purposes should influence how states adopt global health recommendations as well. Political leaders have to decide whether external principles of governance are useful for their state and whether these principles match their ideational commitments. Inasmuch as the external organizing principles of health governance happen to be antithetical to the nature of domestic political authority and ontological security, political leaders will not adopt external standards of AIDS governance without serious reservations.

I start this chapter with a theoretical statement explaining why using constructivism is more fruitful than applying realist, liberal, and Foucauldian perspectives to examine the core goals of the state and stipulate their implications for the study of health governance. Then I explain how the constructivist take on the core goals of the state improves six main models of global diffusion and highlight how social purposes might influence norm diffusion processes. Finally, this chapter considers a variety of commonly mustered additional explanations that shed light on peculiarities of health governance in Russia and South Africa.

DISTINGUISHING THE PERSPECTIVE

Realism, liberalism, critical approach, and constructivism offer distinct ways to think about the goals of the state and the ensuing governmental responses to HIV/AIDS. In this section, I distinguish between these perspectives and justify why conventional constructivism, properly refined, provides usable analytical insights.

The Realist Approach

Realists commonly define the state as a utilitarian and unified agent pursuing state building and security as its core goals. Military security is indispensable, as its absence undermines the state as an autonomous political organization and hinders the survival of society. Security in this case is an integral part of political authority because legitimacy of the rulers critically depends upon their effectiveness in providing it. However, military security is by no means the only subject matter that can function as a legitimate social purpose. The tide of globalization has transformed the meaning of security, summoned elites to address other challenges, and put elites to nontraditional tests of their ability and resourcefulness. Coming to grips with the actual goals of the state, therefore, requires an additional theorization that realism cannot provide.

Applied to the threat of HIV/AIDS, realist thinking implies that the state should protect both its armed forces and its law enforcement agencies by providing at least some basic level of treatment and by promoting the general health of its citizens. In theory, although there is no hard evidence of higher levels of infection in the armed forces compared to the general population, HIV and the ensuing opportunistic diseases can affect military preparedness and law enforcement. Overall, maintaining a healthy population is desirable in the event of a large-scale military conflict, because the government will likely require a large number of healthy and able conscripts. Arguably, it was the concern about the armed forces' health and preparedness that factored into Uganda's decision to fight AIDS at the outset of the spread of the disease. Some countries clearly prioritized providing treatment to the armed forces, the policy behavior most consistent with realism. However, it is now clear that the pandemic of AIDS does not challenge international security and does not provoke state collapse.[1] Realist logic, then, because it rules out humanitarian reasons, cannot explain why developed states continue to sponsor efforts to eradicate AIDS and provide generous health assistance abroad.

Alternatively, realism can explain why during the 2000s the discourse of HIV/AIDS as a threat to security spread widely and quickly among many nations across the globe. In practice, leaders of the developing world overstate the arguments portraying AIDS as a security issue and deploy them to attract external resources with the aim of scaling up the response to the pandemic.[2] Resource-limited and even middle-income countries seek to satisfy their material interests by absorbing external resources. Adopting external health norms increases the chances of gaining some material benefits and logistical support to deal with local problems. Challenging and resisting international health norms simply impedes developing nations' ability to acquire these resources. For this reason, the state-sponsored hostility to international health norms is a hard behavior to explain. This anomalous behavior, of course, could result from various cognitive problems that limit the rational thinking of high-powered decision makers. Although this is always a possibility, arguments about misperception undermine the main advantage of realism—its compelling parsimoniousness. Once that powerful and elegant simplicity disappears, there is no reason not to consider the other contingent and actor-specific justifications and rationales for health policy making. As realism does not provide a secure grip on these actor-specific reasons, we need to keep searching for a different set of conceptual lenses.

The Liberal Approach

Liberalism, another major theoretical framework, interprets the state as an institution that represents a variety of interests, often promotes economic welfare, and protects society from falling back into underdevelopment. Policy makers can secure these core liberal objectives by making sure that the spread of human immunodeficiency virus is contained and remains minimal. This means that governments must invest in the health infrastructure, provide modern health care, develop or purchase the appropriate pharmaceuticals to combat disease outbreaks, spend money to promote healthy lifestyles, and so on. The aggressive evidence-based fight against HIV/AIDS might save the government the resources that are necessary to execute other social policies. At minimum, states are likely to realize the value and effectiveness of proven solutions. These solutions, however, do not exist as an essential constitutive feature of the state, unaffected by time and place; they are, on the contrary, contingent. The state, after all, does not have to commit to developmentalism or respect evidence-based medicine and science. Leaders can make health available in a variety of different ways. In order to protect the welfare of the population, they can resort to holistic healing, traditional and alternative medicines, or quarantine and deportations.

The liberal tradition looks at states as rational, self-interested, but not unitary actors. Elites, firms, policy networks, hospitals, agents of change, activists, norm entrepreneurs, and other societal actors all have their own interests, the configuration of which determines the systems of governance. The liberal-pluralist state is not supposed to endorse the ontological values of any social actors but rather resolve social and political conflicts that emerge around those values.[3] Social actors often disagree about the principles of public health, especially when different pathways to health are available. These kinds of disagreements are not particularly unique or rare. They feature heavily in both the global North and the global South. Two obvious examples include the clash between traditional/holistic healing and evidence-based medicine in South Africa and the collision between punitive strategies and harm-reduction measures in Russia. In these circumstances, the state should remain impartial and operate on the principle of neutrality, aggregating preferences and adjudicating domestic conflicts arising out of ontological incompatibility of coexisting beliefs and values. Although the state is supposed to establish a set of neutral and fair procedures to adjudicate the aforementioned conflicts, both South African and Russian states chose which ontological values to uphold and then acted on their own beliefs.

In short, the liberal approach cannot explain whether the state's desire for health as a precondition of attaining wealth will involve the proven solutions advocated by multiple international actors. Many health policies that we empirically observe today are compatible with the liberal tradition. This fact, however, does not make them the natural norm or even the only way of policy making. Liberalism thus requires an additional theorization in order to explain where main governing ideas come from and why leaders commit to them.

The Foucauldian Approach

Scholars applying the concepts of critical, or Foucauldian, theory usually design their studies to reveal persistent inequalities and expose the sources of human disempowerment and alienation. They seek to unveil the deep-seated underpinnings of governance and reveal intricate and subtle ways in which loosely defined power operates and how it disadvantages some human subjects. In general, the Foucauldian notion of governmentality is supposed to describe the extant rationales of governing while avoiding the trap of imposing exogenous preferences and values on the studied governments and societies. It also posits that the global liberal order fosters voluntary compliance by limiting the conceptual parameters of appropriate governance methods that collectivities subsequently internalize as normal.

As valuable as these insights are, the overall effectiveness of this perspective is paralyzed by its poststructuralism, that is, the confidence that an immutable global order invariably constrains agency. First, the assumption that individuals and societies across the globe are guilty of restricted reflexivity and limited intentionality leads to a conclusion that people primarily reproduce the dominant rationalities of governance. This assumption simply ignores the significance of recurrent domestic debates about the appropriate techniques of governance and the variety of governance methods governments actually employ. Second, the assumption that liberal (or neoliberal) governing methods have already taken a firm hold of the world dismisses the myriad tensions, contradictions, and compromises about social practices and organizing principles that define present-day international affairs. In summary, without denying the validity of the empirical observation that globalization diffuses Westernized and liberal principles of governance, I assert that it should be precisely the task of a researcher to inquire how these principles interact with the locally crafted goals of the state, goals that in many cases remain in flux. Further, while critical scholars profess their own inability to study global structures independently of the conceptual constraints they impose on a scholar, such an epistemological position is hardly helpful for doing normal social science.

Equally problematic is the application of the Foucauldian analysis to the issues of health governance. In critical theory, biopolitics is primarily about production and/or reduction of life as a mechanism of exercising power. In this perspective, governments can equally secure human life and the physiological necessities of populations, or, conversely, governments can destroy and limit life in order to keep the population in conformity with their values and designs. In another version of Foucauldian analysis, the state shapes the conditions of life, makes bodies conform to normality, and centralizes various institutional techniques to punish and correct what it perceives as the abnormal.[4] In this context, AIDS is presumably an emblematic case for probing the hidden workings of power relations. Health services and institutionalized AIDS treatment are the key social mechanisms that rulers deliberately deploy to sustain or stabilize domestic power relations.[5] As attractive as these propositions might be, they are unfalsifiable, since any kind of biopolitical action can be interpreted as consistent with the Foucauldian vision of how the state decides to maintain its power.

Scholars who wish to establish what states see as normal and abnormal should not infer these categories from states' actions and the outcomes of health governance. In addition, critical scholars have demonstrated a blunt unwillingness to distinguish between states with obviously different types of political authority. For instance, it appears that there is no distinction between the apartheid state and the postapartheid regime, as they both exploit the politics of death in order to attain their political goals.[6] In order to avoid this deficiency, the Foucauldian perspective requires making use of an additional theorization pertaining to the set of politically and historically contingent ideas about the objectives of the state and abandoning its universalistic focus on the application of bioviolence as the basic implement of the state. But this intellectual move undermines the political and intellectual appeal of the critical paradigm.

The Constructivist Approach

Constructivists made significant progress by postulating that core goals of the state emerge out of the state's justifications for its own existence and rationales for sovereignty. The state officialdom has to unpack its own raison d'être in domestic political discourse and validate it as a categorical commitment in social practice. The obligation to act on the specified range of ideas subsequently imposes limits on the elite's interpretive flexibility and instrumental rationality. Sophisticated constructivist accounts offer explicit answers about what social purposes might look like and what their implications could be. Christian Reus-Smit finds that the purpose of the modern state is to enhance individual intentions and potentialities.[7] Rawi Abdelal discusses social purposes in conjunction with how postimperial states endeavored to assert their nationhood as a natural locus of political authority.[8] Contrasted with rationalist paradigms, these two constructivist studies in principle allow delineating the core goals of the state with precision, although both Reus-Smit's and Abdelal's accounts are too restrictive to offer politically and culturally contingent characterizations of a political space. Reus-Smit, for instance, limits the contemporary conception of the state to its liberal iteration. Given the heterogeneity of the social relations in modern states, it is likely, however, that while the modern state actually follows specific justifications for its own existence, the content of those justifications (a range of ideas that individualize a given political community) is unique and varies from country to country. To have a solid conceptualization of the social purpose of the state, it is therefore pivotal to reveal which specific ideas about the core goals of the state express the elite's governing obligations and to show that these ideas gain strong social traction in a given political space. The necessary caveat is that certain groups of states might embrace fundamentally similar social purposes.

My approach focuses on elite groups that develop politically meaningful ideas and commit a significant amount of resources to act on them. Elites, placed high on the social and political ladder, construct and choose the ideas regarding the goals of the state and the common good. Then, elites unfold identity arguments that assert some ideas as suitable for domestic systems of governance and rule out others. Identity arguments are very important. They communicate meanings and stabilize normative expectations. Without a coagulating force of identity arguments, elements of political representations will continue to "float freely" in societies and are not likely to acquire autonomous and intersubjective conceptual power.

The collapse of Communism challenged the Russian elite to rethink the role of the state. That the weakness of the Russian state in the 1990s necessitated efforts to restore its capacity and develop its quality is obvious. In theory, the Kremlin could have internalized Westernized and liberal rationales of governance. But Vladimir Putin steered the country in the opposite direction. He was determined to revive the strong centralized state, eliminate any alternative spheres of authority, resurrect the government as a transformative force in the economy, and reinstate Russia in the position of a great power in the international system. To be sure, these choices were far from the only possible response to the intensifying governance problems, and they ignored the hard-hitting lessons of history. Continuous failures of the Soviet administrative-command economy showed that controlling the commanding heights was not tantamount to economic boom and prosperity. Despite its self-glorifying image as the challenger to the American hegemony, the Soviet empire proved to be an unattractive colossus with feet of clay. In short, the profound transformations of the late 1980s and early 1990s have shaken the historical durability of statism in Russia. While few would deny that a strong and effective state is a necessary prerequisite for the quality of governing, Putin's elite has failed to internalize values of a modern pluralist state and instead has revived the comatose conceptions of authority equated with statism.

In South Africa, Mbeki hoped to defy the Western neocolonial stereotypes about the native incapacity to govern. He envisioned a successful leadership of the former liberation movement based on three normative pillars of the African Renaissance: indigenous authority, marketization as an appropriate way of economic empowerment, and the status of moral leader in global politics. While for an external observer the African Renaissance is a confusing salmagundi of themes, the notion of indigenousness is the pivot around which its core meanings and supplementary sensibilities turn. Public intellectuals and governmental representatives alike claimed that the emphasis on indigenous knowledge was counterhegemonic and anticolonial in nature and therefore affirmed the values of the African Renaissance. They also claimed that no Western policy models were able to provide working solutions to South Africa's problems. Although officials sustained their rhetoric of devotion to democratic values and a liberal-pluralist conception of the state, it was surely secondary to the emerging themes as described above.

In the two emergent powers, politicians and key decision makers approached a looming health crisis using social purposes as their conceptual lenses. Domestic responses to AIDS were confluent with the embraced standards and principles of governance that rested on the normative foundation of social purposes. Since Russian social purpose was primarily about statism, it becomes clear why the country's government vigorously responded to the outbreak of AIDS but failed to remove barriers to prevention among vulnerable populations or involve nonstate stakeholders in AIDS governance. Since South African social purpose was primarily about erecting and upholding indigenous principles of governance, it becomes clear why Pretoria became obsessed with finding local solutions to the epidemic and made an effort to resist external recommendations and practices that did not fit the preconceived notions of suitable models of health governance.

Summary

In this section I have selected a proper theoretical perspective for the next step in my investigation. All four of the approaches I have outlined above provide conceptual lenses with which to examine the cardinal goals of the state and parse their influence on health politics. The major analytical shortcoming of rationalists of varying provenance (both realists and liberals) is that they strongly commit to the assumption that the state operates on exogenously attributed goals (utility maximization expressed in the pursuit of, respectively, security and wealth). Their theories, therefore, remain indeterminate as to why decision makers select one policy course over its alternatives. The most fundamental objection to the intellectual opponents of rationalists—critical scholars—is that their conceptual models are hard to falsify. While the Foucauldian notion of governmentality is loosely similar to what constructivists call the "social purpose," ideological predilections espoused by critical scholars wear out the analytical efficacy of their theories. These shortcomings invite a scholar to ponder other avenues of theorizing how state goals crystallize and how they influence domestic systems of governance. Compared to the three aforementioned intellectual paradigms, constructivism, with its focus on the cardinal goals of the state stemming from the specific raison d'être of a given political unit, offers adequate conceptual lenses to explain how officials politicize health governance. In the next section, I put social purpose in the context of norm diffusion models, summarize the core argument of the book, and then discuss several alternative explanations.

SOCIAL PURPOSES IN GLOBAL DIFFUSION

In the globalized world, the spread of norms, ideas, and policies is a pervasive, ubiquitous, and perhaps normal mode of interaction among states. Some governments might find it a relatively mundane task to tailor their metanorms to spreading liberal governmentality or to adjust their social purposes to external principles of governance. Others might find this task more difficult. What sets the latter group of states apart is that they champion unique normative orders. South Africa's conception of the African Renaissance and Russia's uncompromising "sovereign democracy" are two cases in point. An exciting task is to inquire how and to what degree the normative content of domestic political authority influences norm diffusion processes. Situating social purposes in the context of the six main analytical models explored below—learning, coalition building, substitution, socialization, competition, and norm congruence—offers an improved explanatory strategy, one that is useful for highlighting how domestic structures of authority influence domestic adoption of international norms. These models are obviously ideal types. Some specific approaches, such as the renowned "spiral model," for instance, combine elements of more than one model and are not examined here.[9] Below I argue that it is useful to bring social purposes to the analysis because doing so sharpens or alters our theoretical predictions.

Learning

Among all the models discussed in this section, the learning model provides the most "rationalist" and utilitarian portrayal of norm diffusion. It implies a rational process of selecting helpful governance solutions and discarding useless ones. That governments might adjust their causal beliefs about a necessary policy course and follow external advice is clear. Although there are many nuanced forms of this model, it can be simplified as follows. Domestic leaders, decision makers, and politicians consider all the available information in order to solve a problem at hand. They tend to appreciate foreign models if adopting external alternatives has a significant advantage over doing business as usual. They follow external advice if the benefits of international policy are tangible and the information about policy success is confirmed elsewhere. Cultural openness to external arguments and unusual opinions matters, but persuasive data should speak for themselves. Vibrant epistemic networks and communities of experts act as interlocutors: they facilitate obtaining and interpreting external information and alleviate potential cognitive distortions.[10] Repeated exposure to international organizations and sustained interaction with external and transnational actors that advocate new alternatives are important prerequisites for learning. While an isolated country might not be able to get new information, a full-blown pariah status, either self-imposed or externally induced, characterizes only few countries. Even when leaders either stay passive on the international stage or remain alienated from the outside world, most states can borrow something useful from the outside world. All of these considerations make the learning model appropriate to explain the diffusion of health governance norms across the globe.

AIDS governance hinges on technological, evidence-based solutions, such as the life-saving medicinal properties of antiretroviral cocktails and the harm-reduction programs that have rapidly become part of the international mainstream. Since it is reasonable to expect that a government will adopt useful new policies and effective innovations, what happened in Russia and South Africa is counterintuitive. Was the learning process broken there at some point? South Africa and Russia could have either bumped into some serious obstacles while interacting with their international environment, or failed to grasp the available technical and epidemiological information, or drawn wrong conclusions about best practices and international advice, or lacked an adequate degree of bureaucratic competencies to process the incoming information.

But the available evidence does not support these propositions.

During the time of the pandemic, neither country found itself isolated from international experiences and advice. Technological expertise and help, especially since the early 2000s, became increasingly available. Information about policy baselines and epidemiology spread rapidly across the globe, providing many opportunities for learning. Very few international policy participants debated the nature of the human immunodeficiency virus and/or misunderstood the implications of AIDS for public health. For instance, there were enough technical data that showed that utilizing antiretrovirals for HIV treatment and promoting harm reduction to control the spread of infection among intravenous drug users help mitigate the spread of HIV. Despite this, these two governments purposefully looked for alternatives that were less compelling from a technical viewpoint but agreeable with the normative tastes of their rulers. For instance, Pretoria actively looked for alternative international health guidelines that could be compatible with domestic policy choices on traditional healing. Despite the World Health Organization's cautious recommendations and the World Bank's half-hearted embrace of traditional knowledge, the South African government tried to elevate these international guidelines to a prescriptive status. Pretoria thus tried to justify its drift away from antiretrovirals to traditional medicines and challenged Western medicines with an alternative treatment agenda.

Of course, learning about external practices depends on the timing of the information processing. In either country, the timing was right. Since the late 1990s, Russian state officials and bureaucrats could not have missed the fact that HIV/AIDS was a looming health crisis. The official reports compiled between 1999 and 2001 indicated that the number of those infected increased sixteen times. Preoccupation with the looming epidemic featured prominently in health bureaucracies. Similar concerns unfolded in South Africa. According to the South African Department of Health, by 2002 HIV prevalence reached 26.5 percent among antenatal clinic attendees and around 11 percent in the whole population. HIV stabilized only by the year 2004. But for many critical years, decision makers remained uninspired by external cases of success.

The main shortcoming of the learning approach is that it focuses on the spread of technical solutions and standardized practices and thus overlooks the potential significance of the deep-seated principles of governance that guide leaders in their attempts to use or reject external fixes. In the Russian case, for instance, harm reduction, elsewhere a cardinal component of good AIDS governance, was a novel and uncomfortable concept. To adopt it was to bridge the gap between international validity of the underlying organizing principle of human rights and the habitual domestic opposition to it, which crystallized as elites and opinion leaders were actively cultivating domestic intolerance to Western-style liberalism. While the unrefined learning model can thoroughly explain the process of technical policy adjustments (or lack thereof), it remains vague about "true" learning, the notion implying a dramatic shift in normative orientations and abrasion of previous commitments.[11] To correct this shortcoming one has to focus on leaders' normative obligations rather than highlight their ability or failure to understand technical information and act on it when necessary.

Put differently, although elites certainly recognize the existence of international approaches, they are not necessarily inspired to adopt new norms without necessary qualifications. On the one hand, when external organizing principles of governance do not impinge on the ideas elites hold dear, rulers will be more likely to consider the available information and embrace change. On the other hand, elites firmly committed to a certain range of ideas do not welcome changes that seem inappropriate overall. They might revile external norms, after all. In many cases, ruling groups will adopt only a subset of the available practices, those that are consistent with internalized perceptions of the core goals of the state and comfortable understandings of the appropriate role of the state in solving domestic problems. As I show in my empirical chapters, Moscow and Pretoria have been inclined to adopt recommendations and best cases on a selective basis. As a result, systems of health governance in Russia and South Africa do not simply reflect what leaders have learned about the available technical solutions to address an intensifying health crisis at home.

Coalition Building

Coalition building is the most "political" and common mechanism of global diffusion. It typically gives us a persuasive portrayal of policy transfer. Movements, activists, celebrities, parties, and subsets of state officials might prefer solutions incompatible with the traditions with which governments seek to solve a problem. All these actors, especially if they "have pursued, but never achieved a particular institutional solution to an important political problem," are minority traditions.[12] In certain contexts, minority traditions enjoy some domestic support; their representatives can occupy powerful policy positions. In most cases, however, to achieve change, minority traditions need influential and authoritative external actors (outsiders) to boost the norms they advocate. Outsiders empower, sponsor, and simply encourage domestic minorities. As a result, governments choose to adopt external norms and advice if they feel they have to broaden their support, reach out to additional would-be followers, and cement prospective support groups together. While this portrayal is certainly plausible and in many cases empirically accurate, probing social purposes tightens a conceptual grip on what happens in domestic arenas. Importantly, the conflict between minority traditions and governments is not just a disagreement about the technicalities of a policy reform but also a normative clash stemming from a deep devotion to incompatible conceptions of the state and its cardinal goals. This clarification has profound implications for the study of norm diffusion.

When the contestation between governments and minority traditions has normative underpinnings, the role and intensity of identity arguments are likely to increase. Identity arguments often look like sophisticated versions of ad hominem attacks, which challenge the credibility of those domestic actors that champion alternative principles of governance. In short, aggressive identity arguments have the discursive power to turn minority traditions into the offenders against the common good; they portray the proponents of alternatives as actors subduing the state's raison d'être and thus being a source of ontological danger to the very existence of the political unit. Government-friendly opinion leaders spin the image of domestic minority groups as illegitimate puppets who propose inadequate and pernicious governance methods. Simultaneously, governments impose legal constraints on policy actors so that the enacted systems of governance conform to expectations as they are expressed in the dominant conception of the social purpose. Whether this imposition is successful or not depends on other factors as well, including the coercive capacities of the executive and ruling groups' abilities to deploy a compelling discourse of blame and accusation. As a result, despite all the external support potentially thrown in favor of minority traditions, ruling elites will not join coalitions with those actors that undermine the nature of their authority. Reaching out to the principled nonsupporters is undesirable. Contrastingly, coalitions with those subnational groups that share the elite's commitments are likely to be deemed appropriate and useful.

The foregoing considerations help explain why the South African Cabinet burned its bridges to the increasingly powerful "protreatment" coalition. Building a partnership with protreatment activists and groups would have been beneficial for the Cabinet in general and Mbeki personally. But the energetic proponents of conventional treatment supported policy solutions that went against the normative ideas expressed in the African Renaissance. On the other side of the globe, the Kremlin's success in unfolding identity arguments amplified the coercive power of the Russian government. In Russia, no minority tradition, especially those domestic organizations that advocated harm reduction based on human rights principles, had a chance to promote itself as a socially responsible and commonly esteemed governance participant. Although for a while some representatives of domestic civil society harbored the illusion of their importance and independence, the Kremlin accepted nongovernmental organizations as subordinate actors only if their activity and service did not impinge on the principles of sovereign democracy. State officials kept tightening control over domestic movements, parties, and nonstate associations.

In sum, coalitions might pave the road for foreign norms and practices to shape domestic governance systems. However, if social purposes really matter, we should expect a government to stick to the localized interpretation of a norm and pursue selective policy promotions even when that government is in danger of losing the support of the advocates of change.

Substitution

The norm substitution model posits that outsiders intervene directly while applying raw power (coercion) and dispensing soft pressures (financial incentives and conditionality). Outsiders can intrude with some combination of new agendas, material incentives, intellectual resources, and so on. In certain circumstances, external actors are determined to achieve domestic change and possess adequate material leverage to impose specific policies and norms.

Financial incentives and conditionality surely matter. The global North's development assistance that changes domestic approaches to health in resource-poor environments is a case in point.[13] Recipient states with meager administrative capacities and paltry resources seek generous influxes of financial aid and thus try to avoid challenging external arrangements and health norms. Substitution may work in some individual cases, such as Zambia and Mozambique, where a domestic response otherwise would not exist the way it currently does. Quite simply, many states do not possess enough resources to muster unique solutions to domestic policy problems and cannot institutionalize alternative methods of health governance even if they desire to do so in principle. It is clear that Russia and South Africa are the emergent regional powers in which radical norm displacement is not likely to happen. Without some degree of extant domestic interest in adopting foreign norms, outsiders are not likely to make governments replace their internalized principles of governance. Thabo Mbeki, for instance, was able to withstand the global opprobrium he received for his unorthodox biomedical views; the country's leaders dismissed many pleas to expand access to essential medicines.

Even when we encounter some evidence of full or partial norm substitution, we should overestimate neither the overall power of external agents of change nor the chances of outright norm replacement. In the South African case, financial incentives offered by the U.S. President's Emergency Plan for AIDS Relief (PEPFAR) were the main force that accelerated the national rollout of an antiretroviral treatment.[14] But this did not deracinate Pretoria's commitment to traditional medicines. In the Russian case, generous external funding of the early 2000s pushed Russian bureaucrats to treat domestic nonstate actors with some degree of respect and tolerance. But taking domestic NGOs more seriously than before did not make state officials internalize the principle of nonhierarchical and nonstate governance. Nor did Russians abandon their conceptual proclivity to privilege state-centric solutions as the tool to address all social problems.

In short, if social purposes do not matter, we should expect national elites to interact with outsiders strategically. Elites can certainly calculate both the benefits of conforming to external influences and the potential costs of challenging them. This means that elites will adopt international norms if a deviation from the global baseline causes opprobrium or financial losses. But governments are likely to oppose external pressures if those pressures challenge normative underpinnings of domestic authority, even when the costs of noncompliance are high. Thus, if social purposes matter, we should expect a discriminating adaptation of external demands and selective resistance to external pressures.

Socialization

Another well-investigated mechanism of norm diffusion is socialization, which constructivists commonly define as the internalization of new values and novel norms. For the purposes of studying global diffusion, it is fruitful to characterize socialization as compliance with outside norms when joining international political communities, intergovernmental institutions, or international regulative regimes is highly desirable.[15] In essence, external persuasion is important, but domestic actors often take the legitimacy of international norms and practices for granted and start emulating them. It is not by chance that the vast literature on socialization emerged in conjunction with the Europeanization of the former Soviet satellites in eastern Europe. This mechanism explains how and why central and eastern European countries came to adopt the European Union's norms in the process of democratic transition. These countries had to adjust to fundamentally different principles of governance in order to be able to join the emergent European suprastate. It is possible to argue, moreover, that it was the initial sense of belonging to the international society of European states and ontological compatibility with them that in part drove the eastern European inclination to being socialized.

To make the socialization approach work for countries other than those discussed above, a scholar must first identify the formal or semiformal "commonwealth" of countries that attract new members and then demonstrate that prospective members link the perspective of joining the club or staying in it to the unavoidable normative adjustments. An attractive hegemon can offer a lot to those international actors that are willing to join its system. While it is feasible that small nations would see many tangible benefits as a result of joining the leading nation, it is less likely for a massive state to embrace external values with the same ease. Both Russia and South Africa aspired to become regional centers of attraction and involve their small neighbors in their political and economic orbit. Quite simply, the role of the follower, the disciple, and the aspirant in the international system was not for them. Immediately after the collapse of Communism in Russia and apartheid in South Africa, these big but somewhat peripheral countries clearly drifted toward the liberal-democratic core. But after the turbulent period of transformation was over, playing new uncomfortable roles or internalizing alien norms became less attractive. As Russia and South Africa drifted away from global socializing agents, Putin and Mbeki envisioned their states as regional powers defending a multipolar world where alternatives to Western paths of development and political values had a full right and an opportunity to flourish.

Any scholar systematically ransacking Russian newspapers will quickly discover the ambivalence underlying the way Russian officials cope with external actors. The swelling number of politicians and opinion leaders argue against any external practices that do not fall into the arbitrarily constructed comfort zone of authentic Russian values. Officials often accuse their critics of groveling before the West. At the same time, the same officials crave an unqualified external respect. Several prominent members of the United Russia lamented that the West did not understand Russia's soul and did not appreciate the country's fundamental affinity with the West.[16] But Russia also sought to generate external respect by creating the image of a committed upholder of international norms and laws that the West was intentionally manipulating for its own advantage. In short, as the Russian conception of the social purpose matured, the desire to internalize available international norms decreased. This general observation applies to Russian behavior in regard to adopting global health norms.

Competition

Governments compete with each other for scarce resources, favorable international regulation, regional leadership, global recognition, and so on. To remain competitive within the global power hierarchy, governments must select a governance course attuned to external practices that have proven their efficacy. The explanatory power of world economic competition as a diffusion mechanism is apparent when applied to the global spread of economic liberalism. Because indicators of economic success speak for themselves and because strong liberal orders support economic efficiency, competition uproots those domestic policies and norms that lead to economic decay and an inability to compete. Although countries remain culturally different in many ways, the imperatives of global competition make no allowance for heavy normative idiosyncrasies.

To make this explanation work for global health, one should expose clear rhetorical evidence that governments understand health as a development issue, as well as reveal how exactly changes in AIDS governance models could be effective to win economic competition. Because health is a precondition to development, it becomes a significant dimension of the global power hierarchy. On the other hand, some governments understand their position in the global hierarchy not as an outcome of genuine competition but rather as a result of their ability to resist externally induced change at home and their capacity to promote domestic rules abroad. Winning the competition to promote ideas, engage people, and attract capital was the stated goal of Putin's vision for Russia's global ambition.[17] Although both countries are likely to be sensitive to external recommendations and assistance, both Russia and South Africa chose to act as international leaders in response to HIV/AIDS. Russia and South Africa both attempted to promote their policy tastes in response to HIV/AIDS, thus pitching themselves as proactive international norm entrepreneurs. The Kremlin wanted to assert itself as a regional rule giver and sponsor of regional health. In similar but more exotic ways, Pretoria tried to promote traditional healing after South Africa's engagement with the counterepistemic community of health dissidents dissolved.

On balance, although strategic considerations matter, and health, therefore, can be a practical foreign policy tool, states are gradually finding out that it is difficult to use external health assistance as leverage. It is therefore difficult to explain the aforementioned choices without paying attention to states' ideational commitments. It is also now clear that the purposes behind the external health ambitions of such different powers as Brazil, Russia, India, China, and South Africa were diverse. Health assistance increased the Brazilian humanitarian reputation, upheld American moral values, sustained Indian loyalty to South-South solidarity, and served Chinese economic and strategic interests abroad.[18] These considerations warrant exploring the influence of social purposes on competition as a mechanism of global diffusion.

Norm Congruence

The congruence model generated much consideration in constructivist international relations. Constructivist scholars assert that the process of norm diffusion depends in one way or another on the similarities between domestic and international norms, ideas, and identities. In turn, domestic norms and values that fundamentally contradict external advice generate obstacles on the course of policy diffusion. However, if norm congruence is absent at the beginning of the interaction, it might emerge once credible messengers (advocates, norm entrepreneurs) develop matches between external norms and broader domestic values.[19] To describe this process, constructivists sometimes employ somewhat confusing terminology. Suffice it to say that grafting, pruning, transplanting, and other gardening metaphors describe the activities through which external agents of change penetrate policy arenas and transform domestic norms.

This model is promising, but it has to be refined. Sometimes the fundamental norms and organizing principles that constitute normative orders are obvious (democracy, the rule of law, freedom from torture, nonintervention), but sometimes they are not. If the latter is indeed the case, then a scholar who wishes to make use of a congruence argument should offer a solid theory about what constitutes the underlying appropriateness of the targeted polity and why.[20] The inability to address this weighty analytical concern has three broad shortcomings.

First, because domestic norms and ideas are always many, a congruence argument is in danger of setting up only haphazard connections between certain cherry-picked domestic orientations and international principles. The plurality of competing domestic norms, contesting sensibilities, and clashing ideational proclivities is an ordinary state of affairs in any nontotalitarian society. A scholar should not simply conjecture which norm will have causal consequences for global diffusion; theoretical and empirical work is needed. In addition, this line of reasoning fails to distinguish whether domestic leaders strictly follow the principled standards of appropriate behavior or, on the contrary, conduct noncommitted business as usual. For instance, Russia's permissive and modestly favorable material conditions prompted leaders to increase public spending to improve health infrastructure and medical services. This behavior seemingly reflects Russia's recognition of the global norm of universality of treatment, but because norms should not be inferred from behavior, some critical thinking piece is lacking here. Ultimately, those who uncritically use the norm congruence argument will falsely recognize norm diffusion to have taken place when in actuality it has not occurred.

Second, if there is an initial fundamental harmony (equivalence, match) between internal and external normative orders, then the process of framing external advice to match the domestic values of the targeted polities is trivial. If enacting a new course of governance is not overly costly for elites, then agents of change can alter the minds of domestic decision makers, who eventually will recognize the validity of external norms. Norm entrepreneurs can also portray best practices and external norms in such a way that they begin resonating with the local normative context of the targeted polity. This insight sounds fairly straightforward and accurate, since norms describe only the horizon for appropriate behavior. But norms are not infinitely flexible and boundlessly malleable. Further, some metanorms might foreclose the debate on appropriate methods of governance, while others might stimulate discussion and adaptability.

To be theoretically compelling, then, this approach must ascertain extant width or narrowness of normative horizons, as well as the stability or volatility of domestic normative devotions. If domestic horizons are prohibitively narrow, then domestic decision makers will not buy into various norm congruence arguments supplied by the proponents of change. Theorizing the distinctions between constitutive norms (sometimes called fundamental norms or metanorms), organizing principles, and standardized practices is a conceptual move that allows separating domestic metanorms as a variable that sets conceptual parameters of domestic normative horizons.[21] Scholars commonly try to avoid such theorizing by using the notion "lifeworld" as a conceptual shortcut. This notion implies a significant degree of initial (cultural) proximity between interacting agents. However, that working assumption about the common normative structure undergirding different political places is not as credible as it might appear. Statements about the shared lifeworld (civilization) are often attempts to shape it and bring it into being.[22] Instead of making sweeping statements, investigation of metanorms requires a thorough ransacking of domestic discursive formations. In short, without knowing the limits of normative horizons (which ultimately depend on the underlying normative orders), expectations about the ease or difficulty of norm diffusion will be imprecise.

Third, if no external principles seem intuitively appropriate, and if there is no overlap between external and internal normative orders, then trying to harmonize an external norm with domestic values requires localization. Localization is often necessary because alien political, economic, and social concepts require an adequate "translation" in order to be understood. But a thoroughgoing localization of external norms that goes too far creates domestic simulacra of external standards of appropriate behavior. For instance, in Russia, the current standardized practice of elections bears a resemblance to Western practices, but it is localized to the degree that it defies the organizing principle of democracy. After all, new norms should remain "different" and uncomfortable because they are supposed to fix something broken or something lacking in domestic contexts. Politicians and decision makers can certainly challenge external advice if the externally proposed fixes are not capable of solving problems at home. In principle, leaders must engage in a sensible discussion about a governance strategy and its underpinnings as part of the policy process. But without understanding the broad normative context, we will never know whether this discussion is genuine or duplicitous, whether localization is a form of adoption or an erosion of external models. The rhetoric of unsuitability and the necessity of norm localization can imply that leaders either do not want to solve the problems at hand (because the leaders do not acknowledge the existence of these problems and do not believe they require fixing) or do not agree with the underlying organizing principles that the seemingly technological policy fix entails. In sum, the localization model is valuable in principle, but it often fails to capture the deep-seated dynamic of norm diffusion.

Scholars often try to correct the shortcomings of all three versions of the norm congruence model by making use of additional variables that will do most of the conceptual work. Explanations revolve on the pivot of material leverage, conditionality, international opprobrium, the power of policy gatekeepers, and the qualities or characteristics inherent in or ascribed to international norm advocates and domestic norm takers. Using additional variables is not a telltale sign of an impaired research strategy, but to develop a genuinely constructivist argument we should concentrate on the autonomous power of norms, that is, on the conceptual power of the intersubjectively shared ideational elements. All too many scholars have shied away from this task and thus have failed to spotlight the normative underpinning of global diffusion.

My study addresses the aforementioned concerns. I argue that the concept of the social purpose captures the preexisting normative order around which additional regulative norms and standards of behavior revolve. Because social purposes set the parameters of domestic appropriateness, examining social purposes helps explain the deep-seated reasons why domestic ideas frustrate or facilitate norm diffusion. In different countries, variations in the content of social purposes politicize international guidelines differently; varying degrees of consensus around those purposes define the strength and attractiveness of such politicization. In this book, the metaphor of "filtering" indicates the process by which leaders recognize the standards of appropriate behavior, cherry-pick compatible external initiatives, and develop alternatives to those external norms that do not match the underlying domestic metanorm. The horizon of domestic appropriateness depends, first, upon the content of the social purpose and, second, upon the degree of its legitimacy. It is clear that in recent years the horizon of appropriateness has narrowed consistently in Russia, while it opened up in South Africa after Mbeki's removal from power.

Summary

There are many reasons why governments decide to adopt or challenge international advice and policies. Because we cannot directly observe either international or domestic norms, demonstrating their clash is not as simple as it might seem. So much is clear. The foregoing discussion established that probing social purposes improves our analytical expectations regarding the available norm diffusion models. The ensuing sections first present a skeletal explanation of how and why Russian and South African politicians qualified and even opposed international guidelines. I then appraise five additional explanations.

THE ARGUMENT IN BRIEF

Since the early 1980s, scholars, practitioners, and domestic policy makers have discussed the multiple implications of the AIDS epidemic for human rights, economic development, military preparedness, and international security.[23] Without denying the complexity of the pandemic and the diversity of policy responses, scholars have tended to think that a global consensus on AIDS governance has indeed materialized. For purposes of clarity, it is obligatory to reiterate both the current standards for AIDS governance and the set of organizing principles that underpin them. Framing HIV as a public health issue, using conventional antiretrovirals, expanding treatment to all who qualify for it from a medical standpoint, offering prevention services adequate for the local epidemiology (whether harm reduction or newer tools of biomedical prevention), and building robust partnerships with all relevant stakeholders are these standardized procedures. The acceptance of medical evidence-based solutions, the recognition of treatment as a public good, the respect of human rights, and the acknowledgment of external and domestic nonstate actors in nonhierarchical governance are the corresponding organizing principles of AIDS governance. Table 1 summarizes the organizing principles and the standardized procedures of AIDS governance. The introductory sections of chapters 4, 5, and 6 describe these principles and procedures in detail.

The necessary caveat is that the exact phrasing of the standardized practices and their precise combination are analytical constructions. According to Evan Lieberman, for instance, the main features of the global consensus highlight the necessity to assemble competent and independent bureaucratic authority, broadcast prevention strategies, provide treatment and support of HIV-positive people, and protect human rights.[24] Doubtless, the international consensus on AIDS governance will change along with developments in life sciences, patent laws, available resources, and so on. That the organizing principles and standardized procedures evolve in the governance process is normal and expected. The point that bears emphasis here is that the broad consensus on the main practices and principles of governance should remain intact.

First, international policy consensus is about treatment. Here and below, the term antiretrovirals (ARVs) describes a combination of safe and effective drugs that suppress the human immunodeficiency virus. Antiretrovirals are life-saving medications; they turn what used to be a death sentence for infected individuals into a chronic but manageable condition. A decision maker who questions the

Table 1   Conceptualizing AIDS governance

Core questions	Organizing principles of governance	Standardized procedures of AIDS governance
How do governments understand a matter of common concern, and how do they frame the nature of the crisis at hand?	The state should frame AIDS as a public health issue and accept evidence-based medicines	• The epidemic should be addressed as a public health crisis • The state should enforce the standardized protocol and discourage alternative (substandard) medicines • The state should secure the supply of generics and monitor the global pharmaceutical industry's activities
What is the core set of activities that governments should undertake in order to solve the issue at stake?	The state should recognize health as a common good imbued with strong human-rights connotations	• The state should remove barriers to prevention services to any vulnerable group • Ideally, governments should put all eligible individuals on treatment and mobilize finances to HIV-related programs
How should states interact with other participants in social practice?	The state should commit to the principle of nonhierarchical and nonstate governance	• Elites and ruling groups should not hijack independent AIDS bureaucracies • Governments should involve private actors in partnerships • The state should include civil society in the policy-making process • The state should maintain partnerships with the mainstream international AIDS organizations

life-saving properties of ARVs raises doubts about the causal links between HIV and AIDS and enforces the substandard protocol, in fact, deviates from the global consensus. As unambiguous as all this technical information might be, the organizing principle undergirding international recommendations—the medical evidence-based solution to the public health crisis—may raise concerns at home.

While Russian state officials never challenged the notion of proven medicines, the Kremlin's approach to HIV nevertheless was quite unique. Members of the Russian elite came to understand and frame the disease as a challenge to the state as an ultimate value. Fighting AIDS gave the Russian government an opportunity to communicate its desired public image of a successful and functional state. The Kremlin's overreliance on the governmental mechanisms of delivery combined with the limited administrative capacity of the state machinery engendered negative externalities in terms of bureaucrats' inability to sustain the standardized protocol. Moreover, in order to showcase Russia's reinstated global power status in the international system, its leaders nurtured unrealistic ambitions to develop a number of evidence-based innovative drugs. Welcome as they are, efforts to bolster pharmaceutical research and development critically depend on advanced industrial capabilities, technological sophistication, and economic productivity. Although these prerequisites were by and large absent in Putin's Russia, ideational devotions to "pharmaceutical sovereignty" prompted the government to pursue that route.

In South Africa, President Mbeki immersed himself in the public conversation about the toxicity of the antiretrovirals, arguing that the epidemic was about development and local knowledge. The stress on indigenousness (sometimes referred to as nativism or Africanism, or anticolonial sentiment) as the core goal of the state fueled a disbelief in proven Western biomedical products. Pretoria emphasized the use of complementary, alternative, and traditional medicines for the treatment of both HIV and its opportunistic diseases. This impinged on the standardized protocol in treatment and created a permissive environment in which multiple producers peddled substandard medications without any conventional proof of their safety and efficacy. The pursuit of alternative medicines was equally about implementing the state's mission to restore the local cultural heritage and about deploying local solutions as a cardinal tool of health governance.

Second, international guidelines make clear that the failure to provide universal coverage and remove barriers to prevention impedes efforts to contain the disease. On the one hand, governments should ensure access to treatment to all who qualify for it from a medical standpoint. To mobilize the necessary amount of resources requires governments to address the issue of life-saving pharmaceutical products as a matter of noncompetitive consumption of the public good. On the other hand, universality of access to prevention is equally about the principled ideas and values regarding human rights. Without prevention programs, such as harm reduction and opioid substitute treatment, governments will not be able to solve the HIV/AIDS health crisis. As no vulnerable populations should be excluded from adequate prevention services, the principles of human rights need to be observed and implemented, even if this entails removing legal and cultural obstacles to prevention. Under certain circumstances, however, domestic metanorms are incompatible with the principles of human rights in particular or the provision of the public good in general.

The Kremlin challenged human rights principles, dismissed Western advice on harm-reduction programs, and neglected to take seriously those evidence-based claims that highlighted the importance of needle exchanges and opioid substitution. The emphasis on statism and great power status thwarted adoption of human rights principles, since these principles, in the eyes of Russian leaders, were subversive. At the same time, the Russian government was ready to provide treatment as a public good. As the Kremlin came to see itself as an engine of economic development and the enforcer of social justice, it increased public spending for health care and the treatment of infectious diseases and strove to make universal medical coverage available. Not surprisingly, the Kremlin relied solely on state mechanisms to do so.

In South Africa, the picture was quite different. The Cabinet was not ready to recognize treatment as a public good. The South African stress on market-centered empowerment (economic neoliberalism) questioned the validity of the extensive rollout of antiretrovirals in the public sector and affirmed the necessity to protect the private sector from sharing the burden of health governance. But policy makers tried to abide, albeit with limited success in regard to the epidemiological outcomes, by the principles of human rights and to apply these principles to preventive services.

Third, partnerships with civil society, the private sector, and international organizations are a matter of good governance. Governments alone cannot attune health programs to diverse conditions in various parts of the country, while civil society often diversifies services, improves outreach, supports vulnerable groups, spreads awareness, raises additional funds, and so on. Restraining partnerships and excluding relevant stakeholders creates an unhealthy governance environment. However, the existing norms of state-society and state-business relations might not reflect the organizing principle of nonhierarchical and nonstate governance. For instance, it is clear that in modern capitalist states, state-society and state-business relations are noticeably different from those that exist in patrimonial states. Further, these norms might not arise out of structural conditions but rather reflect those fundamental domestic ideas encompassed by the country's social purpose. When governments handpick certain stakeholders and give them a privileged position in the enacted system of health governance, the health partnership acquires situational and local characteristics. Inasmuch as social purposes include ideas about legitimate standards of governance, they affect the styles of partnership in health policy making.

In Putin's Russia, the *siloviki* (law enforcement agents and prominent politicians with a background in the so-called power ministries), joined by conservative church functionaries, captured the policy debate on HIV/AIDS and framed it according to their ideas and organizational mission. This behavior went against the international notion that competent health and AIDS bureaucracies should independently perform the routine tasks related to their own purview. As Russian leaders drifted toward a developmental state autonomous from society, they ceased to view civil society and the private sector as equal partners. To weave domestic stakeholders into the top-down power hierarchy, Russian leaders used both the carrot of generous state funding and the stick of punitive laws, thereby skillfully reducing the autonomy of the fledgling civil society. The Kremlin also embraced the idea that Russia was a great power. Delusional as this self-image might be, it certainly affected the Kremlin's behavior. Supplied with windfall mineral rents but lacking an adequate and modern health-care industry, Russian leaders chose to act like donors in the international arena and fended off the expertise and resources of well-established international health organizations.

In Mbeki's South Africa, the assault on those competent health agencies that resisted Pretoria's challenge to conventional medical approaches amplified Pretoria's negativity toward the principles of scientific regulation of medical issues. Civil society was not left alone either. A standard account of the state-society relationships in South Africa is likely to tell the story of the epic clash between the recalcitrant government and modern civil society. Overly sensitive Thabo Mbeki and his umbrageous health minister did not take criticisms of their policies and leadership lightly. It surely was some degree of personal animosity that factored into frustrating the partnerships with protreatment stakeholders. Despite the broad international support behind protreatment activists, Mbeki's administration was willing to support the nonstate advocates of alternative medicines and complementary diets. This choice entailed no clear political benefits besides encouraging those organizations whose missions were similar to the vision of the African Renaissance. Pretoria's commitment to exercise moral leadership on the continent prompted the country's leaders to challenge the authority of international organizations and welcome the counterepistemic community of AIDS dissidents. (The notion of "counterepistemic community" describes the community of scientists and experts who rely on other than evidence-based practices and wish to countervail dominant international regimes.)[25]

In either country, the enacted patterns of health governance were not preordained. As several policy experts indicate, prior to 1998, Pretoria followed international prescriptions. More specifically, the 1994 National AIDS Plan received accolades as the ideal policy-drafting process that reflected the majority of international prescriptions on how to curb the pandemic.[26] In the early to mid-1990s, Mbeki, eager to compensate for Mandela's lack of leadership on the issue, publicly demonstrated a strong interest in spearheading the fight against AIDS. His early vision impressed both Peter Piot of UNAIDS and AIDS activists.[27] In other words, the preconditions for adopting the external solutions were all in place. But this was before the African Renaissance took hold of the South African elite. Once the second president became committed to the new vision for the country, he seized the opportunity to employ traditional medicines, believing that utilizing these medicines would ultimately prove the capacity of the former liberation movement to govern and invalidate Western neocolonial stereotypes about the failure of the Africans to solve domestic policy problems by themselves.

Unlike many other states, the Russian government never denied the threat the disease posed. Even as other pressing problems overwhelmed Russian politicians, Boris Yeltsin pledged to donate his autobiography's royalties to fight HIV/AIDS.[28] In 1989 and 1990 Yeltsin decided to spend his remuneration for paid lectures and speeches in the United States and Japan to buy disposable hypodermic needles for Soviet hospitals.[29] In the 1990s the federal legislature enacted a stream of AIDS-related laws and programs, including a provision for free access to treatment. Despite overwhelming financial shortcomings and the meager administrative capacity of the state, the preconditions for learning about human rights standards and the efficiency of evidence-based prevention strategies were all in place. However, once external standards of AIDS governance became antithetical to the sovereign democracy's statism and its antiliberal impulse, the expected norm diffusion slowed down and became paralyzed.

Some features of AIDS policy making in the two countries turned out to be inadvertently delusive and resulted in misguided governance choices. Yet for a while the postapartheid elite believed—and the Russians still do—that their course of action was quite normal and to a large degree desirable. However, while citizens do connect to the articulated ideas in principle, the consequences of these ideas in practice might belie the generated expectations. A failure to fulfill societal expectations might trigger a split in the ruling group, widen social unrest, and impede leaders' legitimacy. This is precisely what happened to Thabo Mbeki, who invested too much of his credibility and personal reputation into pursuing alternative solutions to the health crisis. Once in full swing, South Africa's AIDS policy disaster sobered even those who had favored the African Renaissance as a grand rejuvenating idea. For instance, Phumzile

Mlambo-Ngucka, Mbeki's second deputy president, although sharing the predilections of her boss, in the concluding years of Mbeki's administration became compelled to transform the existing structure of health governance. In Russia the existent administrative capacity of the state did not match the extensive promises of the country's government. Although the political consequences of this divergence are yet to be seen, the failures to deliver have begun tarnishing Putin's shining armor.

ADDITIONAL EXPLANATIONS

So far I have provided a skeletal explanation. This section discusses several additional explanations. (Other considerations appear in the appropriate chapters.) First, although the literature on South African responses to AIDS strongly emphasizes individual-level variables, the determinants of leaders' behavior cannot be reduced to personal idiosyncrasies. Second, a variety of scholars imply the possibility that some initial conditions—either dearly held premodern biomedical ideas or the inheritances of Communist and apartheid health systems—heavily constrain health governance in the two countries. These types of conditions surely undermine good health governance, as they can generate powerful incentives to ignore modern evidence-based medicine and dismiss international best practices as irrelevant to local epidemiological circumstances. But these conditions are not inviolable; leaders do not have to treat them as unbreakable. In the following subsection, I discuss the role of material interests that might warp normal health governance and undermine the interests of public health. In the concluding subsection, I comment on the surge of antineoliberal alarmism, which overstates the power of neoliberal ideology in global health governance.

The Role of the Individual

Individuals, especially high-powered ones, matter. So do their health-related ideas. Some leaders certainly promoted some random and odd ideas to solve important domestic problems. Turkmenistan's Saparmurat Niyazov was, perhaps, the best embodiment of the notion that leaders sometimes impose the quirkiest policy solutions for the strangest possible reasons, or for reasons that defy a commonsensical explanation. He fired much of the country's health-care professionals and thought to replace them with conscripted soldiers. This behavior, of course, is an outlier that tells us more about the raw autocratic power of an unhinged leader than the independent impact of a state's ideas about a particular course of governance.

Mbeki's case is different. His ideas are an instance of something more than just individual-level compulsions, although it is easy to believe otherwise. Let me set the record straight. There is no dispute that Mbeki personally contributed to and perhaps amplified the country's inconsistency with regard to international best practices. Mbeki's policy blunders included his public denial of the causal links between HIV and AIDS and the courting of AIDS dissidents. All this is well documented. In the early 2000s, international journalists and academics exposed South African HIV/AIDS policy blunders to international audiences. They provided strong evidence that President Mbeki questioned the relationship between the human immunodeficiency virus and the acquired syndrome of opportunistic diseases. They also exposed his resistance to roll out universally adopted life-saving antiretroviral treatment therapy. These actions went against the key guidelines and evidence-based recommendations of the core international health actors, including the World Health Organization and the professional health-care community. This critical exposure, of course, followed the rules of its journalistic genre. The intention was to focus public attention on some severe shortcomings in the provision of HIV/AIDS medications in South Africa. At the same time, it was not the job of either the mass media or health activists to construct or test any theories designed to explain the puzzle of Mbeki's counterintuitive and disastrous policies. As a result, it was easy to end up with an impression that it must have been idiosyncratic factors such as Mbeki's personality and his leadership style that could explain what was going on in South Africa.

This personality-oriented theme became rather popular and took on many variations. Mbeki's opponents underscored his "contrarian streak," criticizing his taste for going against prevailing notions and ideas, his injudicious use of Internet resources of dubious expertise, and his beliefs in various conspiracies that allegedly aimed to undermine South African political and economic development. Critically minded health policy scholars and domestic treatment activists continuously expressed a high degree of outrage, if not undiluted hatred, for the president and his key political allies who were in charge of AIDS policies. Mbeki's supporters, contrastingly, admired how their president crafted his domestic policies. They touted his intellectual sophistication and unwavering dedication to a thoroughgoing analysis of complex issues. In their eyes, the president's style of health policy making confirmed his reputation as an independent thinker in search of sensitive, innovative, and unorthodox approaches. Not surprisingly, they argued, Mbeki's detractors were not able to grasp his conceptual maturity, complex sensibilities, intricate policy making, and desire to break the Western monopoly on scientific truth. Even after the president's downfall, commentators praised Mbeki's fight to think independently of Europe and the United States and glorified his deliberate battle with the international pharmaceutical industry. In a series of newspaper articles, Frank Chikane, Mbeki's director general in the presidency, indicated that it was Mbeki's "intellectual prowess which sank him."[30]

Was Mbeki then too conceptually complex to perform the pragmatic tasks of public administration?

Thabo Mbeki is indeed a person of many colors: his stress on Africa's return to its roots does not preclude him from injecting profusely long quotes from assorted Victorian poets in his political speeches and having his wardrobe stocked with standard British business suits. An internal cable report from the U.S. ambassador, Delano E. Lewis, to Washington, D.C., on February 23, 2001, was broadly reproduced in the South African media and exposed Mbeki's intolerance to alternative viewpoints and criticism.[31]

Mbeki, of course, is not the only leader or celebrity who has heavily influenced domestic health policies. George Bush, Bill Clinton, Kofi Annan, Yoweri Museveni, Fernando Cardoso, Lula da Silva, Vladimir Putin, and Bono have all put their stamp on AIDS campaigns and health initiatives in a variety of ways. I assert nevertheless that an unqualified stress on personality as a key explanatory factor oversimplifies and obscures a more complex story of AIDS governance in South Africa. Simply put, pointing fingers at some leaders' policy triumphs, failures, mistakes, or breakthroughs does not provide a compelling explanation. More important is that the president was not acting alone or only at his own whim. A significant number of domestic constituents were not against Mbeki's health governance. Provincial-level health administrators, for instance, echoed Mbeki's views by restricting the use of antiretroviral therapy, in several cases refusing to prescribe it. Consistent with Pretoria's stress on ethnomedicines, local healers flooded the market with various alternative medications, indigenous concoctions, and dietary supplements. The ruling party's leadership had a mixed record of views regarding the mainstream and heterodox views on HIV/AIDS treatment.

Lest we suppress all these facts, observers and scholars alike should broach the issue of whether the roots of Mbeki's behavior lie beyond his personal compulsions. Constructivist insights steer keen observers of AIDS politics to pose questions about the consistent rationales and normative underpinnings of unorthodox governance models. Suffice it to say that while ideas may pass through some individuals' mental processes, those ideas still are social phenomena and not the property or attributes of individuals, agencies, or collectivities.

Premodern Collective Beliefs

Various premodern biomedical beliefs about the disease and traditional healing powerfully reverberate across the globe. Here I define beliefs as internalized ideas spread throughout a population. The adjective "premodern" means that these beliefs are not evidence-based and that their policy utility from a technological standpoint is futile. Intuitively, collectively held premodern biomedical beliefs and ideas generate implications for health policy at home and barriers to external influences. If a policy maker believes in something, he or she is less likely to want external advice about the necessity of change. However, the links between HIV-related interventions and premodern sensibilities are not self-explanatory. Consider the following examples.

Traditional medicines symbolize the resistance to the ways in which the industrialized world dispenses health science across the globe. The recurring pleas to support solutions rooted in the local culture features prominently, for instance, in Gambia and Nigeria.[32] The most noteworthy example includes Gambian president Yahya Jammeh, who reinvented himself as a traditional healer. Jammeh claimed to possess the Allah-sanctioned mandate to cure AIDS, asthma, high blood pressure, and infertility with some secret Koranic herbal-based medicine. Jammeh's actions are best explained by his psychological traits and popularity concerns. But it is hasty and unfounded to assume the independent impact of premodern beliefs about the disease and healing, whatever those beliefs are. Moreover, since the Gambia is not isolated from the rest of the world, conventional medical beliefs are not conceptually unavailable to the country's leaders.

Discrepancies in Jacob Zuma's beliefs and behavior are a good case in point, too. As the deputy president of the Republic of South Africa (1999–2005), Zuma headed the National AIDS Council and the Moral Regeneration Campaign. At that time, his words and actions abundantly displayed his embrace of premodern health beliefs suffused with Mbeki-like denialist attitudes. One of the most telling episodes occurred when he invited members of the African National Congress (ANC) to join him in a candle-lighting ceremony outside the lower house of the Parliament, during which two HIV-infected teenagers claimed that although they had been taking no antiretrovirals, they nevertheless were quite healthy. Zuma pointed these two teenagers out as an example that one can be healthy, happy, and productive while taking no HIV medications at all.[33] Another illustrative episode happened when Zuma had to defend himself against rape charges in court. He offered highly controversial comments about his hygiene choices regarding HIV prevention.[34] This blunder prompted a famous South African cartoonist, Zapiro, to draw Zuma's satirical character from then on with a showerhead protruding from his cranium. Although there is no evidence to suggest that Zuma radically altered his beliefs after assuming the highest office in the country in 2009, his presidential record on health policy has been much more in line with that of the international mainstream. The plausible explanation is that internalized premodern beliefs by themselves do not overdetermine health governance, especially once leaders assume high-powered policy positions.

Premodern beliefs and quackery of various sorts flourish not just on the African continent. On the other side of the globe, in the Russian Federation, "people's healers," sorcerers, homeopaths, and faith healers time and again promote various sorts of folk medicine and telepathic cures. Miracle workers Anatoliy Kashpirovskiy and Alan Chumak keep popping up on national TV, praised by the grateful cured. Fused with the worshiped secrets and esoteric powers of cutting-edge science and technology, premodern beliefs transform into a variety of wild claims of genetic restructuring, organ and bone regeneration, and long-distance laser-based cancer cures. These claims featured heavily in the commercialized healing projects of Petr Garyaev, who, on top of everything else, claimed fake institutional affiliations and boasted academic credentials he had never acquired. Yet various outbreaks of quackery in the country, even while erratically endorsed by high-power politicians, are generally met with hostility and do not define the official approaches to health governance. For Russian health governance, premodern beliefs were nonessential and irrelevant. These ideas simply never fell in the range of Russian policy makers' commitments. On the contrary, the government legislated against various self-promoted healers and psychics.[35]

In sum, there are obviously many obscure biomedical ideas circulating in different political places. Ordinary citizens and powerful leaders might or might not hold them true and dear on the individual level. But governments, policy participants, and opinion leaders can put premodern and alternative beliefs under control no matter how popular they are. My contention thus is that personal and collective beliefs in some questionable health notions will not acquire independent causal power, unless these notions are confluent with the dominant social purpose of the state.

Legacies as Obstacles

Politicians and observers alike often admit that massive health systems generate legacies that inhibit change. Confessions of this sort can mean many things, including politicians' mental inability to embrace change, their unwillingness to upset their constituents, or their reluctance to pay the costs associated with changing policy course. Surely, structural constraints of health systems might be difficult to breach, especially if the system is not underperforming or is not crumbling. Otherwise, the opportunity for change is ripe.

During its first two decades of independence, Russia tried to break free from the Soviet approach to health and attempted to follow external best practices. As critically minded observers note, these efforts were disorganized, improperly encouraged, and poorly enforced. Mixed results of the reform included some notable examples of success (e.g., the liberalization of pharmaceutical markets). Gradually, however, external ideas ceased to be a source of inspiration and innovation in health governance. Although the necessity to reform the health sector had been widely acknowledged, the transformation of health care stagnated. Under Putin's second administration and Medvedev's interregnum, state-centric imperatives prevailed over the liberal approach to health. Domestic reaction to moderate social unrest, such as the ill-received monetization of previously offered in-kind health benefits, can explain only a few aspects of the backpedaling in health policy making.[36] A dramatic turnaround from espousing liberal principles to rejecting them warrants examining how ideas about appropriate standards of health governance change in tandem with political orientations.

It is possible to argue that perception of the enduring legacies of the past affected South Africa's turn to indigenous medical treatments. Apparent and justified is policy makers' hostility toward colonialism and tropical medicine, which were based on Western models of public health. That Mbeki and his entourage decided to question the motives of the pharmaceutical firms and the former colonial powers is not surprising.[37] But these pernicious legacies by themselves would not have preordained the future styles of health governance in the country, which remained conceptually open.

Another dimension of the South African approach to health—domestic appreciation of traditional medicines—is not a natural outgrowth of the medicinal

and cultural activities that lasted for centuries. The history of traditional healing was less straightforward and suggestive for postapartheid health policy than
one might believe.[38] Large-scale cultivation, valorization, and commercialization
of indigenous plant resources with potentially high medicinal values are recent
phenomena. Equally recent is the desire to elevate these resources on the national agenda, even though politicians and health administrators might attempt
to do so under the disingenuous guise of a sacred and inviolable tradition.

On balance, it is tempting to overestimate the power of historical legacies. It
is also enticing to retrofit select features of contemporary health governance into
some multifaceted historical phenomena while ignoring others. In some ways,
historical inheritances usually matter, but how policy makers interpret and deal
with them matters more. My line of reasoning, therefore, suggests that normative debates about the state's social purpose might play a key role in manipulating these legacies to attain particular political goals.

Material Interests

Were the leaders unwilling to accept external norms because they were busy
chasing their own material interests? The taste for enrichment can surely impede learning about best international practices. The taste for easy money can
also prompt unscrupulous politicians and greedy bureaucrats to design or maintain systems of governance that facilitate looting resources rather than improve
public health. The question considered here is if material interests and commercial considerations charted the course of HIV/AIDS policy making in the
two countries. The dominant groups (the *siloviki* in Russia and the Mbekiites
in South Africa) could have made use of AIDS control to line their pockets. The
available evidence, however, points in a different direction.

As the Russian government allocated a considerable amount of resources
in the state sector, firms and individuals closely connected to key public officials found many fraudulent ways to enrich themselves. In South Africa, the
state-sponsored support for traditional healing practices incentivized many proprietors to seek enrichment at the expense of the sick. Given the admitted levels
of corruption in Russia and South Africa, the use of grand ideas to disguise personal gains is plausible. In both cases, however, evidence showing the material
gains of key state officials who were responsible for policy formulation remains
rather weak. Below I consider some examples, substantiating my reasoning.

In Russia, according to the investigative reports published in the influential domestic newspapers, public health, along with weaponry procurement and construction, was one of the most corrupt and inefficient areas of public administration. During the massive federal purchases of high-tech medical equipment in 2008–10, various forms of financial schemes, bribes, and kickbacks (*otkaty*) resulted in the loss of nearly half of the disbursed public funds. The scandal about the massive fraud in purchasing magnetic resonance imaging (MRI) machines implicated the entire system of state contracts as highly inefficient.[39] Similarly, contracts to build new medical centers across the country presented opportunities for fraudulent enrichment.[40]

When some of these facts became widely known in 2010, Medvedev attempted to quash corruption and stop inefficient allocation of resources in the health-care sector. That Medvedev failed in his endeavors tells volumes about the weak administrative capacity of the state and the government's failure to manage its overextended economic obligations. Importantly, corruption will not be cleaned out unless the Russian government terminates its commitments to uphold the state's autonomy from society and sustain the state's role as the main economic actor. But these deeply internalized commitments are the very reasons that Putin and Medvedev have held for differentiating their Russia from other political units. In this context, material interests alone cannot explain the multiple defects of Russian health governance. In addition, there are reasons to believe that industrial lobbyists benefit from the preference for import substitution, but restricting imports of modern pharmaceutical products and medical devices as a conscious policy materialized precisely at the time Russia picked an ideational confrontation with the West.[41]

In South Africa, the industry of traditional medicines generates somewhere between four billion and eight billion rand per year. Pretoria's preoccupation with localized solutions opened the window of opportunity for those domestic and international actors who were willing to exploit it. Unscrupulous business entrepreneurs did not hesitate to utilize local sensibilities, fears, and biases in order to enhance their advertisement campaigns and to achieve their selling targets.[42] Healers' prominence in the growing multibillion-rand industry of traditional medicines implicates some individuals as aggressive profit seekers, whether or not they genuinely opposed colonial medicines and believed in the healing effects of their compounds and concoctions. Although the official backing of that industry might implicate some decision makers in pursuing material interests, there is little evidence directly incriminating key decision makers in crafting health policies in order to line their pockets.

Mbeki's distrust of pharmaceutical companies and his emphasis on local so-lutions attracted and emboldened many an unscrupulous entrepreneur. It is not by chance that Matthias Rath, a German pharmaceutical proprietor, came to South Africa in 2004, when the domestic search for local alternatives for the evidence-based treatment therapy was in full swing.[43] Much reviled for ped-dling his merchandise as a full-blown substitute for licensed biomedical prod-ucts, Rath nevertheless enjoyed the support of those who cherished nostrums and complementary medicines. Since Rath portrayed himself as a crusader against global pharmaceutical companies, Dr. Mantombazana "Manto" Edmie Tsabalala-Msimang, minister of health from 1999 to 2008, fell for the curing promise of his vitamins and micronutrients. However, her connections to Rath and Roberto Giraldo, yet another shady peddler of unproven cures, suspicious as they were, produced no definitive evidence suggesting that she empowered these proprietors for her personal financial gain. More warranted is the conclu-sion that the government supported such healers because of its principled com-mitment to promote indigenous health governance.

In summary, I am not aware of any explicit evidence suggesting that policy makers specifically designed health policy for personal gain. Unless I am wrong on this account, it certainly would be a mistake to insist that neither the Afri-can Renaissance nor sovereign democracy had an independent policy-making impact.

Neoliberalism and Global Health

Michel Foucault inspired many scholars to situate the discussion of health poli-tics in the macrostructures of global capitalism and enterprise society "based on the market, competition, inequality, and the privilege of the individual."[44] Fol-lowing this injunction, many health activists and policy-oriented scholars as-sert that the spread of neoliberal ideology, promoted by the all-powerful World Bank, World Trade Organization, and pharmaceutical firms, shapes trans-boundary and domestic responses to HIV/AIDS.

According to its critics, macroeconomic ideas of neoliberalism, now widely spread across the globe, undermine the capacity of the state and weaken the gov-ernmental commitment to provide health care. Neoliberalism enhances the po-sition of the private sector in global health governance and reduces state author-ity over the health sector. In addition, the private sector commodifies both the very process of knowledge production and the result of this process—the unrestricted availability of essential life-saving medicines. The state further rolls back its commitments to provide medicines as basic public goods.[45] Structural threats, which arise from the unequal access to medicines and health care, the uneven and conditional distribution of foreign aid, drastic cuts in public spending for social services, and parochial interests of donors, are specific expressions associated with neoliberal globalization. Neoliberalism worsens social determinants of AIDS and intentionally scathes public health.[46] Moreover, leftist academics and activists alike view neoliberalism as the hypocritical tool of imposing the Western hegemonic order on the rest of the world. David Roberts asserts that supranational neoliberalism "dictates specific national policies in developing countries that are quite at odds with successful (and for the most part ongoing) state social practices in Europe and North America."[47] To some degree, this argument implies that the state is efficient and, quite simply, the best form of governance currently available. It also supports an unwarranted confidence that redistributive strategies and large-scale spending would imminently recover public health in the Third World. Although this antineoliberal alarmism strikes a chord with any individual committed to upholding social justice, as a scholarly explanation it fails to capture the complexity of domestic health policy making, let alone the fact that in many cases, the Russian one included, the state itself is the root problem of many dimensions of poor health governance.

To be fair, many scholars have provided nuanced and insightful portrayals of the impact of neoliberal ideas. Michael Bosia, for instance, has documented how the adoption of neoliberal guidelines—cutting social spending and making blood products profitable—has inadvertently contributed to the spread of AIDS through the national blood supply.[48] Although using different terminology (ethical mission and moral ambition instead of the notion of the social purpose), Bosia has tackled the French attempt to redefine or alter the accepted conception of the common good and move away from an excessive governmental presence in the economy and public health. This transition was happening not only in times of great uncertainty about the control over the pandemic but also in the context of a profound gulf between the elite's and activists' views about whether or not neoliberal ideas should underpin the policy environment. Thus, the French understood contamination of the blood supply in connection with the challenge to the "ethical mission" (social purpose) of the republic, not as a stand-alone crisis. Consequently, instead of fixing a policy tragedy to achieve mutually desirable policy goals, policy participants entered into bitter contention around the principles of public health.

But in general, is it correct to assert that the unfolding processes of neoliberal globalization undermine both international and domestic commitments to fight the epidemic? Even the sharpest critics of neoliberal governance have to concede that a rather progressive international health regime has been emerging.[49] Indeed, nothing in the set of international HIV/AIDS policies and guidelines is inconsistent with the goals of enhancing domestic well-being and health. Just the opposite: achieving positive results in public health became directly associated with the understanding that the state ought to provide health care and strive to reach the universal level of treatment coverage. AIDS policy entrepreneurs have successfully shaped the global perception of antiretroviral drugs as a classic public good and convinced the top donors to focus their foreign assistance on AIDS.

On balance, while it is important to remain aware of the actual challenges neoliberalism poses to public health, arguments about the power of neoliberal thinking and its multiple pernicious effects should be qualified. The extant policy consensus regarding HIV/AIDS policy norms does not rest on neoliberalism. Despite the pressures of neoliberal globalization (most importantly, approaching health care and access to medicines as a trade issue), international health policy actors have come to agree that governments have responsibility to provide antiretroviral treatment, ensure the universality of access to it, and bring together all relevant stakeholders in the policy-making process.

Summary

Although a number of propositions can explain bits and pieces of the available evidence, to connect them in a coherent picture requires offering a holistic answer. The additional explanations discussed above fail to perform better than my own proposition that the views on the appropriate ways of national renewal were pivotal for shaping the systems of AIDS governance.

CONCLUSION

Very few prominent political leaders doubt that their governments should curb the spread of human immunodeficiency virus and sustain treatment programs. Their general lack of doubt that action should be taken nevertheless leaves the question as to the appropriate course of health governance unanswered. How exactly governments decide to respond to the contagion requires an explanation. This book ascertains how and why debates within a state about its core goals and the common good provoke interest in adopting external norms, trigger hostility to the external principles of governance, or prompt their selective adaptation. Tackling this question is helpful to develop thinking about the variation in across-case health governance without relegating the observed variations to a plurality of situational and individual-level factors. In short, social purposes filter the global flow of policy initiatives, recommendations, and standardized practices on the grounds of their compatibility with the underlying normative underpinnings of domestic political authority. As evidence suggests, sometimes the effects of deploying social purposes are subtle and indirect and sometimes tangible and overt. On balance, the concept of the social purpose of the state should join a set of common factors and variables that scholars make use of to explain health politics. Before returning to the structured, focused discussion of AIDS politics in the two countries, the following chapter discusses the advent of social purposes in Russia and South Africa separately from international norms and domestic AIDS governance.

CHAPTER 2

Assembling the Purpose

State Goals in Putin's Russia and Mbeki's South Africa

SOMETIMES BOTH A STATE'S CAPACITY to perform its administrative functions and an elite's ability to maintain adequate justifications for a state's existence fail. The old ideas and norms appear vacuous. Ultimately, this is a twin decline of both coercive power and the legitimate social purpose. Trying to rebound after periods of political disorder, politicians, state officials, and opinion leaders usually aspire to regain full political authority. They seek not just raw power but compelling and satisfying ideas. In South Africa after the collapse of apartheid and in Russia after the fall of Communism, politicians and opinion leaders sensed the ontological need to redefine their ideas about the core tasks of the state. This chapter tackles Russian and South African quests to discover and promote these ideas. Once elites started treating their ideas as obligations, a distinct social purpose had a chance to materialize in either country. As these ideas spread through the structures of discursive communications and as they took hold of wider collectivities, social purposes acquired independent conceptual power and became social facts.

The analysis of each case is broken down into five subsections. The first subsection discusses each country's elite and its commitment to the distinct goals of the state. The obvious difference between the two cases is that in Russia the group that had climbed to the commanding heights weeded out other justifications for the country's existence as a distinct political space. In comparison, although the South African elite was committed to the ideas that I describe under the heading of the African Renaissance, these ideas failed to become the only collectively approved raison d'être of the country. The three subsections that follow explore the systems of representations through which top politicians and opinion leaders circulated their views. In the Russian case, I survey the elite's focus on state autonomy (statism), state-led developmentalism, and great power status as three cardinal ideas that captured the public mind. In the South African case, I explore indigenousness, market-centered empowerment, and the external ambition of the moral leadership—three ideas that represented the chief obligations of the postapartheid state. The fifth subsection documents domestic identity arguments. These types of arguments constitute only a part, albeit a very significant one, of internal debates about the core goals of the state. Specifically, identity arguments are fundamental for communication between elites, their opponents, and wider audiences. Identity arguments send powerful messages about the essentialized negative characteristics of the ruling group's opponents and therefore have the ability to persuade listeners that the alternative principles of governance are not legitimate and should not be acted upon. I conclude the chapter with some conceptual clarifications that help us think about social purpose as a variable that is applicable beyond the two cases discussed in this book.

PUTIN'S SOVEREIGN DEMOCRACY

After the collapse of Communism, Russian politicians failed to formulate and explain the nature of the state they were trying to erect. They found themselves amid an overwhelming normative disorientation, which characterized the tumultuous politics of the transition to democracy in the 1990s. The first president of the newly independent Russia, Boris Yeltsin, based his political authority on his personal popularity rather than on a compelling and intersubjectively shared social purpose. Nevertheless, after the collapse of Communism, Russians engaged in normative debates about the common good and the nature of social order and political authority. These discussions gave rise to many eclectic proposals that fused various (sometimes barely compatible) ideologies and ideas, although none of them was able to capture the Russian political and social imagination in full. Opinion polls suggested an increasing public preference for stability and order, a tougher realpolitik in the international arena, and ideological certainty. Yet these polls clearly implied that neither a return to the moral ambition of building "developed socialism" nor a further extension of the official half-hearted embrace of Western-style human rights would be popular and desirable. By the late 1990s, many Russian citizens had expressed generally favorable popular attitudes to democratic ideals and simultaneous distrust in nearly all decision makers and political institutions.

Although anti-Communist sentiment was broadly articulated in the popular culture, including movies and literature, it did not turn into a consolidated national purpose. Liliya Shevtsova argued that Yeltsin either was not interested in the normative debates or did not grasp their critical importance for state building. Instead, he wasted precious time and then moved on to transform the economy using unreformed institutions.[1] Kathleen E. Smith attributes Yeltsin's failure to embed proliberal political ideas to his entourage's neglect of highly important symbolic national events.[2] Be that as it may, the failure to elaborate a coherent system of meaning about the state should not be taken as evidence of the absence of a political desire to do so. Once the proponents of retrograde social arrangements started gaining the upper hand in their conceptual assault on the principles of democracy, liberalism, and the free market, Yeltsin realized the necessity to refute them by articulating an attractive normative vision for the country. To do so, he appointed a task force in charge of formulating the concept of "the national idea for Russia." The assembled group limited itself to taking stock of all ideological discourses and political ideas flowing in the society.[3] Because that initiative did not bear fruit, Yeltsin's successors had to start their search for the normative foundation of the emerging political order in Russia almost from scratch. Vladimir Putin's efforts turned out to be quite successful, as he was able to generate clear expectations about the nature of political authority and, with the help of Kremlin-friendly opinion leaders, to stabilize those expectations.

The first subsection discusses how the *siloviki* developed their vision for the core goals of the state. The second subsection explores the principled ideas embraced by Putin concerning the state's autonomy from society. Such autonomy is the first crucial dimension of internal sovereignty, which posits the state as the ultimate and exclusive locus of authority. The third subsection discusses political commitments to the developmental state, the second important dimension of internal sovereignty, which highlights the state's right to select the course and methods of domestic economic development. The fourth subsection explores the meanings encompassed by the Russian interpretation of its external sovereignty. In a nutshell, autonomy from external normative influences gradually became the main vector of Russia's external ambitions. The term "sovereign democracy" captures these principles. The final subsection traces the identity arguments that developed scorn for the liberals as the offenders of the common good.

Committed Elites in Russia

During the second half of the 1990s, a sizable number of *siloviki* began to ascend to the top ranks of the Russian political elite. Although some representatives of the *siloviki* became prominent during Yeltsin's rule, their full-blown political domination did not materialize until Putin became president. The term *siloviki* describes individuals with backgrounds in the so-called power ministries, including operatives and functionaries of law enforcement and especially the Soviet secret police.[4] Internal conflicts and variance in the organizational culture of different enforcement agencies notwithstanding, scholars agree that an emphasis on the *siloviki* as a coherent social group is instructive. According to some estimates, in the 2000s the *siloviki* comprised up to 42 percent of the federal elite as compared to 13 percent in the 1990s. The necessary caveat is that the available data are tentative, since the résumés of most Russian midlevel bureaucrats are not readily available. In a narrow sense, the *siloviki* were the true ideologues of the coming political changes. Sergey Ivanov, Viktor Ivanov, Igor' Sechin, Nikolay Patrushev, and Viktor Cherkesov were the most important members of Putin's inner circle. All these individuals share a similar background and have occupied various key advisory and regulatory positions in the state hierarchy under Putin. Gradually, they have acquired and retained informal and formal powers to promote their conception of the state among various state institutions and in society. Importantly, the trend of staffing high public offices with *siloviki* has never stopped.[5]

The *siloviki* spearheaded the formulation of the new conception of the public good and linked it to their sense of agency. They have overstressed the necessity to revive the strong state, eliminate any alternative spheres of authority, enforce punitive laws, and restore Russia's great power status. They have also triggered an obsession, bordering on paranoia, with the threats to the territorial integrity of the country and its sovereignty. They have attacked the liberal outlook and human rights as inconsistent with their core beliefs. The *siloviki* have explicitly styled themselves as the national saviors and the sole champions of the political existence of the country.

The most noteworthy statement of their creed belongs to Viktor Cherkesov. In his newspaper article "Warriors Should Not Become Merchants," the head of the Russian drug enforcement agency averred that the *siloviki* saved the country after a prolonged economic crisis and political chaos had been inflicted on the nation by liberal antistatist forces during the 1990s.[6] Domestic observers tended to downplay the importance of this article and interpreted it as Cherkesov's attempt to gain the upper hand in some nontransparent business conflicts among various high-powered groups. Nevertheless, the principal metaphor used in his public utterances was very clear. Cherkesov portrayed the *siloviki* as state-building "warriors," in contrast to the subversive "merchants" (meaning oligarchs and liberals), who had to be reined in. In a metaphorical form, this statement confirmed the indispensable role of law enforcement agencies as Russia's backbone, the primacy of state power over the free markets and political freedoms. After this publication, Cherkesov gradually lost his political standing and ended up running for the State Duma on the Communist ticket. Conventional wisdom attributes this ironic twist of fate to Putin's aversion to any internal squabbles made public rather than to his disagreement with Cherkesov's ideas. Despite Cherkesov's misfortune, the *siloviki* did not lose their centrality in formulating and promoting their vision of the core goals of the state.

The *siloviki*-generated images permeated Russian society and crystallized the ways Russians interpreted the core goals of the state. At first, the dominant party, United Russia (Edinaya Rossiya), pleaded with its members to not formulate any "official state ideology" at the expense of solving "real" problems.[7] The chairman of the High Council of United Russia and the Duma speaker, Boris Gryzlov, mused that various restyled ideological orientations were harmful to political and economic development.[8] Very soon, however, Russian politicians chose to abandon this outlook.

Gradually, throughout the 2000s, various political forces conceptually converged around state centrism. The merger of the strictly Putin-oriented party, Unity (Edinstvo), and its former rival, Fatherland/All-Russia (Otechestvo–Vsya Rossiya), into the mammoth United Russia consolidated the domestic elites. Between 2005 and 2008, an internal political discussion flourished within the State-Patriotic, Liberal-Conservative, and Social-Conservative Clubs, which operated as informal discussion divisions or wings within the ruling party.[9] Despite superficial differences, there is no evidence to suggest that these clubs embrace incompatible ideas. Their blurred titles illustrate the absence of any clear-cut normative distinctions.

All this suggests that the elite united around the *siloviki*-generated agenda. That consolidation happened both inside the ruling party and across party lines. Throughout the 2000s, the Kremlin sponsored the formation of several political parties, but their political sensibilities by and large mirrored the Kremlin's normative predilections. For instance, Sergey Mironov's party, A Just Russia (Spravedlivaya Rossiya, founded in 2006), puts a social democratic spin on Putin's hard state and argues (perhaps more vigorously than United Russia) for extensive redistribution of wealth. But the principled ideas the party espouses hardly challenge the parameters of the ideational mainstream. Similarly, Vladimir Zhirinovsky and the members of his Liberal Democratic Party of Russia endorse the values of the strong state and great power status as the pillars of Russian political authority. All-Russia People's Front (founded in 2011 and headed by Vyacheslav Volodin, currently Putin's first deputy chief of staff) is a Kremlin-sponsored movement that unequivocally backs any and all of Putin's ideas and sensibilities.

In short, all formally independent political parties operate within the conceptual confines of the Kremlin-generated interpretation of the core goals of the state and are organic parts of the domestic power hierarchy.[10] Despite the differences in outlooks and varying degrees of political shrewdness, all these forces converge around and depend upon Putin.

Upholding State Autonomy

Whether celebrating or lamenting the rising discourse of statism, observers and scholars alike have agreed that Putin's political agenda hinged on it.[11] The Russian understanding of what the state is like diverges from the liberal-pluralist conception of the state that aggregates preferences and adjudicates domestic conflicts. That understanding implies that independent social life outside the state's control is a hindrance for the survival of the country. Simply put, the state is tantamount to its officialdom; high-powered rulers possess a right to remove any nonstate actor from the governance process.

It is often noted that Putin began his presidency using eclectic, pragmatic, and situational approaches to governance that did not map neatly onto any traditional ideological platform. At the same time, he never concealed his true ideational predilections. In a lengthy newspaper piece, "Russia at the Turn of the Millennium," published in 1999 on the eve of his rule, Putin described the commendable role of the state as "the source and the guarantor of the order, the initiator, and the principal force behind any change."[12] The absence of a strong state threatened Russia's stability and its survival as an autonomous political organization. The extent to which Putin internalized these ideas is illustrated by the fact that twelve years later he reiterated the main points about the centrality of the strong state with the same vigor. The value of state autonomy was indeed at the conceptual center of his political outlook. Heeding Putin's vision, top bureaucrats worked hard to insulate themselves from society and agreed to be accountable only to their boss.

Many opinion leaders elucidated and specified Putin's general thoughts.

Among them, Vladislav Surkov commands special attention. From 1999 to 2011, Surkov served in the Russian presidential administration and fancied himself as a political innovator and the conceptual architect of Putin's regime. But the ideas he offered were hardly original, despite their ornate form of delivery. He contrasted state-centric Russia to other countries that had never been proponents of the statist idea.[13] In 2007 he glorified the state: "Strong central authority for centuries collected, bonded, and developed a huge country that was widely spread in space and time. [Strong central authority] implemented all the important reforms. . . . Today, as power shifted to the center, it stabilized society, created the conditions for victory over terrorism, and sustained economic growth."[14] No less important was Surkov's claim that any nonstatist and liberal values were subversive and antithetical to Russian political culture. These values, in his opinion, threatened the country's stability, growth, and prosperity.

A close reading of the Russian discourse shows that the desire to have a strong state went hand in hand with justifications that rationalized the ontological need to curtail the power of society. By definition, any nonstate actor poses a challenge to the exclusive authority of the state. A strong autonomous state must eliminate internal political threats and purge alternative loci of authority. Not surprisingly, in his May 2004 address to the Federal Assembly, President Putin portrayed nonstate organizations as hungry for foreign money and uncaring about domestic problems.[15] Transnational groups seemed to be the prime target of Putin's antipathy, but domestic NGOs were under attack as well. From then on, independent civil society and liberally minded individuals who fought the exclusive power of officialdom to decide any important issue became the state's antagonists.

This belligerent attitude portended punitive legislation. In January 2006, the State Duma approved the infamous amendments to Federal Law No. 7, "On Noncommercial Organizations" (1996). The amendments imposed strict bureaucratic control over civil society in Russia. The government forced NGOs to undergo complicated registration procedures and pressured them to submit frequent and lengthy reports.[16] Using the new legislation, the government was able to close down around two thousand nonstate organizations within the next year or so.[17] No less serious was an excessively heavy taxation that burdened the majority of NGOs. Instead of nourishing civil society, Russian politicians created the Public Chamber, a paraconstitutional body intended to replace the genuine civil society and assume its functions.[18] Even though the Public Chamber was designed to be a simulacrum of societal control over the government, it was able to draw public attention to the most odious initiatives of the Kremlin and even make their implementation difficult.

The public reaction to these punitive initiatives neatly reflected the split between the Kremlin-friendly opinion leaders and their liberal opponents. The proponents of sovereign democracy praised these restrictions; the Kremlin-friendly opinion leaders regurgitated the unreasonable arguments about the subversive role of civil society. In contrast, liberal observers and commentators interpreted these legislative restrictions as another step on Putin's path toward autocracy. Over time the number of individuals who spoke of a liberal civil society with unqualified suspicion and unconcealed animosity escalated; myriad accusations of intimate and unnatural liaisons between domestic nonstate actors and Western intruders spread in the mass media. The Russian public failed to protect its fledgling civil society.

But this was not the end of the story. The Kremlin's assault on civil society was part of a sweeping political reform that attenuated individual liberties and further diminished the quality of democratic procedures. As the tendency to attenuate democratic accountability continued, the legislators proposed new, intentionally imprecise amendments to the law on NGOs. Any noncommercial organization that posed "a threat to the sovereignty, political independence, territorial integrity, national unity and unique character [*samobytnost'*], and national interests" of the country was to be denied registration. By definition, then, any innovation or proposal to change how things are done in the country goes against Russia's unique character. These wooly definitions arbitrarily "criminalize" a wide range of activities; they also describe the kind of civil society the Kremlin deems desirable. In 2013 the government crowned its previous initiatives with the suggestion that any noncommercial organization sponsored from abroad be deemed an agent of foreign influence. Proposals to shut down any domestic organization that received foreign grants ensued.

As Putin was returning to the highest office of the country, the Russian government moved further to obliterate the remnants of political and financial independence of domestic NGOs using the sticks of severe bureaucratic restraints and the carrots of generous funding available to the approved recipients.[19] All things considered, while the Russian government detested the idea of civil society as norm entrepreneur, it did not rule out the necessity to collaborate with noncommercial organizations in principle. But in making the decision to award financial support, the Kremlin evaluated domestic agents of change on the grounds of whether their missions, styles, and strategies were compatible with or hostile to the goals of the Russian state. Although main grant operators that distribute governmental moneys could not hitherto have cut all prominent liberally inclined organizations from sources of internal financial support altogether, the orientation to sponsor organizations that either deliver specific social services or advocate the newly designed traditional values is apparent. The Russian system of grant distribution in its current form hardly nourishes society's autonomy from the state and instead puts noncommercial organizations at the mercy of a nontransparent system of financial decision making that the state can easily use to its advantage.[20]

It should be noted that the only attempt to make the government transparent and to curtail the excessive power of officialdom was associated with Dmitriy Medvedev's sensible efforts to create the so-called big, or open, government.[21] As his one-term presidency was coming to an end, Medvedev promised that his government would rely on the input of the representatives of civil society, various experts, municipal authorities, and ordinary citizens. He also promised that civil society would participate in the decision-making process, while officialdom would heed societal feedback. In reality, Medvedev's resolve to enforce transparency was weak, and his conception of "big government" looked good only on paper. Although he invited many experts, most notably Igor' Yurgens and Yevgeniy Gontmakher from the Institute of Contemporary Development, to offer a road map to the "open state," no practical suggestions were implemented. It should not be surprising that as no significant steps were taken, the inspiration of the moment passed quickly.

It becomes clear in retrospect that Medvedev's transformative ideas failed to break free from the conceptual straitjacket of statism. Instructive was his constant recursion to the value of the strong state. After all, in his first foundational public statement, Medvedev, even more unequivocally than Putin on the eve of the new millennium, dismissed any principle of social organization that contradicted the devotion to hierarchical and state-centric governance.[22] But those dissatisfied with the main direction of Russian politics were all too eager to overlook Medvedev's conceptual inconsistencies and his inability to follow through on any of his seemingly invigorating ideas. In the end, since Medvedev only adorned the core tenets of sovereign democracy with some progressive-sounding language, the autonomous state as the sole locus of authority retained its status as a core component of social purposes.

In summary, Putin's conception of the state was designed neither to help adjudicate domestic conflicts nor to aggregate the interests of multiple societal groups. On the contrary, the Kremlin vigorously argued against a liberal-pluralist conception of the state. Officialdom detested politically active civil society as a champion of liberal nonstate values and took a scunner against transnational actors operating at the whim of foreign puppeteers. Malevolent nonterritorial agents of change had to be reined in.

State-Centered Developmentalism

Russian officials averred that only the developmental state could improve the Russian economy and elevate living standards for ordinary citizens. While there is no single definition of the term "developmental state," in this book I use it to refer to a state bureaucracy intervening in and guiding the direction and pace of economic development, single-handedly reallocating resources across industries, and protecting national economic interests in the capitalist system of the world economy. Similar but not identical terms are "hard state" and "state capitalism."[23] Leon Aron summarized the implications of developmentalism: "the reemergence of the state as the most powerful actor on the economic stage, serving as both the initiator and implementer of economic policy[, which causes] the slowing down or freezing of structural liberal reforms . . . [and the] rapid expansion of the state sector of the economy."[24] The necessary caveat is that the adjective "developmental" need not be understood as having only positive connotations. At the end of the day, politicians can use redistributive practices to ensure their political survival instead of genuinely increasing domestic levels of social development.

The stress on the state as the vehicle of economic growth and the state's obligation to deliver permeated Russia's political discourse. Putin's key ideas on how to run the national economy focused on the governmental use of mineral rents. These ideas originated in Putin's *kandidat nauk* (a rough equivalent of the American PhD degree) dissertation, which he defended in 1997 at the National Mineral Resources University in Saint Petersburg under the title "Strategic Planning of the Reproduction of Mineral Resources of the Region in the Context of Market Relations: Saint Petersburg and the Leningrad Region." Hardly conceptually fresh, it nevertheless provides an insight into Putin's thinking about the proper principles of economic governance and the means to achieve the economic and social transformation. Putin's subsequent stand-alone publication is a good primary source of the ideas that he had put on paper in his thesis two years earlier.[25]

Later on, Putin unpacked his evolving vision for a wider audience. He stressed the role of government as "the leader in the creation and application of high technologies, in providing a high standard of people's well-being, in the ability to protect the safety and defend national interests on the international scene."[26] He emphasized the responsibility of the federal government to deliver, as well as the responsibility of business to pay back what it owed to the country. Over time, the rhetoric of social injustices perpetrated by big business during the turbulent 1990s heightened the actual tendency of the government to restrict the independence of the private sector. Boris Gryzlov stated that building a socially oriented economy was indispensable to keep the nation united.[27] This obligation also appeared in speeches of such key political players as Yuriy Luzhkov (mayor of Moscow, 1992–2010) and Sergey Mironov (chairman of the Federation Council and the leader of Spravedlivaya Rossiya, 2001–11). In a similar vein, Surkov claimed that only clinging to statism could secure the steady flow of reforms needed to sustain Russia's economic growth. Economic freedoms were deemed subordinate to the requirements of internal and external sovereignty.[28] For many years, Yevgeniy Primakov, former prime minister of Russia (1998–99) and president of the Russian Chamber of Commerce and Industry (2001–11), advocated state intervention in the economy as necessary to improve markets and increase levels of competitiveness. In his outlook, any neoliberal economic prescriptions were a roadblock on the way to Russia's prosperity.[29]

The creation of the National Priority Projects (NPPs) was a case in point. Russian leaders designed the NPPs as the mechanism of an intense and "smart" investment to prompt economic development in certain areas and improve social services. Putin formulated the core purpose of the NPPs: "Concentration of budgetary and administrative resources on the improvement of quality of life of citizens of Russia is a necessary and logical development of our economic policy, which we have been implementing over the last five years, and we shall be implementing in the future. It is a guarantee from inert spending without any palpable feedbacks. It is a policy of investment into an individual, which means an investment in the future of Russia."[30]

By the end of Putin's second presidential term, his bold political ambition to erect a "hard" developmental state had come into full existence. Since the state sector had swelled to about half of the national economy, the state reemerged as the most powerful economic actor. Developmental ideas justified the personal right of the president to single-handedly make economic decisions and the exclusion of business from policy making. In 2008 the newly elected president, Dmitriy Medvedev, seemingly dropped the discourse of a state-led economy in favor of a progressive-sounding narrative of "modernization." The alliteration of institutions, investments, infrastructure, and innovations seemingly broke up with Putin's hard state.[31] Some political observers rushed to predict the end of governance methods stipulated by the sovereign democracy, of which Medvedev had been publicly critical on several occasions. But these predictions reflected liberals' wishful thinking, underlined their inattention to the deep-seated logic of Putin's economic thinking, and highlighted their inability to grasp the crystallizing normative order. Importantly, over the course of Medvedev's presidential term, Putin was not conceptually idle. He continued to develop and propagate his own ideas on economic strategies for Russia, while Medvedev kept twisting his ideas to suit all political forces, which were often at opposite ends of the ideological spectrum. In the end, Medvedev's pledge to economic modernization turned out to be short-lived, while Putin's ideas of the state's social responsibility and massive state-led development survived and flourished.[32]

In summary, the discourse of state-led development was more than a vote-seeking gimmick; the overwhelming majority of Russian voters came to share favorable views on the unshakable role of top bureaucrats in making economic decisions and redistribution in economic life. The discourse of the state as the dominant economic actor builds on the widespread disappointment with Yeltsin's inability to cushion the negative externalities of his shock therapy on the populace. The Russian political elite claimed that all previous problems in economic development had resulted from weak governmental regulation. In this mind-set, uncontrolled markets and the laissez-faire ideology trigger an avalanche of economic troubles and lead to social collapse. It is not surprising, then, that in 2012, on the eve of becoming Russia's president yet again, Putin pledged to provide equal and just distribution of income in the interests of ordinary people.

The Kremlin's External Ambitions

In the 1990s the political elite preferred to downplay the discourse of Russia as a great power in the international arena and shied away from touting its external exploits. In the second part of the 2000s the discourse changed. In a bitter and self-serving reaction to the national humiliation of the 1990s, domestic elites claimed that a core external task of the Russian state was to restore the country's sovereignty and great power status (*derzhavnost'*). Whether reasonable or not, that claim became an integral part of the Russian social purpose.[33]

For Russian politicians, *derzhavnost'* implies "the modern appreciation for material power in world politics while reproducing the recognition of international norms of sovereignty."[34] The Russian rendition of sovereignty entails (1) a coterminous portrayal of authority and territorial rule, which requires protecting the impenetrable hull of state-centric authority; and (2) an assertive participation in global affairs, which implies the necessity of spreading Russian norms and fending off international values. As this understanding of the external tasks of the state prevailed, the Kremlin acted to establish its presence abroad and sought to curb the activities of international organizations in the country. The evolving system of representation enabled and legitimized the mental progression toward a more adversarial view of international actors.

At first, reasserting Russia's sovereignty and great power status was somewhat consistent with interpreting Russia as a European state. Some commentators opined that Russia and Europe shared a common cultural and historical background, including similar values and legal doctrines. But this argument remained short-lived. The Kremlin's increasingly isolationist and hostile discourse now highlights Russia as the defender of conservative values that oppose the moral and religious bankruptcy of the Western world, immersed in sin and deviance. The younger generation of opinion leaders claims that Russians have nothing to learn from the West anymore.

Typical of the evolving discourse were the arguments presented by Alexey Chadaev, the author of *Putin: His Ideology*. In 2005–9 Chadaev served in the Public Chamber, and in 2010–11 he was an ideologist in United Russia's propaganda unit. He defined sovereignty as a state's ability to deflect any foreign influences on domestic political affairs and, in turn, to promote itself as a norm-giver in the international arena. The lack of great power status enables other great powers to change the domestic political regime and impose external governance (*vneshnee upravlenie*). Leaders who adopt any foreign practices abrogate the sovereignty of their countries.[35] Chadaev's book presented a relatively neutral way to think about sovereignty and great power. Quite soon, however, political debates about sovereignty revived the old-school imperial sensibilities. Russian elite and opinion leaders argued that in promoting democracy and human rights, Western countries invariably use double standards and undermine international law.[36]

In the context of Putin's stress on shielding the populace from any external political influences as a fundamental goal of the state, the Color Revolutions (Orange in the Ukraine, Rose in Georgia, and Tulip in Kyrgyzstan) pushed Russian political debate to its livid extreme. The Color Revolutions had profound importance for Russian politicians and opinion leaders because they illustrated the fact that external norms (free and fair elections) challenge state autonomy and sovereignty. A prominent domestic political observer, Vyacheslav Nikonov, opined that the Color Revolutions were "technologies aimed toward weakening the country and building the mechanisms of influence on Russia, not at democracy promotion."[37] Similarly, Zhirinovsky claimed that democracy promotion was a tool of dismembering the polity and prompting interethnic conflicts.[38] Other Kremlin-friendly opinion leaders surmised that the Color Revolutions would destabilize Russian statehood, abrogate national sovereignty, and undermine the country's territorial integrity.[39]

To survive as a country, one prominent political commentator proclaimed, Russia must exercise influence on the "canonic territories" of the country's historical presence.[40] In the context of his bid for a third presidential term to start in 2012, Putin endorsed that view. He expressed his goal to reintegrate parts of the post-Soviet region under Russia's patronage.[41] The annexation of the Crimea in 2014 is a tangible consequence of this discourse.

In general, while the idea of being a great power is surely old, it regained a new vigor during Putin's rule. As high-powered politicians came to agree that the normative hull of the state needed protection, they contended to insulate Russia from foreign influences. Today international norms and international organizations that promote these norms are less welcomed in the country than a decade ago.

Identity Arguments in Putin's Russia

Boris Gryzlov, the speaker of the State Duma from 2003 to 2011, described the Russian self as nationalist, evolutionary, and conservative and the Other as foreign inspired, revolutionary, and liberal.[42] Two years later, a prominent political operator, Vladislav Surkov, said that liberals must not to be allowed to climb to any political position of prominence.[43] These portrayals set off numerous identity arguments that depicted liberals as politically dangerous, economically irresponsible, and culturally alien. The intention of these utterances was to impair the value of alternative spheres of authority and inspire a longing for normative autarky.

A conservative observer, Aleksandr Tsipko, vilified the liberals as an ontological threat to the state, as they conspired "to bury the remnants of the national self-identification . . . so that Russia would never be Russia again."[44] Other commentators claimed that the so-called limousine liberals (i.e., liberals whose experiences and lifestyles were insulated from the hardships of the ordinary people) slavishly followed the external agenda and inspired the West to keep imposing alien sensibilities. These detestable characteristics pale in comparison to Putin's ability to burn the brand of the subversive Otherness into the flesh of the liberals. At a political rally at the Luzhniki stadium in November 2007, Putin lashed out: "They need a weak, sick state. . . . They need a disorganized, disoriented, and divided society. And unfortunately, there are also those inside the country who beg like jackals at foreign embassies and diplomatic offices and who count on the support of foreign foundations and governments but not on the support of their own people."[45] Recently, even church functionaries joined the secular voices in exposing the liberals' proclivity to adopt dangerous foreign norms and disdain good moral values. On many occasions, His Holiness Patriarch Kirill I of Moscow and All Rus' has opined that liberalism is antithetical to the survival of modern civilization and has criticized human rights as an ominous expression of decaying ethical standards.

As Putin's presidency unfolded, the ranks of those who allegedly undermined the Russian state expanded. This sordid Other lumped together various political actors whose political agenda was not truly homogeneous. The camp of Others included the real proponents of liberal ideology, former anti-Communist dissidents, and human rights activists, as well as Yeltsin's political advisors and some members of his government and political activists of various persuasions. This is not to say that all prominent liberals in the executive fell into the category of the subversive Other. After all, many so-called systemic liberals, including Aleksey Kudrin (finance minister, 2000–11), German Gref (minister of economic development and trade, 2000–2007), and Mikhail Zurabov (minister of health and social development, 2004–7), never challenged President Putin's self-righteousness. The aforementioned individuals tended to support Putin's course while slowly losing their independent, agenda-setting power. They also failed to follow up on the liberal reform program and acted more like "technocrats" than political players in their own right.

While the public skepticism of liberal ideals has a long pedigree, Putin's loyalists intentionally manipulated the social ambivalence regarding liberal ideas and artificially augmented it. Their tongue-lashing rhetoric built on the widespread hostility toward all economic reformers of the early 1990s (most notably, Yegor Gaidar and Anatoliy Chubais) and their foreign advisors (Anders Åslund and Jeffrey Sachs). Since the early 1990s, aggressive narratives have proliferated. The loyalists anathematized the reformers' predisposition to adopt foreign economic recommendations without the necessary adjustments. At the same time, Russian elites and opinion leaders tended to misrepresent the course and outcomes of the economic reforms.[46] These allegations conveniently leaped over the terminal ailments of the Soviet economy, complicating Yeltsin's reforms. The Kremlin-friendly opinion leaders masterfully used the objective vulnerability of the liberals' appeal, highlighted the mixed record of their governance, underscored their inability to resist special interests, and emphasized the inadequate levels of their economic sophistication. But this criticism was surely warped: while the looting of state property was widespread after the collapse of Communism, only the liberals got berated for it.

By the end of Putin's second presidential term, numerous journalists and propaganda-like talk shows had augmented official statements to create a broader platform for identity arguments. Arkadiy Mamontov's series of biting broadcasts and Vladimir Solov'ev's heated talk shows, aired on the state-controlled TV, are illustrative examples of the evolving discourse. On these shows, any social actors who did not embrace statism were deemed enemies of Russia. Domestic political elites and spin doctors masterfully "exposed" the liberals' secret plot to subvert the Russian political system and attacked young Russian liberals as foreign spies. A tide of loyalists lamented the despicable role of liberals while suppressing the rich tradition of Russian liberalism and its numerous achievements dating back to the nineteenth century. In this convoluted outlook, anything but statism was simply wrong and unfit for the country.

The liberals gradually lost their ideational grounds and succumbed to the ideas of statism, the developmental state, and great power. Liberals' partial acceptance of responsibility for economic hardships and massive social dislocation has played into the hands of their opponents. In 2004 imprisoned oligarch Mikhail Khodorkovskiy published his essay "The Crisis of Liberalism in Russia" in a prestigious newspaper, *Vedomosti*. Khodorkovskiy lamented that liberals ignored, "first, some important national-historical features of development of Russia, and, second, the vital interests of the overwhelming majority of Russian people." He also grieved that in the 1990s the desire for self-gratification and quick enrichment destroyed the value of socially responsible politics. Whatever the author's motive was, this compunctious opinion piece shored up Putin's evaluation of liberals as subversive and irresponsible Others. In the same pessimistic way, a prominent "first-wave" democrat, Yuriy Afanas'yev, opined that the liberals had set about transforming Russia while being conceptually imprisoned by completely inadequate alien ideas and thus discredited the ideals of democracy and liberalism among their Russian audience.[47] Many other liberals took a clearly defensive stance about their policy mistakes, whether actual or retrofitted, and thus discredited their own ideas about the cardinal objectives of the state.

After the liberals had dissipated as a prominent force in Russian politics, further rhetorical attacks on the liberals served no other purpose than shaming and humiliating the political Other for the pleasure of the state officialdom. It seems that by 2013 the high-powered politicians had come to believe that Russian citizens unanimously supported their normative predilections and universally reviled any external norms. This belief is best expressed in the ballooning use of the term "the overwhelming majority."[48] This term describes the state of affairs when a state does not have to take into account any alternative viewpoints precisely because those viewpoints express the position of the minority. Although this term overstates the degree to which Russian citizens have internalized state-centric sensibilities, it nevertheless reflects an adequate understanding of the widespread popular support of the extant social purpose.

In short, identity arguments sustained and communicated the message that any models of governance not premised on the hardening statism would be subversive. Vigorous and perfervid identity arguments shored up Putin's vision for the cardinal goals of the state. They also prepared Russian citizens for the coming normative autarky.

Summary

The discourse of sovereign democracy encapsulates three cardinal themes: the ultimate political value of statism and state autonomy from society, a stress on economic delivery in the context of the state-led economy, and the necessity to reassert sovereignty and actively exercise Russia's great power status in the global power structure. Not only do these themes clearly stand out as the three most prominent components in the Russian political discourse, but they also have matured into intersubjectively shared core tasks of Putin's Russia. Antiliberal identity arguments have depleted the liberal appeal; Putin's state has become impervious to the principle of nonhierarchical and nonstate governance. As Russians internalized the view that restoring and sustaining the state autonomy was the prime goal of the state, they failed to foresee any negative implications. Very few political observers came to realize that the elite's insulation from society and their insensitivity to alternative political ideas could lead the country to social decay.[49]

While a discussion of the provenance of Russian statism, which certainly has a long pedigree, is beyond the scope of this book, suffice it to say that the consensus on the core tasks of the state emerged out of conscious and intentional efforts that took more than a decade. Without the forceful activities of Putin's elites and the Kremlin-friendly opinion leaders, the result, the social purpose of the state, would have been different. While for the Russian elite it can be difficult to break free from the conceptual jail of its cultural resources, the available evidence suggests that it can be done.

MBEKI'S AFRICAN RENAISSANCE

In South Africa, during the time of political transition to the majority rule in 1990–94 and later during Nelson Mandela's presidency, political leaders and intellectuals discussed several proposals in order to determine the cardinal goals the renovated state would perform. All of these proposals, of course, defied the apartheid ideology. Prominent participants of the liberation movement promoted the ideas of Pan-Africanism, Africanism, nonracialism, and class- and ethnic-based conceptions of the common good. The Pan-African Congress touted a Pan-African national identity from Cape to Cairo. The ANC's Africanism envisioned a common supraethnic nationhood of all black South Africans. Less feasible proposals included ethnic-tribal nationalism (the Inkatha Freedom Party) and radical, class-based nationalism advocated by the members of the South African Communist Party, including Jabulani "Mzala" Nxumalo, Joe Slovo, and the charismatic Chris Hani.

It is understandable that throughout the years of Mandela's presidency, all the aforementioned proposals remained somewhat vague. But it is clear that the country was trying to come to grips with its own raison d'être and rationales for sovereignty. Among multiple possible versions of different social purposes, the conception of the Rainbow Nation was most prominent. Its champions aspired to rebuild, reunite, and heal the nation in the context of profound ethnic, racial, gender, and class gulfs. Mandela's vision and Desmond Tutu's proposal for a multiracial, multicultural South African nation briefly peaked in popularity and then tapered off all too quickly. Thabo Mbeki's poetic and emotional "I Am an African" speech, delivered to celebrate the adoption of the South African Constitution Bill in 1996, was his only public utterance that can be interpreted as his devotion to the goals of the Rainbow Nation.[50]

Once Mbeki became the head of the country, he embarked on a different course for national renewal, one that he and his supporters called the African Renaissance. "The agenda of the African Renaissance," explains Moeletsi Mbeki, a prominent public intellectual and Thabo's brother, "is to restore Africa as a contributor to, as well as a beneficiary of, the achievements of human civilization."[51] In July 2002 the National Executive Committee (NEC), the chief executive organ of the African National Congress, held a meeting that succinctly summarized the substance of the African Renaissance and prepared the agenda for the Fifty-First National Conference, which convened in December of that same year in Stellenbosch. Reestablishing African prominence was deemed possible by "rediscovering Africa's creative past to recapture the people's cultures, encourage artistic creativity and restore popular involvement in science and technology," thus overturning the world image of Africa as an incapable "historical curiosity."[52] In other words, the idea that local solutions can address local problems better than imported ones became the main conceptual pillar of Mbeki's program for national renewal. No less seminal were the ruling party's aspirations to improve South Africa's place in the world by embracing the global neoliberal economy and by enhancing the country's role in "the global system of governance in all fields, including politics, the economy, security, information and intellectual property, the environment and science and technology."[53]

The narrative below unpacks the South African conception of the core tasks of the state. The first subsection briefly discusses the rise of Mbekiites. The second subsection explores the principled ideas concerning the role of indigenous knowledge systems. The third subsection discusses the commitments to market-centered empowerment and its general implications for selecting governance methods. The fourth subsection explores external ambitions as related to the social purpose of the South African state. The final subsection traces the identity arguments that developed scorn for the Afro-pessimists but at the end of the day failed to delegitimize principles of governance alternative to those based on indigenousness.

Committed Elites in South Africa

In South Africa, the leading role in articulating social purpose belonged to the so-called Mbekiites, a relatively cohesive group of politicians who sometimes called themselves nativists for lack of a better term. Unlike the Russian *siloviki*, Mbekiites for the most part lacked a common political background and corporate solidarity, and thus they came together mostly on the situational basis of being Mbeki's loyal followers. These differences stipulated the internal fragility of the committed elites.

Thabo Mbeki consolidated his rule by expanding and strengthening the role of the presidency and the executive power. While under Nelson Mandela the presidential office was rather small, Mbeki created additional internal bodies such as the Coordination and Implementation Unit, the Policy Coordination and Advisory Service, and the Presidential Support Unit.[54] Beyond their instrumental role in formulating and coordinating domestic policies, these units also promoted the presidential vision for national renewal. Essop Pahad, for instance, openly asserted that the office of the presidency was the ministry of the African Renaissance. According to Frank Chikane, a team of senior advisors turned the deputy president's vision of the African Renaissance into an operational plan on how to transform the country.[55]

Informally, the strengthening of the presidency relied on the growing role and power of President Mbeki's inner circle of advisors. South African columnist Richard Calland's list of the most important individuals includes Joel Netshitenzhe (member of the ANC National Executive Committee and allegedly the president's chief political strategist), Trevor Manuel (minister of finance, 1996–2009), Mojanku Gumbi (legal advisor to the president), Phumzile Mlambo-Ngucka (deputy president, 2005–8), Essop Pahad (a minister in the presidency, 1999–2008), Aziz Pahad (deputy minister of foreign affairs, 1999–2008, and allegedly Mbeki's personal friend), Smuts Ngonyama (head of communications for the ANC), Titus Mafolo (Mbeki's political advisor), Cunningham Ngcukana (deputy executive director, New Economic Partnership for African Development [NEPAD]), and Bheki Khumalo (presidential spokesman, 1999–2005).[56] These individuals belonged to the president's inner circle and led the powerful cohort of loyalists. Until 2008 Mbeki enjoyed a power-based consensus on the cardinal goals of the state. To enforce the consensus, Mbeki's loyalists teetered and maneuvered, conducted intricate administrative games, sponsored bitter personal attacks in the media, and opined about multiple conspiracies to overthrow the presidency.

Mbeki and his supporters promoted the African Renaissance as a dominant proposal for national renewal. After the Fiftieth National Conference in Mafikeng, when the ruling party adopted the "African Renaissance" as its ideological master narrative, this phraseology became very common in myriad documents, statements, and official publications. The ANC statements included multiple references to the African Renaissance as one of the core strategic tasks of the ruling party. According to an important official statement, the main mission of the ANC was "to discharge its own obligations to the cause of the complete emancipation of the peoples of Africa."[57]

It is important to remember that the ANC keeps crowding out the other political parties.[58] Although attempts to build a nonracial opposition to the ANC occur regularly, in the first decade of this century no political force could seriously challenge the dominant party. The electoral prospects of the Democratic Alliance remain modest given its history, which dates back to the apartheid era minority rule. On the eve of Mbeki's departure, Mosiuoa Lekota proposed to launch a new party, uniting those Mbeki loyalists who were dissatisfied with the ANC. But the enormous electoral success of Lekota's Congress of People (COPE) in 2009 was not repeated. Hitherto, the Congress of South African Trade Unions (COSATU) has supported the ANC, and the prospects of a new trade union–based party are not clear. The ideas that currently dominate the ANC are most likely to be the basis for a power-based consensus about the core tasks of the state.

Upholding Indigenous Values

President Mbeki was not the first leader or the only politician to consider the appropriate role of indigenous knowledge in the postcolonial context. Yet his bet on indigenous knowledge as the pillar of political authority was novel and unique. Equally daring was that he downplayed the discourse of human rights and the vision of the Rainbow Nation as the potential program for postapartheid transformation. In a nutshell, Mbeki's foremost ambition was to develop governance principles consistent with indigenous values and contextualized systems of knowledge. In his speech "The African Renaissance, South Africa and the World," Mbeki visualized myriad "modern products of human economic activity, significant contributions to the world of knowledge, in the arts, science and technology" as an outcome of the country's renewal.[59]

Conceptually, Mbeki's vision was reinforced by the authors of the occasional papers that were published by the Foundation for Global Dialogue, which promoted attempts to abolish any institutions and customs that "promiscuously copied" Western ones. More than four hundred acknowledged African intellectuals who convened for the African Renaissance conference in September 1998 advocated similar ideas. Select proceedings of that conference were published as an edited volume, whose contributors advised the president on a wide variety of significant issues. Most importantly, the authors converged on the idea that only by applying indigenous knowledge to practical matters of governance could the continent reach its counterhegemonic and anticolonial goals. According to Pitika Ntuli, director of the African Renaissance Institute at the University of Durban-Westville, Eurocentric knowledge continues to dominate African sciences, culture, and education and thus inhibits domestic ability to formulate innovative and workable governance models.[60] Another conference participant, Githae Mugo, called for African education as a "system of knowledge, theory and practice, informed and shaped by a content and form that are definitive of African space as well as the indigenous experiences of Africa's people and diversity."[61] Some intellectuals equated the revival of Africa to the European Renaissance, which restored the grand cultural models of the great ancients. But, the narrative went on, contrary to Europeans, who used their revival to conquer and subjugate other nations, South Africans would not use the spoils of the achieved level of economic and technological sophistication to subjugate less advanced nations.

Later, the 2002 national conference in Stellenbosch resolved to develop indigenous sports, protect cultural heritage, support heritage sites to establish historical memory at the local level, and promote indigenous knowledge systems.[62] Throughout his tenure, Mbeki publicly extolled traditional institutions for securing the cardinal goals of the state, developing communities, and stimulating the new common ground. Early in his presidency, Mbeki and the president's office helped create the National House of Traditional Leaders, the Programme of Support for the Institution of Traditional Leadership, the Traditional Leaders Conference, and the African Renaissance Festival. The Cabinet supported traditional leaders financially and logistically and recognized the role of traditional governance in rural reconstruction and development, as well as in sustaining cultural, linguistic, and religious communities.[63] After 2004, the strategy to promote native medicines as an integral part of indigenous knowledge gained momentum. The Cabinet invented and began observing African Traditional Medicine Day, which highlighted traditional medicines as dearly held values. Not surprisingly, all these developments had significant implications for health governance.

Indispensable to genuine revival was the task to discover and employ the forgotten traditions of the past. Scholars and commentators alike welcomed the emergence of Afrikology as a special discipline. The publications of the Human Sciences Research Council (HSRC) glorified African intellectual traditions and treated authentic customs as inspirational and stimulating further progress. The newly produced narratives, which illuminated cultural landmarks, included, among others, *The Subtle Power of Intangible Heritage*, with Harriet Deacon as the lead author (2004); *The Meaning of Timbuktu*, edited by Shamil Jeppie and Souleymane Bachir Diagne (2008); *The African Intellectuals in the 19th and Early 20th Centuries*, edited by Mcebisi Ndletyana (2008); and *The Deaths of Hintsa: Postapartheid South Africa and the Shape of Recurring Past* by Premesh Lalu (2009). Publications streamlining and valorizing African intellectual traditions contributed to the popularity of the Renaissance as a legitimate political notion. The *International Journal of African Renaissance Studies* has accumulated many arguments that advocate epistemic pluralism and develop a new paradigm for pan-African knowledge. Although the aforementioned publications appeared relatively late, they were surely based on Mbeki's foundational ideas and fleshed them out for a variety of interested readers. Similarly, national parks and natural wonders were considered to represent Africa as the cradle of humankind and thus highlight Africa's everlasting significance for humanity.[64]

In sum, the South African political elite placed a strong emphasis on the necessity to uphold African knowledge systems and to produce and advance indigenous science, technology, and education. The devotion to an authentic Afrocentric knowledge was the main justification for the existence of the South African state as an individualized and distinct political space. As will be shown later, attaining this core task of the state legitimized blurring the boundaries between scientific, evidence-based knowledge and indigenous approaches to it. In general, a focus on "local solutions for local problems" is not antithetical to the principle of nonstate and nonhierarchical governance. But it is definitely adversative to an uncritical adoption of external governance methods.

Market-Centered Empowerment

Vusi Mavimbela, a political operator and intelligence advisor with a rich and diverse work history, envisioned the African Renaissance as the third moment in the African liberation struggle. To push that third moment forward, no less foundational than political independence and democratic reforms was the economic empowerment of the African people. Viewed from the official perspective, economic empowerment was tantamount to marketization and antithetical to redistribution. Mbeki welcomed market-centered empowerment as the cardinal goal of the postapartheid state because it represented the unequivocal reversal of the apartheid era argument that black people were incapable of providing for themselves economically.[65]

Reaching the consensus on marketization as the core goal of the state was not predetermined and materialized only as a result of protracted political and economic debates among the members of the ruling party and opinion leaders. In the late 1980s, the ANC briefly entertained the idea to style the country's economy after the Communists. To that end, the party's members examined the performance of the Soviet, Chinese, and Cuban economies. Yet, with the demise of all of the administrative-planning systems of eastern Europe, clinging to Marxist economic tenets became not that smart. In addition, the main champion of socialism and nationalization in South Africa—the Communist Party—remained too radical to fit in the globalizing world.[66] Not surprisingly, Nelson Mandela publicly distanced himself from the ideas of nationalization.

Although the ANC left ideas of redistribution out of its policy documents as early as 1992, the alternative ones did not vanish right away. The leaders of the prolabor COSATU supported the African Renaissance, but they also struggled to spread the values of job creation, redistribution, and antiglobalization as the necessary orientations of a successful postapartheid state. The COSATU-aligned Industrial Strategy Project (ISP) and Macroeconomic Research Group (MERG) remained faithful to the idea of industrial interventionism, protectionism, and a hard developmental state.[67] Leftist individuals and alarmist groups blamed neoliberal ideology for the catastrophically low rates of employment and ongoing social distress.

Even though radical proposals for economic development were off the table, scholars still dispute the reasons how and why marketization prevailed as a core normative principle of economic empowerment. Hein Marais, the author of perhaps the most solid account of the politics of economic reform in South Africa, drew attention to a unique combination of structural and institutional factors.[68] According to William Gumede, a keen observer of politics and a columnist with several newspapers, the high-powered representatives of international financial institutions conceptually seduced the key leaders of the ANC and, in the course of a few years, fully socialized them in the neoliberal orthodoxy. It is also possible that leaders chose a promarket orientation because of overpowering fiscal constraints. Perhaps material incentives mattered as well: the strong consensus about marketization among the political elite emerged when the successful transfer of assets created the first generation of wealthy black entrepreneurs.

Be that as it may, commitments to the free market, privatization, and cuts in public expenditures accompanied the slow erosion of the socialist-inspired Reconstruction and Development Programme (RDP). In around 1996 the ANC started underscoring economic growth through deficit reduction, tight monetary policy, and trade liberalization, all in line with the core tenets of the Washington Consensus.[69] The Growth, Employment, and Redistribution (GEAR) policy and the Accelerated and Shared Growth Initiative for South Africa (ASGISA) concluded the drift from the idea of redistribution to the principles of neoliberalism. While this shift increased both economic growth and inequalities, it alienated COSATU as an unconditional supporter of the government. In the end, the internal normative debate shaped the resultant economic outlook, and the outcome of that conceptual contestation defined the "soul" of the ANC.[70]

In South Africa, the normative nature of market-centered empowerment goes well beyond its instrumental value as a response to intensifying economic problems. The debate has very distinct undertones. For instance, at a University of Transkei fund-raising dinner on April 30, 1998, Mbeki challenged the devotion to the hard state as unpatriotic and tantamount to national failure:

> What remains is for us all to invest the government with the heavenly powers which would enable it to say—I am the Deliverer and none exists but I. Cursed are those who worship at the feet of idols, because it is I and only I, the democratic state, that will deliver you from your misery! And so you and I can see these masses at the feet of the Deliverer, hands held out in supplication, incarnating in unison—Deliverer, deliver! Is it correct that we preach such a message of disempowerment of the people, predicated on the notion of a deliverer and a recipient?[71]

Despite the ornate and sardonic form of his delivery, Mbeki's key message was loud and clear: it was not the task of the government to deliver; instead, the economic success of the country would be based on the "abandonment of the concept of the Deliverer with its corollary of the Entitled Recipient."[72]

Phumzile Mlambo-Ngcuka and Pallo Jordan (who for more than two decades served as a member of the National Executive Committee and was minister of art and culture during Mbeki's second presidential term) claimed that South Africa had become fully committed to market-friendly values and thus stimulated attempts to frame market-based empowerment in terms of indigenous values. The minister of environmental affairs and tourism, Marthinus van Schalkwyk, asserted that South Africa "fused African wisdom with Western business, to offer business unusual to the world."[73] According to Eddy Maloka, a prominent researcher and chief executive officer of the Africa Institute of South Africa, various talks and discussions linking economic development and the African Renaissance occurred regularly on radio and television programs and in newspaper and magazine articles. The highly regarded *Professional Management Review* bestows the prestigious African Renaissance Award to businesses supposedly successful in contributing to black economic empowerment.[74]

Quite simply, Pretoria tried to put a local spin on marketization using the notion of *ubuntu*. Like many cultural concepts with vague meanings, the interpretation of *ubuntu* is highly malleable and thus can be used to justify or frame different ideas and sensibilities. Two astute observers of the South African economy, Hein Marais and David McDonald, provide crucial evidence that, since the early 1990s, academics and business leaders in South Africa have been promoting *ubuntu* as a homegrown management philosophy. This philosophy allegedly improves corporate governance and social responsibility while safeguarding the principles of the market economy. As a result, the corporate sector came to use the language of *ubuntu* widely to market local products and to endorse market-centered strategies as the way to do business.

In short, with Thabo Mbeki's ascension to the presidency, market-centered empowerment was culturally tailored to fit traditional African values.[75] It also makes sense that breaking free from the inheritance of colonial pathologies requires eliminating state control over the private sector. Empowering businesses is, therefore, the crucial task for economic development. The devotion to neoliberal ideas determined the friendly, albeit fragile, relations between Pretoria and the private sector. Although currently post-Mbeki Pretoria is largely staying the course, economic populism is gaining momentum. Leaders of the ANC Youth League (ANCYL), for instance, have consistently promoted the idea of state appropriation of land without compensation. Controversial Julius Malema, the organization's former head, is now leading his own party, the Economic Freedom Fighters, represented in both houses of the South African parliament. Although his chances to become a dominant political force remain unclear, he might ignite populist sentiments and thus undermine the future of market-centered empowerment in South Africa as one of the cardinal goals of the state.[76]

In summary, despite sharp domestic debates, Mbeki's new vision for the

South African social purpose embraced markets and spurned redistribution. In the next section, I discuss how the African Renaissance oriented the leaders of that emergent power toward pursuing its external ambition.

Pretoria's External Ambitions

The discourse of the African Renaissance was central to Pretoria's external ambitions. A succinct formula offered by the NEC in 2000 highlighted the necessity to strengthen South African independence from global powers and to take part in establishing rules for the global system of governance. When Thabo Mbeki's embrace of Afrocentrism and anti-imperialism replaced Nelson Mandela's emphasis on human rights and the promotion of democracy, the fundamental shift in South Africa's external aspirations became tangible.[77] In addition to continental solidarity and self-reliance, a resistance to Western neocolonial imperialism features prominently in Pretoria's external outlook. Uncertainty about the benefits of promoting human rights and democracy and confidence in the sense of agency premised on finding local solutions to African problems contributed to that shift. As South African leaders viewed their state as the primary and, perhaps, the sole expresser of a continental solidarity, they came close to imagining South Africa as a benevolent hegemon that countervails the global power structure.

Some observers claimed that South African elites deployed the notion of continental solidarity in order to maximize South Africa's foreign policy options in Africa and shore up Pretoria's aspirations to take a permanent seat in the United Nations Security Council.[78] Yet these strategic considerations do not undercut the national commitment to moral leadership as an integral part of social purposes. The minister of foreign affairs, Nkosazana Dlamini-Zuma, interpreted South African foreign policy as a logical extension of the domestic struggle for a just world. South Africa, Dlamini-Zuma's argument went, had the moral responsibility to spread the values of good governance, people-centered development, partnership, and so on.[79]

Among many important international initiatives, NEPAD occupies a place of paramount importance. Heavyweight members of the South African political elite Jacob Zuma, Essop Pahad, and Frank Chikane have promoted the crucial role of NEPAD in implementing the conception of the common good across the continent. The minister of provincial and local government, Sydney Mafumadi, asserted that NEPAD presented "a framework for a break with the unequal and exploitative economic and political relations that manifest [themselves] in the causal connection between development in the North and underdevelopment in the South, of which our continent is an intimate part."[80] Frank Chikane, a member of the ANC National Executive Committee and director-general in the presidency (1999–2008), claimed that the deployment of NEPAD would put Africa on equal terms with the West: "[It] is about restoring the dignity, respect, pride and ubuntu of the African people. . . . From a South African perspective, NEPAD is seen within the context of the development of the vision of the African Renaissance. . . . NEPAD has changed the nature of the relationship between the donor and the recipient, the developed and the developing countries. It has contributed to a partnership of mutual trust, respect and responsibility."[81]

The assertive formulation of the notion of moral leadership implies South Africa's indispensable role in fighting Western neocolonialism (liberal imperialism). To protect the new South Africa is to expose the legacies of racialism, oppression, and domination, which have continued to thrive in the global arena. Further, in his September 2007 lecture, delivered on the thirtieth anniversary of the death of Steve Biko, Mbeki offered a radical critique of the global power structure. He borrowed Biko's main point about the irreconcilable differences with the West and contrasted the Western preoccupation with technological progress and the military with the African emphasis on the spiritual dimension of global human development. African progress in technology and economic development would challenge the perpetuated "global apartheid."

Defending these seminal ideas and acting on them often put Pretoria in an awkward international position. For instance, because Mbeki interpreted the Western critique of African political mismanagement as an assault on the continent's resistance to the legacy of colonialism, he was to defend those African rulers, including Robert Mugabe, who, in Mbeki's mind, were under attack.[82] Although Pretoria's support of Zimbabwe's octogenarian leader damaged Mbeki's international reputation, he did not find it important to distance himself from Zimbabwe on ideational grounds. Instead, he had to confront what he saw as typical imperialist, double-faced criticism for daring to fight enduring inequalities. Mbeki was not the only one whose interpretations regarding the extant power structure were of that kind. The new generation of South African leaders openly asserted solidarity with Mugabe's governance style. Malema, for instance, interpreted Mugabe's disastrous land reforms as a bold opposition to the new global apartheid.

In summary, Thabo Mbeki and his entourage embraced the goal of transformative leadership and sought to make use of anticolonial discourse in order to assert the country's rightful position in the international system. At the same time, certain expressions of global politics were interpreted as ominous for South Africa's transformative place in the world. Taking practical advantage of the best achievements of global civilization and assimilating sophisticated economic knowledge, which originated in the industrialized world, was not tantamount to carelessly accepting any global norm.

As enticing as it might be to succumb to one-dimensional portrayals of South African normative sensibilities, no simplified explanations will do justice to the domestic systems of governance that emerged out of them. As the following chapters show, while Mbeki's Pretoria resisted Western medical colonialism, it also continued to grant an excessive amount of pharmaceutical patents; while the government was skeptical about the new generation of global health organizations and their recommendations, it also accepted external funding provided by them. Choices that seem to be inherently contradictory in Pretoria's collective mind were quite coherent and, as argued in the relevant chapters, were stipulated by its social purpose.

Identity Arguments in Mbeki's South Africa

The African Renaissance was not simply a list of practical economic steps and political items on Pretoria's agenda. Deep personal loyalty to this program was deemed the core marker of the emerging South African identity, which differentiated the bearers of the optimistic vision for the African future from the "unbelievers" and detractors who intentionally stymied the country's progress. Most importantly, the official representations steered away from the civic conceptions of national identity, instead premising a new political identity on the commitment to indigenous systems of knowledge. Nevertheless, right from the onset, identity arguments were conceptually clear but politically not that suggestive.

There are strong identity connotations inherent in all three substantive components of the emerging social purpose. First, the ability to uphold the value of indigenous knowledge and apply this knowledge to practical matters of governance highlights the worthiness of a creative and unique self and stands in opposition to the Other, who does not believe that South Africa can offer anything of significance and value to the world. Indigenousness became the core marker of South African ingenuity, a defining characteristic of South Africans, and the cornerstone of their identity. Presidential spokesperson Mukoni Ratshitanga argued in 2007 that despite the efforts of colonial and apartheid regimes to obliterate the

African cultural milieu, the values of traditional culture "served both as a shield and weapon of struggle."[83] Although racial sensibilities featured prominently in Mbeki's speeches, Pretoria-friendly opinion leaders underscored that the new national identity had to be learned and could not be simply inherited with the color of a person's skin. Indigenousness is a conscious cultural choice based on learning and loyalty to Africa: "Africanness is neither a pure matter of pigmentation, nor a question of geographical or ethnic belonging. . . . [I]t is a cultural choice and commitment, something which is acquired, gained, a matter of deep feeling and concrete behaviour. . . . [E]verybody who feels our continent in the depth of her or his soul and in each beat of her or his heart, can legitimately be considered an African."[84]

Second, another core component of the social purpose of the South African state, marketization, is about an individual who can provide for himself or herself and who rejects both exploitation and redistribution as practices that deny a South African well-deserved subjectivity and autonomy. The Other claims that a South African is hostile to market principles, that Africans are incapable of dealing with pressing local problems. Mbeki's statement in the National Assembly entitled "Reconciliation and Nation Building" in 1998 was one of the initial attempts to develop a compelling identity argument. Despite all its political achievements, the deputy president argued, after four years of freedom the country remained split into two irreconcilable nations, each embodying conflicting values. The unity of the nation was menaced by those who pushed the government to overextend its economic obligations and those who wished to obstruct sustainable economic growth. The same year, Mbeki mocked the proponents of redistribution: "They join the chorus which reinforces that notion that government has legitimacy only to the extent that it delivers. We have a place in society only because we have the miraculous power to deliver. . . . [They pray to a] magnanimous Deliverer who has an exclusive obligation to see to the improvement of the conditions of life of the passive recipient whose only task is to say—give me more!"[85]

Third, the African self enjoys mental and spiritual freedoms, while the Other crusades for "mental colonization." In his diatribe against aloof and cynical observers, Mbeki execrated the Other because he or she is a disloyal Afropessimist.[86] The Other perpetuated the negative construction of a South African and denied him or her a sense of agency. According to Mbeki, "Frightening images of savagery that attend the continent of Africa" span millennia and have to be confronted boldly.[87] Pretoria presented political turmoil on the continent, its violent conflicts, and even the scourge of HIV/AIDS and various natural disasters as obstacles out of which the new Africa will emerge, much as the European Renaissance rose above political fragmentation, armies of mercenaries, outbreaks of pestilence, and climatic instabilities.

Given Mbeki's penchant for writing, the corpus of the texts he penned was quite sizable. His "Letters from the President" appeared almost every week in the online resource ANC *Today*. In these lengthy and sometimes not very lucid contributions, he touched on multiple political topics. As important as his words were, their impact would have been limited without a large number of credible opinion leaders echoing his voice and enacting the same frames of reference. Surely, Mbeki's writings did not appear in an intellectual vacuum. Since 1996 many intellectuals and leaders have shared their thoughts in *Umrabulo*, a journal whose official mission has been "to encourage debate and rigorous discussions at all levels of the movement."[88] The head of the Government Communication and Information Service, Joel Netshitenzhe, and the minister of arts and culture, Z. Pallo Jordan, Mbeki's key supporters, headed the journal's editorial board. *Umrabulo* also frequently gave tribute to the health minister, Dr. Manto Tshabalala-Msimang, defending her controversial health policies. The journal's notable rubric, "Celebrating Our Heritage," emphasized the significance of indigenous values for the country's renewal.

At least two notable attempts were made to create mechanisms to disseminate identity arguments beyond relatively narrow circles of people who followed politics closely. First, the office of the president helped create the Moral Regeneration Movement (MRM), an attempt to propagate the spirit of *ubuntu*, restore the moral fiber of the society, and preserve South Africa's national heritage. Deputy President Zuma and then his successor, Phumzile Mlambo-Ngcuka, led the MRM to create a national consciousness and identity compatible with indigenousness. In 2006–8 Mlambo-Ngcuka delivered several addresses in which she unpacked the meaning of the moral regeneration in conjunction with forming a new South African identity.

Second, the Native Club aspired to consolidate an aggressive core of African Renaissance acolytes. Although initially the club tried to be elitist and operated without much press coverage, South African newspapers came to view the Native Club as an ANC project.[89] This view seems to be warranted: the club was in part sponsored by the Department of Arts and Culture and directed by Mbeki's senior political advisor, Titus Mafolo, and Mbeki's biographer, R. S. Roberts. Predictably, *Umrabulo* favorably covered the club's mission and its agenda for action. Yet the mainstream postcolonial intellectuals and mass media clobbered it as divisive and shallow. Intensifying discussions went public and finally erupted in a minor political scandal, covered by the *Independent Online*, *Mail & Guardian Online*, *Sunday Times*, and *Pretoria News*.

The initial mission of the club was rather extensive. It aimed to develop a progressive force to sustain the African Renaissance, countervail the multiplying domestic critics, shape and define South African identity, and revive indigenous African cultural values and spirituality. Mafolo asserted that the club's goal was to stimulate those discursive resources that would reflect the notion of indigenousness and embed it among wider audiences: "[The club] . . . aims to mobilise South Africans to ensure that the ideas, philosophies, values and knowledge that propel society in a particular direction reflect the indigenous identity of our people. We seek to strengthen our democratic order by interrogating the philosophical framework within which we produce knowledge and within which certain ideas have become entrenched and dominant in our society. This is particularly critical because today, blacks in South Africa are responsible for around only 15% of knowledge production."[90]

On balance, the unfolding identity arguments clearly demonstrated that Mbeki and his supporters indeed internalized the core ideas of the African Renaissance as obligations that had to be validated in social practice. Not surprisingly, they acted on these obligations. But these arguments failed to delegitimize conceptual alternatives to the core goals of the state as encompassed by the African Renaissance. Artificial construction of an Afro-pessimist did not communicate a compelling ontological menace; some loud opinion leaders, like Roberts, never gained popular support and credibility; civil society subgroups and individuals were conceptually and politically free to formulate their own ideas and to act on them. That is why attempts to promote public animosity to civil society groups that did not employ indigenous solutions to the public health crisis ultimately failed. That is why the public did not converge on the understanding that only Pretoria's governance methods were natural and self-evident. It is important to remember, however, that the weakness of identity arguments did not imply that the effects of ideas about the core goals of the South African state on the systems of governance were negligible.

Summary

South African leaders elevated local solutions for local problems (indigenousness), supported market-centered empowerment, and claimed moral leadership as the external ambition of the state. Chief proponents of the African Renaissance deployed identity arguments, as well. They pitched themselves against Afro-pessimists and neocolonialists who schemed to keep South Africa subjugated to the West and denied the country its sense of agency. Domestic audiences, however, were not fully convinced. Criticism and confusion remained widespread. Some observers commented on the African Renaissance as "the new ideology of self-deception, the refusal to acknowledge the current realities that parameter even our own political space."[91] Obviously, this appraisal is too tough and does not give Mbeki's vision full justice. The presented evidence suggests that the evolving discourse of the African Renaissance developed and disseminated very clear reasons that Pretoria held for the existence of the post-apartheid South Africa.

SOCIAL PURPOSE AS A VARIABLE

The previous two sections have empirically described Russian and South African ideas about the cardinal goals of the state. Since in this study social purposes are a causal variable, it would be helpful to summarize how they vary. That in their expressions and contents social purposes heavily depend on unique social and historical contexts is obvious. Less obvious is an adequate typology of the concept. This section aspires to distill generalizable ideal types of social purposes and to devise an adequate terminology to describe what these ideal types are.

These goals require the following moves. First, we should note the extent to which the cohesive dominant groups devote themselves to articulating and employing a coherent justification for the state's existence. Second, taking stock of myriad texts, we should delineate the content of the main discursive stream and ascertain if one elaborate and identifiable set of ideas about the core goals of the state dominates the rest of the alternatives. Third, we should evaluate the extent to which identity arguments—important systems of representation—enhance the legitimacy of some ideas and paralyze the appeal of others. Different combinations of these three parameters are aggregated in four ideal types of social purposes. In table 2 I distinguish between absent, fractured, power-based, and legitimate social purposes. These distinctions are important because they allow me to specify the implications for governance and norm diffusion.

Social purposes become fully legitimate when they take on an intersubjective quality among both high-powered leaders and ordinary people. If social purposes are legitimate, then elites and society share the same ideas about the goals

Table 2   Ideal Types of Social Purposes

Committed elites	Goals of the state	Identity arguments	Implications for governance
		Absent	
The political elite is fractured. Various high-powered groups fail to develop compelling justifications for the state's existence.	Domestic public debate about the cardinal goals of the state is stale; no definite discourse emerges.	Identity arguments are either absent or important only to small-scale subcultures and subgroups.	Ideas about the cardinal goals of the state are not relevant for adoption of the external standards of governance. Elites evoke compliance with the threat of force or direct coercion.
		Fractured	
The political elite is fractured. Competing elite groups express different and conflicting ideas as justifications for the state's existence.	Multiple credible conceptions of the cardinal goals of the state circulate simultaneously.	Multiple identity arguments circulate simultaneously and are equally compelling or equally flimsy.	The impact of ideas about the core tasks of the state on external standards of governance is either limited or situational. Elites evoke compliance simultaneously with the threat of force and on voluntary grounds.
		Power Based	
One clearly identifiable ruling group dominates the domestic political landscape. Political groups that challenge the committed elite do not accept the prevailing justifications for the state's existence.	One elaborate and identifiable set of ideas about the core goals of the state dominates the alternatives.	Elite-driven identity arguments are only partially successful.	External principles of governance are considered inappropriate unless they match the shared ideas about the core tasks of the state. Elites evoke full compliance both on voluntary grounds and by limiting the discretion of dissenting policy participants to decide and act on their own.
		Legitimate	
One clearly identifiable ruling group dominates the domestic political landscape. Political groups that challenge the committed elite increasingly concede to the prevailing justifications for the state's existence.	One elaborate and identifiable set of ideas about the core goals of the state dominates the alternatives.	Elite-driven identity arguments are successful. The elite's opponents are dubbed as subversive Others.	External principles of governance are considered inappropriate unless they match the shared ideas about the core tasks of the state. The enacted system of governance is considered self-evident; voluntary and habitual compliance ensues.

of the state and deem these ideas indispensable for the state's existence and the state's sovereignty. In the narrow sense, legitimacy of social purposes is the extent to which elite-driven ideas about the cardinal goals of the state gain strong social traction. In a broader sense, legitimate social purposes reveal the kind of underlying normative order that leaders and societies desire to operate in. Using constructivist parlance, a legitimate social purpose is a metanorm or a constitutive norm around which additional regulative norms revolve. Social purposes have their own conceptual clout. The degree to which social purposes take on an intersubjective quality determines whether the elite-generated governing strategies will be perceived as natural, normal, and self-evident. In that case, people are less likely to consider the value and appropriateness of alternative methods of governance. Furthermore, habitual or undisputed compliance with core ideas makes it easier for political leaders to escape the blame for the negative consequences of their governance methods and even shift the burden of blame onto other social actors.

Elites, of course, need not possess solid ideational commitments or a coherent conception of the common good: they can rely on coercion and use functioning state machinery for extracting resources or for any other self-serving purpose. State agencies, as well as a society and its various groups, can lack any sense of mission and purpose. In this case, public notions of the common good and purposive conceptions of the state are absent. In other circumstances, objective structural conditions dictate a course of action that makes no allowance for interpretative variation. When these conditions occur, a rationalist conception of the state is sufficient to explain domestic systems of governance.

The aforementioned instances of what social purposes may be like exemplify two ideal types that occupy opposite sides of the spectrum. In between, there are additional ones. First, power-based social purposes emerge when the entire domestic elite or its subgroup is strongly committed to upholding a range of specific ideas and possesses enough coercive and administrative capacity to enforce its normative vision. Although a power-based consensus can influence domestic systems of governance, various social actors, domestic movements, and individuals would do well to challenge this consensus. There are several possible circumstances that maintain the power-based consensus. One plausible situation occurs when the elite is not fully cohesive. One or several subgroups that split from the dominant elite can lack the political or administrative capacity to apply their ideas to practical policy making, although their alternative ideas regarding the nature of political authority can be reasonably compelling.

Another plausible situation occurs when elite-driven ideas acquire only moderate traction in society. This can happen for a variety of reasons, ranging from the elite's ineptness in promoting its vision for the state or when strong traditions of pluralism are reified in domestic institutions. Strong identity arguments usually help the elite justify which of the competing ideas are or are not to be internalized as appropriate, but these arguments are not always successful. As society on the whole fails to internalize the elite-generated social purpose, it is clear that the independent impact of that social purpose will remain limited in time and scope. Power-based consensus is likely to become vulnerable when the adverse consequences of the governance strategies, premised on social purposes, become tangible and when people begin interpreting these adverse consequences as a policy tragedy.

Second, competing groups and individuals simultaneously advocate different justifications for state existence, while no elite subgroup possesses enough resources and capacities to turn its ideas regarding the core goals of the state into the only conceptual underpinning of the domestic systems of governance. While thinking about competition among multiple credible conceptions of the cardinal goals of the state is not quite irrelevant, conjectures about the influence of fractured social purposes on the systems of governance and norm diffusion are highly speculative.

The foregoing empirical discussion makes the point that the social purpose in Russia became fully legitimate while remaining power based in South Africa. In the latter case, members of the domestic elite were strongly committed to upholding a range of specific ideas about the state but, for a variety of reasons, failed to socialize their audiences into their normative outlook. Leaders had to rely on the administrative power of the state. That is why, once Mbeki's allies and unconditional supporters lost their power, their ideas about the cardinal goals of the state lost their status as reasons for action, although the core of the African Renaissance did not fully dissipate. In effect, South Africa's AIDS policies became far more in line with established international norms. In Russia, once Putin is fully out of office and once he loses both formal and informal levers of power, new rounds of discussions about the core goals of the state will billow. The brittle stalks of new ideas already protruded from the asphalt of normative consensus when Putin deceitfully and briefly stepped down from the highest office of the country. However, the fundamental change in AIDS governance strategies will become likely only concurrently with the profound political change caused by Putin's final departure, among other things. At this time (the mid-2010s), Putin's version of Russia's social purpose is preponderant and is not likely to face any serious internal challenges.

CONCLUSION

In this chapter, I have examined the ideas enclosed in the unfolding discourses of sovereign democracy and the African Renaissance. These ideas were more than situational and rational reactions to transitional difficulties. Instead, they represented nascent normative orders and formulated the set of goals the renovated states must follow. In both post-Communist and postcolonial countries, ideas about the state have emerged out of contingencies rather than inheritances, preordaining normative proclivities. The most important contingency was the ascent of both Russian *siloviki* and South African Mbekiites to political prominence. These politicians possessed a unique sense of agency, mission, and identity and developed new sets of meanings about the state in order to break free from the now-discredited previous political ideals and institutions. In each state, the developed systems of meaning and representation turned out to be tangibly different from the previous ones.

Putin, the *siloviki*, and the regime's acolytes claimed that statism was vital for the existence and survival of the country. Liberal approaches to governance in Russia, despite their prominent presence in domestic political debates, have yet to resonate among wider audiences and to appear on the roster of legitimate state goals. At the same time, the internally shared ideas about the core tasks of the state diverged from international organizing principles of governance. For these reasons, the proposition that external principles of health governance are likely to be considered inappropriate in Russia seems quite feasible. In South Africa, a normative commitment to indigenous values constituted the core goal of the state. Although Mbeki's ideas on the core goals of the state resonated with a significant portion of domestic audiences, to a certain extent he had to resort to administrative power to rein in the dissenting voices of domestic civil society and disillusioned politicians. On balance, the African Renaissance did not become fully legitimate, because South African civil society remained vibrant and committed to pluralism.

Because newly formulated goals have to be legitimated and popularized, I have examined not only how committed elites articulated them but also how they unfolded political discourses and identity arguments. The identity arguments worked in Russia better than in South Africa. Putin and his entourage unpacked their ideas and communicated them well. Evidence presented in this chapter suggests that social purposes achieved their full legitimacy in Russia while they remained power based in South Africa. Nevertheless, the internally shared ideas about the cardinal tasks of the state pushed South Africa to question international organizing principles of governance, as well.

The necessary caveat is that both of the notions that I apply to describe the set of ideas about the core goals of the state engendered internal terminological discussions. High-powered politicians at times were uncomfortable using these notions without qualifications. At the same time, they seemed to agree deeply with the meaning and implications of these notions. In Russia, although Dmitriy Medvedev superficially disliked the label "sovereign democracy," he never challenged its substantive contents. In South Africa, there was surely a debate about the meanings and implications of the African Renaissance. Nevertheless, despite initial confusion, the cardinal ideas encapsulated by the discourse of the African Renaissance became clear over time.

On a final note, making predictions about the embraced methods of AIDS governance for any extended periods of time is not easy. Political leaders, opinion leaders, and citizens might reconsider the prevailing justifications for the existence of their state. It follows from the core constructivist assumptions about intersubjectivity that genuinely shared ideas might outlast the political and physical existence of their originators. Not surprisingly, certain ideational orientations survived Mbeki's fall. It also follows that although some leaders stay in office for a very long time (like Putin), the status of their at one moment fully internalized ideas as indispensable components of political authority might be corrected or terminated. In reality, however, the newly designed conservative values have augmented the state's autonomy from society and have justified the state's intrusion into the private lives of ordinary Russians.

The narrative that unfolds in the ensuing chapters is about how the process of developing social purposes under Vladimir Putin and Thabo Mbeki underpinned the systems of AIDS governance in Russia and South Africa.

CHAPTER 3

Facing the Contagion

AIDS as a Problem of Public Health

WHEN GOVERNMENTS FAIL to understand an epidemic as a problem of public health, practices developed to address health issues deviate from the standard repertoire of biomedical solutions. Because understanding issues in a particular way certainly does not preordain the ensuing social practices, no scholar should claim that to analyze issue framing suffices to explain why certain governance choices prevail over others. Nevertheless, a keen observer can discern whether governments address the problem on the grounds of some politicized considerations or not. Governments are likely to address AIDS as a problem of public health only if they fully commit to the biomedical paradigm of the epidemic and rely on competent health bureaucracies that act on the basis of up-to-date scientific discoveries.[1] If that is the case, then political leaders will be likely to adopt conventional medicines, enforce the standardized treatment protocols, and accept the available international instruments that help secure the supply of generic drugs.

To set the stage for the structured, focused comparisons, this chapter first conceptualizes international biomedical approaches to HIV/AIDS. In the first section, I highlight that it is important to frame the epidemic as a public health crisis, pursue standardized treatment options, fight denialism, and be highly cautious about complementary and alternative medicines while keeping tabs on the strategies and actions of the global pharmaceutical sector. The latter allows dealing with HIV/AIDS as an issue of public health rather than a matter of intellectual property rights or an issue of domestic research and development. The following two sections start discussing the systems of AIDS governance in Russia and South Africa by examining how and with what consequences the leaders of these two states came to frame their general concerns regarding the contagion.

For Moscow, the ominous epidemic was a telltale sign of Russia's internal and external weakness. Although this orientation did not challenge the adoption of evidence-based medicines, it indirectly predetermined governmental failure to follow up on all too many obligations (that were supposed to highlight the increasing strength of the Russian state and the exceptional competencies of the country's leaders) and to enforce the standardized protocol in treatment. For Pretoria, the menacing spread of HIV was perceived as a unique challenge to local development and the Cabinet's ability to govern. Because of this, for South Africans to remedy the contagion was to expand the boundaries of knowledge and, instead of treating complementary and traditional medicines as unavoidable cultural obstacles, to engage them as a full-fledged medical alternative that had much to offer for improving public health. Social purposes stipulated how Moscow and Pretoria chose to adjust their pharmaceutical sectors to international approaches to generic drugs. In sum, each government premised its reasoning about the nature of the epidemic and the necessary course of action on an underlying devotion to fulfill the core goals of the state.

INTERNATIONAL APPROACHES TO THE HIV/AIDS CRISIS

Since the 1980s, international leaders and practitioners alike have characterized the HIV/AIDS epidemic as a serious policy challenge. Nonetheless, for most of the 1990s, the lack of effective and relatively cheap biomedical products caused health policy "quiescence."[2] This term describes a situation in which even the most credible and energetic individuals failed to propose a common framework featuring unambiguous and universally agreed-upon solutions to the HIV crisis. The discovery of effective antiretroviral therapies in 1996 turned things around.

The discussion below is organized as follows. The first subsection outlines the prevailing modes of issue framing because they help us evaluate how committed elites and policy participants intend to deal with the AIDS challenge. The second subsection highlights the increasing effectiveness of evidence-based medicines and standardization of the treatment protocol. The cumulative effect of the continuous failures in finding an AIDS vaccine, the decreased toxicity of anti-HIV medications, the explosion of different brands of antiretrovirals, and the availability of pre- and postexposure prophylaxis put treatment at the heart of the global biomedical paradigm. The term "antiretrovirals" (ARVs) describes different combinations of safe and effective drugs that suppress the human immunodeficiency virus. The existence of a standardized biomedical product swept the emotional appeal of miracle cures away and disproved the delusional dissidents and conspiracy theorists who challenged professional conventions. Today, complementary and traditional medicines should belong to the realm of cultural heritage rather than evidence-based health governance. The third subsection explores the methods that powerful pharmaceutical firms use to protect their own material interests. The developing and resource-strapped countries that are committed to addressing AIDS as a public health problem must keep tabs on the global pharmaceutical industry, using the available political mechanisms of protecting the availability of generic products and shielding their low prices. According to the World Health Organization's definition, a generic drug is "a pharmaceutical product, usually intended to be interchangeable with an innovator product, which is manufactured without a license from the innovator company and marketed after the expiry date of the patent or other exclusive rights. Generic drugs are marketed under a nonproprietary, or approved, name rather than a proprietary, or brand, name. Generic drugs are frequently as effective as, but much cheaper than, brand-name drugs."[3] The wide availability of generics has been at the heart of the global contestation.

The Pandemic as a Public Health Crisis

The outbreak of the HIV/AIDS epidemic has forced governments to respond to it as a public health crisis. HIV/AIDS, of course, is about development, military or human security, human rights, demographic crisis, poverty, inequality, intellectual property rights, and so on. However, ignoring a public health approach is the first signal that governments might be inclined to disregard some elements of evidence-based medicine as the organizing principle of health governance. The reason for minimizing the significance of a public health approach might be that governments are preoccupied with other priorities that have nothing to do with protecting the public from the disease.

Important international actors have not always addressed the pandemic as a public health crisis. In the 1980s conservative governments typically framed AIDS in terms other than public health. President Ronald Reagan's administration, for instance, understood AIDS in the context of medical competition with France, an ideological struggle with the USSR, and the diminishing significance of Africa in the competition between two global superpowers.[4] That is a distant memory now; in the mid-1990s, things started to change. The invention of remarkable and life-saving antiretrovirals and the spread of knowledge about their effectiveness were first steps to end the exasperating propensity to address HIV in that vein. The International AIDS Conferences had a fundamental influence on forging the global consensus and spreading the understanding of the contagion as a public health issue. In the early 2000s the advent of a new generation of AIDS organizations cemented the global consensus further as they addressed the spread of HIV/AIDS primarily as a public health crisis, with a strong emphasis placed on the expansion of access to life-saving medicines. Later, in June 2006 and July 2011, the UN General Assembly adopted political declarations that secured the high political status of the extant norm.[5]

By the early 2000s, the health benefits of providing the universal ARV treatment in the public sector became clear due to success stories of the fight against HIV/AIDS in Brazil, Thailand, and Uganda, to mention some exemplary cases. While activists and policy makers typically showcase policy making in these three countries as best practices, a quantitative and qualitative change on a global scale became evident at the XI International Conference on AIDS and STDs in Africa, held in Lusaka, Zambia, in September 1999. At that conference, the majority of African nation-states publicly committed to addressing HIV/AIDS as a public health crisis and pledged to provide life-saving ARVs. Former laggards turned things around by seizing the initiative in arguing for broader international assistance from the developed nations and global health organizations, thus acting as norm entrepreneurs. To use conventional constructivist terminology, it was a tipping point that triggered a "norm cascade."

Today leading actors in global health governance signal their continuing commitment to the public health policy approach against HIV/AIDS. In 2007 the Institute of Medicine of the National Academies of Science published a comprehensive report that praised the President's Emergency Plan for AIDS Relief (PEPFAR)—one of the most significant international AIDS programs—for addressing HIV/AIDS as a preventable communicable disease and a manageable chronic infection rather than as a terminal illness generated by some unique local sociocultural characteristics.[6] Similarly, in 2008 the WHO reaffirmed the importance of framing HIV/AIDS as a public health crisis. In sum, the public health approach to HIV/AIDS "is based on the principles of simplification, standardisation, decentralisation, equity, and patient and community participation, and has been pivotal in unlocking the treatment agenda, and starting to close the treatment gap between rich and poor countries."[7]

Addressing HIV as an issue of public health does not imply that governance methods all over the globe will be uniform. On the contrary, because local epidemiological conditions vary, governments must adjust their policies to the epidemiological trajectory on the ground. Variations in health policies across countries might emerge, for instance, in relation to the change in medical views regarding the minimum decrease of the number of T cells that warrants immediate treatment. Variations might also arise if the epidemic penetrates the generalized population or remains confined to some smaller groups. Conditions on the ground might require setting up particular mechanisms of resource allocation, devising unique strategies of partnerships, and so on. No differences in local conditions justify those local leaders who address the epidemic as a non–public health issue and reject evidence-based policy solutions. No differences in epidemiology can give good reasons for local leaders to deny health services to certain subpopulations. At the very least, the plea to use local solutions should not contravene sensible policy making and good governance. The overuse of the local-solutions rhetoric is a telltale sign that leaders are pursuing their own parochial agendas, which can feasibly stem from prevailing domestic ideas about the core tasks of the state and the common good. The bottom line is that if policy makers do not respond to the HIV/AIDS crisis as a public health problem, they are likely to be at variance with international policy norms.

Standardized Protocol in Treatment

In order to address HIV/AIDS as an issue of public health, leaders should accept internationally approved pharmaceutical products. ARVs are retroviral inhibitors, a class of drugs that suppress the replication of the human immunodeficiency virus in human bodies. Antiretrovirals do not cure AIDS, but they significantly delay the development of opportunistic diseases and prolong the survival of infected individuals.

On March 19, 1987, the Food and Drug Administration (FDA) approved zidovudine (AZT, brand name Retrovir).[8] First synthesized in 1964 for the purposes of cancer research, this monotherapy was toxic and had multiple negative side effects. For a while, the early medications remained prohibitively expensive. A real breakthrough came in the mid-1990s. During the 11th International AIDS Conference in Vancouver, British Columbia, scientists presented an effective fixed-dose combination of protease inhibitors for treating HIV-positive patients. The major biomedical difference from the earlier regimens was that scientists figured out how to contain the infected cell by targeting a different enzyme. Health policy observers could not restrain their excitement about the "treatment almost miraculously restoring the health of many people terminally ill with AIDS."[9] Offered in a combination with other medications, highly active retroviral treatment also diminished chances of developing drug resistance. In addition, treatment-naive patients benefited from the fixed-dose combination, as copackaged drug products alleviated potential adherence problems and simplified the logistical issues of drug distribution. According to the FDA's industry guidelines, "A co-packaged product consists of two or more separate drug products in their final dosage form, packaged together with appropriate labeling to support the combination use. A fixed dose combination product is one in which two or more separate drug ingredients are combined in a single dosage form."[10]

Just one year after the Vancouver conference, the FDA approved Combivir, the first two-drug, fixed-dose combination of lamivudine and zidovudine, offered by GlaxoSmithKline. The recent copackaged combinations usually include lower dosages of the AZT in combination with other drugs. By the end of 2003, the WHO officially recommended seven different three- and two-drug fixed-dose combinations.[11] In 2004 national regulators, representatives of the pharmaceutical industry, health-care providers, and advocacy groups gathered in Gaborone, Botswana, to discuss the scientific and technical principles of fixed-dose ARVs. As a result of these talks, the conference cosponsors, Southern African Development Community, the United Nations Joint Programme on HIV/AIDS, the U.S. Department of Health and Human Services, and the World Health Organization, issued a final principles document regarding safety, quality, and effectiveness of copackaged treatments.

At what point should governments start providing treatment? Quite simply, the early initiation of widespread antiretroviral treatment has obvious benefits for health. The WHO recommends treatment if the count of CD4 cells (i.e., cells that are responsible for immune response) goes below a certain threshold. In 2006 the WHO insisted that treatment must start at a cell count of two hundred; in 2013 its new consolidated guidelines recommended an earlier initiation of treatment if the CD4 cell count was five hundred or below.[12] Currently available antiretrovirals are effective for the suppression of viremia—the presence of viruses in the blood. Antiretroviral treatment sheds the virus in semen and vaginal secretions, increases the number of CD4+ T cells, reduces immune activation, restores lymph node architecture, delays or prevents opportunistic infections, and enhances the overall clinical improvement of HIV-positive patients. The list of approved HIV-related therapies, including information on brand and generic names, manufacturers' names, approval dates, and approval speed, is available on the Food and Drug Administration's information sheets. As of 2014, the FDA had granted tentative and full approvals for 170 generic formulations from foreign manufacturers.[13]

In addition to the described medical breakthroughs, the rapid decrease of the cost of treatment has made antiretrovirals a viable tool in confronting the contagion globally, including in resource-limited settings. Although it has been difficult to estimate the actual costs of treating patients with HIV/AIDS in different countries, the price of treatment came to the colossal sum of roughly U.S.$150,000 per person per year in the early 1990s and then declined to only $15,000 by the mid-1990s. Ten years later, the cost of key drugs was less than one dollar per day per patient.[14] All this emboldened many international organizations to endorse treatment as a feasible centerpiece of the domestic response to HIV/AIDS.

The global understanding of AIDS as a public health issue, however, did not emerge without a challenge. In what follows, this subsection summarizes different arguments promulgated by AIDS dissenters and then describes the limits and challenges of employing traditional medicines to improve public health.

The principal assault on evidence-based medicine sprang from an AIDS reappraisal hypothesis that was generously suffused with conspiracy theories. In the late 1980s, Peter Duesberg, a German-born researcher of cell and molecular biology at Berkeley, opened the controversial debate concerning the nature of the retroviruses and their relation to AIDS. Duesberg's academic credentials and international acclaim for his cancer research seemingly lent credibility to his proposition that the immunodeficiency virus was harmless and that the real cause of a medical condition known as AIDS was the use of drugs. In June 2000 Duesberg addressed a South African AIDS panel with a provocative talk entitled "The African AIDS Epidemic: New and Contagious or Old under a New Name," in which he argued that "American and European AIDS epidemics exhibit the characteristics of diseases caused by non-contagious, chemical or physical factors *not* viruses" and described AIDS in Africa as a "nutritionally or environmentally caused disease."[15] Following Duesberg's claims, dissidents spread the idea of the multifactorial etiology of AIDS and asserted that lifestyle issues and drug abuse could have been the primary cause of the retrovirus.[16]

Other equally outlandish assertions followed. First, the spread and implications of the epidemic have been overstated, while the presented statistical data were not accurate. Second, the purpose of biomedical research was to generate profits for the pharmaceutical firms. Individual "virologists had 'invested' in the HIV hypothesis—not just financially, though this was true in some cases, but personally, professionally, and psychologically."[17] Third, because the human immunodeficiency virus was not a sufficient condition for AIDS, the real cause of AIDS had been misidentified. Since AIDS included many opportunistic diseases, the correlation between AIDS and HIV was an artifact of the definition itself. Fourth, the proponents of the "drug-AIDS" hypothesis stated that acquired immunodeficiency syndrome was "a collection of chemical epidemics, caused by recreational drugs, anti-HIV drugs, and malnutrition."[18] Fifth, the "poison by prescription" argument pointed out that azidothymidine was toxic and dangerous. For this reason, AZT contributed to immune overload and resulted in immune suppression. Dissidents, for instance, attributed the death of the famous dancer Rudolph Nureyev to azidothymidine.[19]

Needless to say, the professional medical community did not endorse these speculations. Since the early 1990s, Dr. Robert Gallo, immunologist Dr. Anthony S. Fauci of the National Institutes of Health (NIH), and many others have repudiated all these claims with absolute certainty. While mainstream health experts and medical professionals did not take Duesberg's conjectures seriously, scores of sensation-hungry journalists, such as John Lauritsen and Celia Farber, joined the movement, whose members proudly described themselves as AIDS dissidents, realists, rethinkers, and heretics.

The heyday of the dissident skepticism was rather brief; many members of the movement did not live very long, as they refused to take the life-saving medications. Nevertheless, the remnants of denialists still harp on their old major themes on the Internet and sometimes come together into such obscure groups as Alive and Well, HEAL, Perth Group, and Group for the Scientific Reappraisal of the HIV-AIDS Hypothesis. Despite their marginal status, under favorable circumstances the AIDS dissidents are able to endorse unconventional views on healing and support obscure local beliefs. They offer fraudulent expertise and self-serving justifications for those governments and state agencies that decide to resist evidence-based medicines. Although the so-called counterepistemic community was largely marginal in the international arena, it outfitted top South African leaders to reappraise the meaning of the epidemic.

Another challenge to the global commitment to evidence-based treatment has emerged in conjunction with the rising popularity of complementary and alternative medicines. The former can be defined as substances that assist a human being's innate healing force used together with conventional medicines. The latter is best defined as any nonconventional medical therapies that are used as a replacement for conventional medicine.[20] While the conceptual borders between these notions are clear theoretically, in practice they are porous and depend on how health authorities decide to use them in their systems of governance. For instance, herbs, vitamins, and nutritional supplements can be viewed and employed as either complementary or alternative medicine. The South African case, discussed below, is a case in point.

The notion of traditional medicine (which I will also refer to as nostrum remedium) can be confusing. The World Health Organization defined it as a comprehensive concept that includes various forms of indigenous medicines, both medication and nonmedication therapies.[21] Intergovernmental organizations converge on the conclusion that promoting indigenous and traditional knowledge contributes to standardizing and commercializing human knowledge about plants. Although the WHO has exhibited an interest in traditional medicines, it has been extremely careful not to overstate their safety and efficacy. While genetic resources and ethnomedicines might be abstractly useful for health governance, none of the credible international bodies suggests replacing modern medical products with either alternative or traditional medicines. Those who wish to consult international documents regarding policy baselines and precise guidelines and use these documents to learn how to use traditional medicines will remain disgruntled. Often, intergovernmental organizations place genetic medicinal resources under the broader rubrics of culture, heritage, and folklore, thereby interpreting them as a form of cultural expression rather than as medicines. The WIPO Intergovernmental Committee on Intellectual Property and Genetic Resources, Traditional Knowledge and Folklore seeks to protect traditional medical knowledge precisely because of its social, cultural, and scientific value and because it is important for many indigenous peoples and local communities.[22]

How to strike a balance between a range of unorthodox medicines and evidence-based products for the purposes of good health governance is a daunting question. Complementary and traditional medicines can be used to compensate for the lack of access to conventional drugs in resource-poor settings. There is also a growing popularity in the so-called integrative approach, aiming at holistic healing. A debate about the spread and use of complementary and traditional medicines in terms of both their impact on individual health and the proper ways of integrating them in Westernized public health systems is prominent in the health policy literature. The central controversy that remains unsolved is about the practical value of traditional healing. Internationally, the use of herbal remedies and plant medicines has become very popular. Naturopathic healers of various convictions contribute to the considerable increase of consumption of various herbal remedies. For instance, Western naturopaths praise the positive medicinal effects of garlic in preventing cognitive decline, sustaining cardiovascular wellness, inhibiting the growth of cancer, reducing drug toxicity, and so on. These opinions do not belong to the conventional medical mainstream. At the very least, the discussion about the medicinal value of indigenous plants and the pharmacological effects of these substances is yet to be resolved. Although many studies on ethnomedicines garner evidence about the medicinal properties of plants, these studies give no definite answer whether nostrums can produce tangible benefits for health. While the proponents of traditional medicines remain uncritical about the medicinal properties of local plants, there are many reasonable concerns about reactions between presumably medicinal plants and chemical compounds in conventional pharmaceutical products. At the very least, governments should welcome the regulation of indigenous knowledge. Qualified regulative bodies should carefully scrutinize the products offered by the purveyors of complementary medicinal products of any sort.

Integration of traditional and conventional medical practices is another contentious point. Emphasizing the desire to integrate traditional knowledge into the modern health-care system is not similar to pinpointing nostrums as appropriate for local health governance. Although there might be a positive effect of integrating traditional healers into modern health-care systems, the negative externalities might outweigh the estimated gains. The empirical findings from the southern African region remain controversial, even though many healers supposedly were willing to learn from medical personnel. The studies of traditional healers documented both accurate and faulty knowledge about the existence of alternative AIDS cures, as well as the diagnosis, nature, and genesis of HIV.[23] For example, the Zimbabwe National Traditional Healers Association joined the Ministry of Health, yet for more than three decades this incorporation did not fully overturn the widespread traditional understanding of the etiology of contagion as a moral disease spreading from the guilty to the innocent. While many traditional beliefs proved to be sticky and difficult to turn around, healers continued to administer highly risky practices that were not based on the evidence of health improvement.

In summary, using evidence-based drug products increases the likelihood of AIDS-free survival. Equally important to manage the antiretroviral treatment properly is to stick to standardized and simplified regimens. Staying away from substandard treatment protocols helps to prevent drug resistance. Fixed-dose combinations and copackaged drug products help practitioners operate in resource-limited settings. Under certain circumstances, policy participants might decide to reject the antiretrovirals as too toxic and ineffective, stress complementary and alternative medicines as the primary substitution for ARVs, or select regimens that are too advanced for the state of the epidemic. Needless to say, undermining the standardized treatment protocol is dangerous. It could compromise the results of treatment and lead to the spread of drug resistance, among other complications. Further, in the developing and resource-limited countries, difficulties of access to the modern health-care system undergird the revival of interest in traditional medicines. However, lessons from the countries that use indigenous knowledge in health promotion are not pointing in the same direction. Any mechanistic integration of the two health-care systems is likely to perpetuate or even aggravate problems related to regimen adherence and drug resistance. Moreover, the lack of quality control leads to understandable side effects with adverse complications for health.

The Pharmaceutical Industry and Generics

The pharmaceutical industry and the global firms that occupy a highly influential position in the global power structure understandably frame the issue of life-saving medicines as a matter of intellectual property rights and international trade. Protecting expensive brand-name medicines and erecting barriers to the wide use of generic medications (when patents to brand-name drugs are not yet expired) are among the main financial and legal holdups on the road to an AIDS-free generation and are to a large extent antithetical to the goal of effective AIDS governance. Luckily, the excessive commercialization of research and development and the commodification of vitally important pharmaceutical goods has diminished, inasmuch as the global players have agreed to integrate public health objectives into trade considerations. In 1999 the World Health Assembly urged its member states "to ensure that public health rather than commercial interests have primacy in pharmaceutical and health policies."[24] This progress, however, does not eliminate the necessity for governments to press further for greater flexibility in intellectual property rules and to protect their use of public health safeguards.

The Agreement on the Trade-Related Aspects of Intellectual Property Rights (TRIPS) is aimed at the protection of patents for pharmaceutical products. Scholars and activists alike often describe TRIPS as a powerful barrier to opening the competitive market for generic life-saving products. In the late 1990s and early 2000s, TRIPS remained a major roadblock, preventing access to generic pharmaceutical products in the developing world.[25] Questionable pricing mechanisms fortified these institutional barriers. Alarmed critics alerted their audiences that TRIPS protected the profit-seeking goals of giant pharmaceutical manufacturers of the industrialized world, such as Merck, Boehringer Ingelheim, La Roche, Bristol-Myers Squibb, GlaxoSmithKline, and others. These corporate actors hoped that the World Intellectual Property Organization (WIPO) and the World Trade Organization (WTO) would regulate antiretroviral medicines solely as a matter of intellectual property.

In October 2001, during multilateral trade negotiations at the WTO, a group of developing countries pressed to correct the stress on intellectual property rights in conjunction with the understanding that a public health crisis and national health emergency might be more important than observing patents for pharmaceuticals. They drafted a ministerial declaration that pushed developed countries "to ensure that medicines for treatment of HIV/AIDS and other pandemics are available to their citizens who need them, particularly those who are unable to afford basic medical care."[26] As a result, the fourth session of the ministerial conference of the WTO in Doha, Qatar, adopted a foundational document that reaffirmed the primacy of public health in dealing with HIV/AIDS treatment. The Declaration on the TRIPS Agreement and Public Health acknowledged countries' rights to acquire certain instruments to protect public health.[27] TRIPS safeguards include research exemptions that permit generic manufacturers to test protected drugs before the patent expires, compulsory licensing of patented products to domestic firms without the consent of the drug originator, and parallel importation of a patented product without the consent of the patent holder. These safeguards allow governments to enjoy a certain flexibility in finding low-cost drugs. Although academics and activists alike were skeptical about the practical ability of developing countries to implement these safeguards, the evidence suggests otherwise.

International policy entrepreneurs and global activists framed the access to life-saving drugs and generics as an issue of public health and thus contributed to the process of integrating public health objectives into trade considerations. On the eve of the Seattle ministerial conference, advocacy organizations began their campaign for equal access to medicines. In 1999 at the Palais des Nations in Geneva the Consumer Project on Technology, Health Action International, and Médecins sans frontières organized the first international meeting dedicated to the effective use of compulsory licensing. The result of this international meeting—the so-called Amsterdam Statement—provided conceptual tools to the global campaign for access to medicines that from then on involved many international and domestic NGOs, including the Treatment Action Campaign of South Africa, Act Up Paris of France, and the Health Gap Coalition of the United States.[28] In 2001 the British charity Oxfam singled out GlaxoSmithKline as the main target of its "Cut the Costs" campaign. The same year, in Washington, D.C., hundreds of demonstrators protested against drug companies' lawsuit to protect expensive branded drugs from being replaced by their cheaper equivalents in South Africa.

That public outrage incrementally attenuated as the private sector expanded its commitments to fight HIV/AIDS. As early as 2001, Glaxo Wellcome, Merck, Boehringer Ingelheim, F. Hoffmann–La Roche, and Bristol-Myers Squibb began offering modest discounts on select antiretrovirals to African nations. They slashed costs for the fixed-dose combinations and offered differential pricing for drugs for select developing countries. Although these actions were situational and perhaps strategic, humanitarian reasons might also be detected here, since big for-profit corporations actually joined global campaigns for access to the life-saving medicines.[29] Since the early 2000s, pharmaceutical giants have pursued many corporate philanthropic initiatives on their own, selling drugs with preferential pricing, providing medicines free of charge, or negotiating special deals with select countries. Launched in 2000, the Accelerating Access Initiative proved to be a notable example of a fruitful cooperation between seven major pharmaceutical companies and five United Nations agencies that resulted in major reductions in ARV prices, sometimes dropping down to 10 percent of their commercial price in industrialized countries.[30]

The argument that patient rights should prevail over patent rights, notwithstanding its undeniable humanitarian appeal, would not have shaped global AIDS governance the way it did if the market had not been opened to generics. The industrial competition initiated by Indian companies Ranbaxy, Cipla, Aurobindo, and Hetero Drugs drove the prices of branded drugs down. Quite simply, Indian producers came to dominate the generic ARV market. In 2001, when the price tag of the branded product was still over $12,000 per patient per year, Indian manufacturer Hetero Drugs offered the world's first triple fixed-dose combination (stavudine, lamivudine, and nevirapine) at less than one dollar per day. In 2008 ten Indian firms manufactured fifty-three generic products, which accounted for more than 80 percent of annual global purchase volumes.[31] As a result, high-quality and safe bioequivalent products pushed drug originators to offer discounts for the branded products. At the same time, the health community reached an agreement on the standards for approval of fixed-dose antiretroviral combinations and agreed on their safety. In 2004 the bioequivalent fixed-dose combinations for the global HIV/AIDS programs started to make their way through the Food and Drug Administration's standard review process for regulation and approval. Since May 2004, the Center for Drug Evaluation and Research (CDER) has also provided further clarifications regarding regulatory requirements for pharmaceutical companies that wish to submit fixed-dose combinations and copackaged drug products for treatment of HIV for review at the FDA. According to one study, from January 2004 to March 2006 generic companies supplied 63 percent of the drugs for sub-Saharan Africa at prices that were on average about a third of the prices charged by brand-name companies.[32]

Importantly, the new generation of AIDS organizations was able to avoid the constraints of the prohibitively high prices of brand-name pharmaceuticals. As early as 2004, almost 60 percent of all treatment purchases supported by the Global Fund to Fight AIDS, Tuberculosis and Malaria (GFATM) were generics. The evolution of PEPFAR's approach to drug procurement shows the indispensable role of generics in the ongoing global health governance. At first, PEPFAR purchased the drugs for Africa from the pharmaceutical giants at the American price and did not allow cheaper generics. Randall Tobias, the first global AIDS coordinator in charge of PEPFAR, argued that only safe and regulated brand-name remedies should be purchased with PEPFAR's money. Given Tobias's prior position in the private sector with Eli Lilly and Company, that attitude was hardly surprising. By 2007, however, a different trend had come into full force. Mark Dybul, in 2006–9 the U.S. global AIDS coordinator, reported to the House Committee on Foreign Affairs that PEPFAR had "increased its purchasing of generic versus branded antiretrovirals from 72 percent from April to September 2006 to 88 percent (by volume) from January to March 2007."[33] While in 2004 only one generic drug was approved for use in PEPFAR, there are now 143 generic antiretrovirals used in its programs. While only 14.8 percent of the antiretroviral packs purchased with PEPFAR funds used generics in 2005, generic formulations accounted for 97 percent of such purchases only five years later.[34] The supply chain management system (SCMS) has become an integral part of how PEPFAR ensures a continuous flow of essential high-quality, cost-effective medications and supplies bioequivalent drugs.

In summary, the progress toward using generic drugs as a standardized practice in AIDS governance is undeniable. So is the international understanding that generic products are of paramount importance. In 2010 UNITAID (a global health initiative established in 2006) set up the Medicines Patent Pool in order to increase access to newer antiretroviral medicines and create competitive markets for generic manufacturers to produce affordable copies of second-line treatments.[35] Several major pharmaceutical companies have already contributed to a pool of shared patents on antiretroviral medicines.[36] However, multiple threats to generic ARVs continue to surface during trade negotiations and show up in bilateral and regional trade agreements. The private sector is not likely to abolish patents and other intellectual property restrictions, avoid the commercialization of biotechnology, and argue against the commodification of antiretrovirals. In 2011, for instance, the United States, the European Union, and Japan moved to strengthen intellectual property laws.[37] Also on the list of challenges is the increasing demand for the newer versions of first-line medicines, as well as the demand for more expensive patented second-line regimens. Creating a competitive market for second-line medications that are protected by patents and matching the supply and incessantly growing demand are daunting tasks as well.[38]

To recapitulate, despite numerous current and future tensions, low- and middle-income countries currently have at their disposal a number of useful legal and political mechanisms to maximize their access to life-saving medicines. In addition, countries and activists can influence the substance of intellectual property rights laws through vigorous protests, mobilization campaigns, and litigation. In certain circumstances, however, governments choose unexpected and counterintuitive courses of action. Pretoria used bitter rhetoric to vilify the global power structure, although the strategy was hardly useful for dealing with the country's looming challenges. Equally frustrating for good AIDS governance was Moscow's desire to overwhelm the global market with mass-produced new molecular entities when both the intellectual and industrial prerequisites of doing so were simply not in place. The reasons why the state might choose these self-defeating paths are revealed in the relevant subsections below.

Summary

Antiretrovirals are essential life-saving products; they turn what used to be a death sentence for infected individuals into a chronic but manageable condition. Although prohibitively high prices remained the main challenge until the early 2000s, the generic supply made widespread treatment possible. Without effective and relatively cheap antiretrovirals, it would be almost unworkable to respond to HIV/AIDS as a public health crisis. The technological breakthroughs in effective medicines and the appearance of high-quality bioequivalent drugs on the market drastically decreased the costs of treatment and allowed an increase in the number of patients receiving treatment. Relatively simple guidelines and tangible indicators of success have eased the process of policy diffusion for the relevant domestic actors. Because the treatment protocol is standardized, it leads to profound similarities in HIV/AIDS policy across countries. Questioning the biomedical consensus regarding antiretrovirals (and the standard knowledge that HIV causes AIDS) and/or enforcing the substandard protocol (any alternative and complementary medicines as partial or full substitutes to treatment therapy) constitute a significant deviation from the standardized policy prescription.

Various factors can stimulate governments to frame AIDS in terms other than those of public health and to avoid conventional governance solutions. Incomplete information about the available medications, faulty knowledge about the level of epidemiological threat, and incorrect attribution of the reasons behind policy successes elsewhere complicate norm diffusion. Nevertheless, the repeated exposure of domestic policy makers to international health developments is likely to eliminate controversial information and facilitate learning about the standards of policy responses. No evidence suggests that Moscow or Pretoria was either unaware of external information about the policy baselines or confused by external standards of good AIDS governance. Rather, the potential adopters had issues with the organizing principles underlying these recommendations.

In what follows, I discuss first Russian and then South African governance efforts to fight AIDS by deploying (or refusing to do so) conventional medicines. In the Russian case, the stress is on the inability to enforce and follow the standardized protocol because of the overextended obligations of the state. In the South African case, the stress is on complementary and alternative treatments as substitutes for ARVs. Each section concludes with a discussion of the methods each government chose to deal with ongoing developments in the pharmaceutical industry.

SUPPRESSING THE VIRUS IN PUTIN'S RUSSIA

Russians framed the problem of AIDS as an important political issue. Because Russian officialdom viewed the outburst of the epidemic as a ramification of the state's weakness, the government responded to the outbreak of HIV as a problem not reducible to a pressing public health issue. Most importantly, the Russian government interpreted the scare of HIV/AIDS in conjunction with the looming demographic crisis (see the first subsection below). Although pervasive state centrism did not rule out the wide use of conventional medicines, it surely complicated the process of purchasing and distributing the medications and undermined the standards of adherence (see the second subsection below). The third subsection discusses the escalating desire to develop original brand-name medicines. The Russian aspiration to bolster domestic pharmaceutical research and development might be commendable in principle, but the lack of prerequisites implicates that desire as a self-serving fulfillment that is not likely to increase Russian competitiveness in the global power structure.

Reappraising the Epidemic in Russia

The scope of Russia's health crisis is staggering. Low fertility, high mortality, high prevalence of cardiovascular diseases, low quality of medical services, and exceedingly high levels of tobacco and alcohol consumption are, without any doubt, gravely challenging the country's prospects for economic development and its security, broadly understood.[39] Adding to all these problems, in the early 2000s Russia's rates of HIV infection grew exponentially. According to the UN-AIDS 2011 World AIDS Day report,

> In Eastern Europe and Central Asia, there was a 250% increase in the number of people living with HIV from 2001 to 2010. The Russian Federation and Ukraine account for almost 90% of the Eastern Europe and Central Asia region's epidemic. . . . There is little indication that the epidemic has stabilized in the region, with new HIV infections and AIDS-related deaths continuing to increase. After slowing in the early 2000s, HIV incidence in Eastern Europe and Central Asia has been accelerating again since 2008. Unlike most other regions, AIDS-related deaths continue to rise in Eastern Europe and Central Asia.[40]

Somewhat unexpectedly for both domestic and external observers, Vladimir Putin raised the issue of HIV/AIDS as a looming security crisis at the State Council meeting in April 2006.[41] Many domestic and international observers publicly lauded—and rightly so—Putin's acknowledgment of HIV/AIDS as a grave threat, as well as his serious commitments to finance the response to the epidemic. Importantly, the resolution to fight HIV/AIDS came right at the moment when Russian leaders became preoccupied with an alarming demographic decline that, in their interpretation, threatened the state's power and the survival of the nation. It is not by accident that even as early as in his 2003 address to the Federal Assembly, Putin linked the impending consequences of the epidemic to the challenges of achieving a strong state. Following this address, several high-powered politicians warned about the negative effects of HIV/AIDS on national security and state survival. On March 30, 2005, Aleksandr Zhukov (then first deputy prime minister) indicated that "the HIV epidemic is far more than just a health issue: in the light of [Russia's] ongoing demographic decrease, it presents a serious threat to Russia's strategic, social, and economic security."[42]

By 2006 Russian opinion leaders of varying ideological persuasions had become obsessed with the pending demographic collapse. An eccentric conservative journalist, Aleksandr Prokhanov, never missed an opportunity to lament that Russia had been losing more than a million souls per year since the inception of the economic reforms. Even Mikhail Khodorkovskiy, former head of a prominent oil company, imagined a strong Russian state inhabited by 220–230 million people, which meant an improbable increase of 90 million individuals.[43] It seemed that Russian elite and opinion leaders of diverse persuasions failed to grasp the long-term trends of the unfolding population crisis, which commenced with the destruction of traditional peasant families during coercive collectivization campaigns and continued through the rest of the socialist era, which failed to stimulate a major baby boom. Instead, in conjunction with the official discourse that demonized the "wild nineties," Russian officialdom viewed the decline in population as the direct consequence of finance minister Yegor Gaidar's shock therapy and the pitiful retreat of Yeltsin's fledgling state. A sizeable portion of the Russian public converged on the idea that demographic challenges threatened the survival of the state.

Vladimir Yakunin, president of the state-run Russian Railways, who fancied himself a major social thinker, pushed that interpretation to the extreme. He opined that mysterious internal and external foes waged "demographic wars" against Russia.[44] These views echoed concerns of the Russian Orthodox Church, succinctly expressed in a report under the telling title "Demographic War against Russia: Demography, Family Planning, and Genocide." The report appeared on one faith-based Internet site that was edited by a prominent church functionary, Tikhon (Shevkunov), and it exposed sexual education and family planning as an American foreign policy tool deployed to subjugate Russia.[45] The spiking epidemic of HIV/AIDS then had nothing or very little to do with public health, according to that contorted outlook.

Ironically, the propensity to reappraise the meaning of the epidemic through the conceptual lenses of statism inhibited the predisposition to combat HIV/AIDS as an urgent public health crisis. The special governmental committee that in theory gathered to formulate a consolidated national strategy to respond to HIV/AIDS as a broad public health crisis has remained largely defunct since its inception. Moreover, I am not aware of any references by Medvedev to HIV/AIDS as a national health crisis. In his multiple newspaper and online interviews, as well as in speeches addressed to the members of the National Priority Projects (NPP) council, this theme remained curiously absent. Even his LiveJournal blog (blog-medvedev.livejournal.com) remained silent on the issue. This lack of attention seems strange, since Dimitriy Medvedev in his capacity as first deputy prime minister (2005–8) was in charge of improving health governance and modernizing public health.

The official statistical data tend to downplay the rate of HIV infection in the country. According to the official estimates, at the time when the Russian government decided to fight the virus, the number of people registered as HIV-positive had reached 370,000.[46] Six years later the total number of registered HIV-infected individuals in Russia amounted to 720,000 people. The majority of independent estimates was less optimistic and doubled the possible number of the HIV-infected population. But officialdom held fast to its own estimates to feed the unwarranted public certainty that the epidemic remained limited to some marginalized groups. While the majority of state officials have acknowledged the continuing growth in the reported new incidences of HIV infection, they have failed to grasp that the epidemic affects a variety of groups beyond marginal and negatively constructed populations. For instance, official references to the feminization of the epidemic—the first signal that the contagion had become generalized—were not frequent.

Moreover, turning a blind eye to the continuing increase in new incidences of HIV infection, the growing number of AIDS-related deaths, and the rising number of individuals who live with the virus allowed politicians to spin the relatively modest success in improving domestic health as an astounding accomplishment. The Russian government understood that the success of vigorous domestic responses to HIV/AIDS would shore up its reputation. Indeed, the Kremlin never shied away from lionizing its own role in stopping the spread of HIV at home. In doing so, Moscow wanted to convince the public of the government's unqualified success in mitigating AIDS and to contrast that success with the global failure to deal with the pandemic. There is clear evidence that the Russian government purposely invented the fictional failures of the international fight against HIV/AIDS to promote its own strategies of health policy making.

Domestic coverage of the epidemic on the state-controlled network TV was impressive. The informative ad campaign "Be in Touch with Your Health," which unfolded on national TV in all Russian regions, featured social ads that educated their audience about the nature of the domestic epidemic. By 2009 the federal and regional TV channels had televised nine educational video clips more than fifty thousand times, while private channel REN-TV aired nine films about real people living with HIV/AIDS. Media campaigns doubtless are important for good health governance. But the state-controlled TV channels tended to highlight the international lack of control over the epidemic in contrast to the Kremlin's successful handling of the contagion. And yet, given the epidemiological reality on Russian soil, it was surely difficult to sell this imagery. As one telling study of ordinary citizens' perception of the official coverage of AIDS puts it, "Russians spoke of the state channels as reducing real and necessary news about HIV/AIDS in Russia by blending it in with HIV/AIDS as a global problem" and "alter[ed] what they know to be true to give a false impression of security."[47] At the same time, the study's focus groups felt that the private coverage of the epidemic was far more accurate and grave than the official communications about AIDS.

Weak critical voices that highlighted the swelling policy shortcomings and contradicted the official grand narrative of unqualified success were never fully deracinated from the public discussion of AIDS governance. Recent hearings in the Public Chamber spotlighted several important concerns.[48] However, broad societal acceptance of the core tenets of sovereign democracy explains the lack of active or militant contestation around the principles of AIDS governance in Russia. Health crisis exploitation perhaps has reached its limits, but it also has become apparent that the public in general is not alarmed by the Kremlin's underperformance.

Despite the mounting tensions around the issues of demographic decline and the relative political urgency attached to the need to fight AIDS, the Kremlin kept downplaying the epidemic as a public health crisis. The reality of the swelling number of new HIV infections contradicts the many celebratory claims of success in fighting AIDS.

Implementing a Standardized Protocol in Russia

The Russian government never rejected the life-saving role of antiretrovirals in principle. The government's response did not deviate from the international consensus that rolling out evidence-based medicines was a vital necessity. At the same time, politicians did not suspend their broader ideational commitments regarding the core tasks of the state. The implemented centralized system of procuring and disbursing drugs was consistent with the embraced ideal of hierarchical state-centric governance. Further, political devotion to the state's autonomy from society impelled top bureaucrats to set policy goals and make important policy decisions without heeding the views and recommendations of the professional medical community. Combined together, these orientations contributed to the failure of good health governance: drug shortages occurred on a regular basis in many provinces, and constant violations of the standardized protocol in treatment persisted across the country. To be sure, the government acknowledged all these troubles when they culminated in too many setbacks in fighting AIDS. But the way top decision makers tried to rectify these failures indicated that they certainly were not aware of the root causes of the government's difficulties. All the proposed and implemented corrections to the policy course, not surprisingly, remained confined to various organizational rearrangements.

In the early 2000s Russia used azidothymidine for monotherapy. After 2006 the Russian government switched to the combination therapy and started its universal disbursement. The biggest scandal erupted in November 2006, when the Ministry of Health (Rosminzdrav) ordered the replacement of relatively cheap first- and second-line drugs with costly medicines. Executive Order no. 785 excluded the first-line Combivir (lamivudine and zidovudine), the second-line Trisivir (a combination of abacavir, zidovudine, and lamivudine), Reyataz (atazanavir sulfate), and Fuzeon (enfuvirtide, T-20). Instead, the new standard included the third-line Prezista (darunavir), which was manufactured by Tibotec and had been approved by the FDA only a few months earlier. Subsequently, Deputy Health Minister Vladimir Starodubov signed an executive order amending the federal standard of HIV treatment. It prescribed treating 50 percent of adult patients and children with this new medication, even though the benefits and adverse effects of darunavir on children were not clear. Some health officials still argued that this drug was experimental.

These decisions did not make sense from an epidemiological standpoint. In

Russia the truly frightening stage of the epidemic began in the late 1990s. Thus, the majority of patients receiving antiretrovirals did not develop any resistance to the prescribed first-line combination of drugs. Besides its partial utility, the third-line darunavir had other limitations, as well. One of the leading Russian epidemiologists, Vadim Pokrovskiy, estimated that among thirty thousand patients receiving treatment, only three hundred could have benefited from the new product, while not more than three thousand could even be treated with it in principle. He concluded that doctors would have trouble including daruna-vir in the individual drugs cocktails. In addition, according to the new standard, the new drug had to be administered in hospitals rather than disbursed for individual treatment at home. On top of all these problems, the cost of treatment was likely to increase by 30 percent. In absolute numbers, the cost of darunavir was about $14,000 a year.[49]

Not surprisingly, medical professionals and the representatives of a group known as Russian People Living with AIDS (PLWA) criticized this decision from day one. After an outburst of public criticism, Mikhail Zurabov (minister of health and social development, 2004–7) flatly denied any wrongdoing and called the decision to change drug treatments an expected and almost unavoidable error.[50] His deputy, Starodubov, said that this decision was supposed to decrease the price on the medicines because foreign companies were willing to manufacture the pharmaceuticals under dispute on Russian soil.[51] These justifications sounded very much like a cover-up of administrative inefficiency. In response to the unfolding discussion, Duma deputy Mikhail Grishankov raised the issues of incompetence and corruption in the Ministry of Health. He asserted that the approved drug list gave huge advantages to a number of pharmaceutical firms and undoubtedly privileged some bidders. He also expressed concerns that these schemes could destroy the presidential campaign for HIV treatment. Subsequently, a group of select State Duma deputies sent a petition to Vladimir Putin and Dimitriy Medvedev with the request to correct the harmful decisions made in the Health Ministry.[52]

This incident of purchasing quite expensive and relatively inefficient drugs was not a stand-alone episode. Seven months later, in June 2007, the WHO informed governments about the global recall of a protease inhibitor called Viracept, some batches of which contained a high level of a cancer-causing substance.[53] This recall brought into the public spotlight yet another staggering fact. The government had purchased enough of this drug to treat as much as 15 percent of Russian patients. For some unclear reason, Viracept cost the Russian government a lot more than the rest of the world. Furthermore, the same recall statement stated that the WHO had already recommended using different protease inhibitors, especially in postexposure prophylaxis packs.

Confusion about the government's modus operandi ensued among key stakeholders, as well. As the representative of PLWA summarized it, "The bureaucrats follow a strange logic, purchasing the least effective pharmaceuticals for the most expensive price. This logic undercuts patients' interests, as opposed to the commercial interests of [trading] parties."[54]

Breaching the standardized protocol is dangerous for both HIV-positive patients and the general population, as it may lead to widespread resistance to the older medicines and the virus's mutation. Decisive for the success of sustaining the standardized protocol is orderly and uninterrupted purchase of the appropriate list of pharmaceuticals, which allows doctors to prepare their combination to match patients' exact needs. In theory, the Kremlin wanted to improve and enforce a centralized and transparent mechanism of procuring the essential drugs.

But excessive centralization made health governance at the provincial level unwanted and burdensome. In the summer of 2006, for instance, AIDS centers in the Moscow oblast, Rostov-on-Don, Bashkortostan, Voronezh, and Khabarovsk, had to interrupt treatment for many patients. Local politicians and bureaucrats responded to an intensifying centralization of health governance by neglecting their direct duties. The governors of the above mentioned regions decided to cut the regional health-care budgets and to rely on the federal supply of antiretrovirals.[55] Ironically, when in 2013 the government decided to revamp the system of drug purchases and allowed the regions to buy medicines on regional trades, the prices skyrocketed and shortages ensued.[56] All too many missteps by Russian authorities undermined good health governance.

The failure to procure the required antiretrovirals was not new or unusual. In March 2006 the Ministry of Health, while having spent more than $13 million on ARVs in general, failed to procure ten out of fifteen essential pharmaceuticals necessary for the combination treatment. The regional disbursement lapsed by two months, and in the meanwhile only the regions assisted by the nongovernmental sector (GFATM's Globus program) had enough supplies to cover the disbursement gap. High-powered health officials acknowledged the "difficulties" and lamented their consequences but did not correct their mistakes. According to the other data provided by NPPs, in 2006 the government failed to procure thirteen out of twenty-six necessary antiretrovirals.[57] Similarly, in 2007 the government was ready to spend more than $25 million on medicines, yet both the promise to procure necessary medications and their disbursement lapsed by six months.[58] In effect, Russian patients who had already started treatment received the cocktail comprised of two drugs instead of three or had to wait for the overdue services altogether.

The commitment to top-down governance did not allow leaders to develop functional solutions to the looming crisis of health governance. Instead of offering different, nonbureaucratic ways out of the permanent crisis that would allow civil society to play a larger role, Medvedev chose simply to reshuffle the mandates of his health agencies. He terminated Roszdrav, the federal agency for health and social development, and put the ministry of health back in charge of purchasing ARVs. These organizational rearrangements in 2008 hardly improved the overall state of the public procurement of medicines.[59]

In short, the foregoing discussion identified policy implementation as the weakest link in suppressing the virus in Putin's Russia. The government failed to sustain an effective and stable system of tenders for drug procurement and thus failed to purchase a sufficient number of life-saving medicines on time. The root of the problem was in the ideas about the dominant role of the centralized authority as the sole provider of the common good in the context of top-down health governance. In addition, because many high-powered bureaucrats insulated themselves from societal influences, the important advice of stakeholders and medical professionals fell on deaf ears. It is unlikely that the government will be able to rectify the aforementioned shortcomings without changing its broader ideational dedications.

Embracing Pharmaceutical Sovereignty

This subsection reveals how the Russian preference for import substitution trumped the immediate concerns of public health. Neither the Kremlin nor key health officials questioned the importance of generic medicines in controlling prices and increasing coverage. Nor did they ever vilify the global pharmaceutical industry. But securing generics or parallel importation has never been the main objective of officialdom. Part of the reason for not raising these issues was that Moscow was keen to maintain a low profile regarding intellectual property rules and thus to ease its delayed ascension to the World Trade Organization. The subsequent events revealed the government's entrenched preoccupations, which had little to do with the global struggle for access to low-cost drugs.

Between 2000 and 2004, many developing countries negotiated ARV treatment at significantly reduced prices, used or threatened to use compulsory licensing, and emphasized the domestic development of generic versions of brand-name drugs. While the ARV therapies in Russia remained costly (about $12,000 per year per patient), the government did not formulate any coherent policy that could have pushed the pharmaceutical companies to slash prices. Moreover, public officials chose not to register generic antiretroviral drugs in Russia, despite massive civil society campaigns. In March 2005 the Ministry of Health and Social Development for the first time negotiated reduced prices on ARVs, slashing the cost of treatment to about $3,000 a year. Welcome as these efforts were, the government avoided talks of parallel importation and the TRIPS safeguards and focused instead on import substitution.[60]

In March 2007 Medvedev announced his vision of a world-class competitive and innovative drug industry. Roszdravnadzor, the federal service on surveillance in health care, recommended substituting as many as 5,351 foreign drugs with domestic ones. The Ministry of Industry and Trade (Minpromtorg) offered a more detailed road map toward "pharmaceutical sovereignty." Its officials specified highly ambitious goals to be achieved by 2020. The first objective was to increase the price share of homemade drugs in the internal market to 50 percent (compared to the modest 20 percent in 2009) and up to 90 percent in the segment of essential medicines. The second goal was to invent up to two hundred domestic innovative drugs and then export them.[61] This number is overwhelming, especially if one surmises that the government intended to create, review, and manufacture new molecular entities rather than some combination of "me-too" drugs (i.e., drugs closely related to the original prototypes but with minor differences) and generics. Three years later, at the Cabinet meeting that was dedicated to issues of the state policy on pharmaceuticals and medical devices, the head of Minpromtorg, Denis Manturov, confirmed the strategic course on import substitution and massive state investments into drug research and development, clinical trials, and technology acquisition.[62]

But the approved state program skated over the otherwise sobering fact that the desired first-rate drug industry had to be built almost from scratch. That the prerequisites of pharmaceutical development were by and large nonexistent was very clear even before the government settled on import substitution as its main objective. Vladimir Starodubov, for instance, acknowledged the dismal state of the industry. He noted that in 2007 only 15 out of the 150 Russian pharmaceutical firms conformed to the Good Manufacturing Practices (GMP).[63] Although the industry and business community welcomed the GMP certification, by September 2012 only 56 out of 454 firms had made a successful transition to new manufacturing standards. Given these facts, achieving import substitution or global competitiveness will remain quite a challenge. However, the critical voices are likely to remained unheeded. After all, it was the core goal of Putin's state that was at stake here.

The available evidence suggests that top Russian leaders and legislators alike nurtured an ambition to develop a number of innovative drugs that could have showcased Russia's reinstated position in the global power structure. Tatiyana Yakovleva, a prominent member of United Russia, offered that Russia's "strategic objective is to overcome the increasing trend of total dependence on Russian drug supply from foreign manufacturers."[64] Although Dmitriy Medvedev had fully supported this strategic course, the key representatives of the industry made no credible progress toward achieving real competitiveness in the global pharmaceutical markets. The ensuing discussion goes into further detail on the government's approach to stimulating the drug industry for global competitiveness.

Medvedev's air castles were fully shared by his new-old boss as well. To regain global technological leadership, Putin candidly stated in 2012, Russia has to prioritize the development of a modern and competitive pharmaceutical industry.[65] It is telling that on the first day of his third term, he demanded the domestic pharmaceutical industry achieve full independence from the foreign manufacturers of essential drugs. Currently, this trend is gaining full momentum and goes well beyond pharmaceutical regulation. In 2014, for instance, the Ministry of Industry single-handedly drafted a proposal to ban purchasing a wide range of medical devices, including MRI machines, from abroad if the same product was available from Russian, Kazakhstani, or Belarusian companies.[66] Given that only two years prior to this initiative more than 80 percent of all medical devices had been imported from abroad, this legislation essentially pushed the idea of import substitution to a dangerous extreme. Although the implementation of the policy was delayed, the proposal was never off the table. It is clear that closing the market is a protectionist orientation that impairs public health.

The idea of the developmental state was also behind Putin's "state corporations," which came into being at the end of 2007. While Medvedev imagined the country as a globally competitive producer of innovative medicines and biotechnologies, state corporations were envisioned as locomotives that would stimulate the national pharmaceutical sector. These entities accumulate enormous amounts of financial resources and consolidate a considerable number of firms and enterprises. Different state corporations hold military-industrial firms, atomic and nuclear plants, shipbuilding and aircraft industries, and transportation. State corporations combine independent management under direct governmental and presidential control with private ownership but without fully privatizing the constituent enterprises.

It is instructive that the idea of state corporations to implement state economic policy belonged to Sergey Chemezov, yet another representative of the *siloviki*. Chemezov was a KGB officer in the 1980s and Putin's subordinate in Saint Petersburg. He currently serves as director-general of the Russian Technologies State Corporation (Rostekhnologii). In 2008–9 Chemezov lobbied to subsume thirty-five state drug enterprises and laboratories under Rostekhnologii.[67] Another *silovik* and former KGB officer, Sergey Ivanov, lobbied to concentrate the drug industry under the state corporation Russian Pharmaceutical Technologies but failed to see his initiative materialized. In the end, the task of developing innovative drugs was transferred to another state corporation, the Russian Corporation of Nanotechnologies (Rosnano), with Anatoliy Chubais as its chief. In July 2010 Russian news agency RIAN reported that Rosnano would invest about $40 million in biomedical projects, including developing treatment for AIDS, hepatitis, and cancer of the pancreas. After the buzz about innovations at home waned, one Rosnano official offered that it was more efficient to buy innovations from abroad.[68] Although Chubais eventually realized that technology transfer is more plausible than developing an innovative and competitive pharmaceutical industry from scratch, conservative opinion leaders derided his public statements as inconsistent with Russia's rightful place in the global power structure.

That "pharmaceutical sovereignty" will not materialize is evident from the blunt fact that state corporations, chosen to spur economic growth, were hardly efficient. Vadim Volkov argues that while state corporations "are expected to deliver tangible results and global competitiveness," no institutional arrangements can prevent Putin's cronies from controlling industries and stuffing their pockets with public money.[69] The allegations of corruption notwithstanding, the major point that bears emphasis is that the grandeur of pharmaceutical sovereignty rested on the perceived role of the state as the initiator and implementer of economic policy and was also consistent with the great power complex.

Summary

The Russian public has expressed a wide variety of ideas about the meaning of the epidemic. For medical professionals, it surely has been a public health crisis. However, top politicians converged on the understanding that the spread of HIV was an expression of the alarming demographic decline that emerged in conjunction with the market-oriented reforms of the early 1990s or even as a result of external actors' subversive activities against Russia. State Duma deputy Mikhail Grishankov opined that the epidemic would have been prevented but for the collapse of the Soviet Union and the fall of the Iron Curtain.[70] Not surprisingly, high-powered politicians responded to HIV as if they defended the state. In addition, Moscow's desire to stimulate import substitution and to penetrate the global pharmaceutical markets highlighted the Kremlin's chase for the self-gratifying image of a great power.

Russian ideas about the core goals of the state did not impinge on the adoption of biomedical solutions as the organizing principle of health governance. However, the focus on state autonomy created an environment in which massive inefficiencies and the misallocation of resources were impervious to societal correction. The leaders' unwillingness to consider better policy led to their inability to ensure the uninterrupted delivery of appropriate antiretroviral medicines.

In sum, Russian leaders followed their own ideas about the core goals of the state rather than accepting the external models of good health governance as their primary stimuli.

MEDICAL PLURALISM IN MBEKI'S SOUTH AFRICA

The primary objective of Mbeki's health governance was to promote medicines developed in Africa for Africa. Doing so would affirm the capacity of the former liberation movement to rule and disprove Western neocolonial stereotypes. The strategy to promote medical pluralism in South Africa was consistent with the government's commitment to uphold the indigenous knowledge system, the idea central to the African Renaissance. First, South African elites questioned the similarities between the South African epidemic and the spread of the virus elsewhere and then challenged the usefulness of the global health guidelines. Leaders framed the domestic epidemic as a problem of knowledge and development. Second, Mbekiites treated the "toxic AZT" with great suspicion, since the colonizing powers would surely pump more drugs into African bodies in an attempt to stifle African development. As a result, elites unleashed a massive assault on Western biomedical products. In contrast to the international consensus, Pretoria promoted a mix of complementary and alternative medicines and later attempted to institutionalize African traditional healing. Third,

Pretoria's hard-hitting but futile rhetoric against the predatory and conspiratorial drug companies was intended to countervail the powerful pharmaceutical
lobby. For a long while, the Cabinet remained insensitive to changing external
circumstances and attempted to neither produce generics nor launch their parallel importation, and it did not use conventional trade mechanisms to tilt the
crystallizing intellectual property regime in South Africa's favor. I explore all
three pillars of South African medical pluralism consecutively in the three subsections that follow.

Reappraising the Epidemic in Mbeki's South Africa

According to Pieter Fourie, the Mbeki administration's response to the HIV/AIDS
epidemic was an ongoing attempt to reappraise the structural variables that
drove the epidemic.[71] This reappraisal highlighted several general themes, variations of which the Cabinet, Mbeki, and his supporters continuously articulated.

In April 2000 Mbeki penned a long letter to world leaders in which he explained his position on AIDS in Africa. The gist of it was very simple: Mbeki
questioned biomedical conventions on HIV and lent his support to AIDS denialists, who were portrayed as the champions of innovative and controversial
ideas that had been rejected by the inert scientific community.[72] According to reports, Clinton administration officials considered this letter so provocative that
they tried not to release it to the media. Leaked to the public on the eve of Mbeki's visit to Washington, D.C., the hard-hitting letter infuriated health activists
and over time triggered an avalanche of international opprobrium. That opprobrium made Mbeki refrain from making overly objectionable health statements
in public but failed to suppress his true devotions. Since 2002 Mbeki and his entourage have continued to promote the same old views but in a furtive manner.
Even after 2007, when the country launched the globally approved, large-scale
national ARV program, Mbeki and his trusted allies shied away from speaking in
public about the benefits of conventional medicines.[73]

The anonymous report with the eccentric title (*Castro Hlongwane: Caravans,
Cats, Geese, Foot & Mouth and Statistics: HIV/AIDS and the Struggle for the Humanisation of the African*) is the well-known epitome of Pretoria's controversial views. Castro Hlongwane was a black teenager who was forced to leave a
school party because of his alleged infection. His name was used as a metaphor
for South Africa, which had been repeatedly suffering "the crimes and falsities
of 'scientific' Eurocentrism." To admit that you have a virus means to invite the

West to treat you as inferior on the pretense of questionable biomedical dogmas. The only way to defeat AIDS was to defeat not the virus itself but the humiliation and dehumanization of the African people.[74] Most likely cowritten by Mbeki and Peter Mokaba, this report is formidable, as it encapsulates and ties together all the central claims made throughout Mbeki's presidential tenure. It remained important long after the date of its original distribution to the party's members at the Fifty-First National Conference of the African National Congress in 2002. When several years later Mark Gevisser asked the president to answer a set of tough questions regarding his health policy, the famous journalist was told to study a copy of the report.

Two themes of the report deserve special attention. First, *Castro Hlongwane* challenged conventional etiological findings regarding HIV. Instead, it spotlighted lifestyle issues, the massive consumption of recreational drugs and narcotics, and the reliance on toxic antiretroviral medications as the reasons behind the origins of the disease and its rapid spread. In this presentation, the virus was simply a carrier of Western drug-related diseases, while in Africa, in contrast, the virus was a combination of extreme poverty and malnutrition. The theme of poverty was central to Mbeki's previous speculations as well. In his address to the ANC Caucus, Mbeki claimed that 90 percent of deaths attributed to AIDS were the result of poverty.[75] Following Mbeki's lead, Sam Mhlongo, head of the Department of Family Health and Primary Health, emphasized the need to alleviate poverty as a precondition for disease eradication.[76] It is true that poverty and malnutrition exacerbate the effects of the virus and make the therapy less effective, but discussing and lamenting the sorry condition of poverty and malnutrition hardly addresses the immediate needs of responding to the contagion as a public health crisis. In addition, the report claimed, because the majority of the diagnoses were inaccurate and unreliable, the number of HIV-positive individuals in South Africa was hugely overestimated. This claim went against the global consensus that the estimates from the prenatal clinics and mortality data in South Africa warranted an expansion of treatment and prevention services.

Second, this report borrowed heavily from the early literature that had discussed the impact of racism and prejudice on the process of collecting and interpreting information on the immunodeficiency syndrome in Africa in the 1980s. For the most part, it repeated the accusations of Zimbabwean scholars Richard and Rosalind Chirimuuta, the authors of *Africa, AIDS and Racism* (originally published in 1987). Racism, Mbeki agreed with the Chirimuutas, had shaped and fueled Western perceptions of African sexual immorality. Neocolonial science used Africans as objects of negative construction, denied them human dignity, and treated them like children.[77] In a racist's mind, Africans were "prone to rape and abuse of women" and upheld "a value system that belongs to the world of wild animals." Thus, the outbreak of HIV/AIDS provided the West with the ideal opportunity to represent salacious Africans as the Other, "lustful, lower order, germ-carrying" blacks, "natural born promiscuous carrier[s] of germs."[78] This theme fit the African Renaissance's mission to spread awareness about racialism and neocolonial sensibilities in the production of knowledge.

Castro Hlongwane, of course, is not the only instance of an intentional reappraisal of the contagion in South Africa. But during his second term, Mbeki had to improve his bad public image. He employed spin doctors, who tried to locate Mbeki's controversial statements in the respected tradition of the "pronative" and anticolonialist thinking of Frantz Fanon. In addition, Robert Suresh Roberts, a member of Mbeki's political-intellectual entourage, linked Mbeki's views to Harriet A. Washington's *Medical Apartheid: The Dark History of Medical Experimentation on Black Americans from Colonial Times to the Present* (2006) and Celia Farber's *Serious Adverse Events: An Uncensored History of AIDS* (2006). Roberts insisted that global science was ridiculing the native quest for African solutions. Trying to placate the media and health activists, Roberts alleged that Mbeki had never been an AIDS dissident and never questioned the value of ARV treatment. According to him, while Mbeki boldly highlighted the shortcomings of Western biomedical science, the president's detractors were spreading false information about his sensibilities in order to defame him politically.[79]

As the external and internal criticism mounted, Mbeki became unwilling to discuss his biomedical views openly. However, in a private letter to Roberts, he reaffirmed his vigorous belief in the counterintellectual deceits of neocolonial science: "The most virulent of the debates, about knowledge, has been the contest concerning the science that informs the global and our own programmes on HIV and AIDS. It is most interesting that the most vocal in this contest centered their argument . . . on the demand that all the discussion must be terminated, and that all that had to be done was to implement what directly and indirectly, the pharmaceutical companies said should be done to dispense the drugs they produce as widely and as quickly as possible."[80]

These themes reverberated powerfully among ordinary South Africans and some nonstate organizations. Nkululeko Nxesi, the leader of the National Association of People Living with AIDS (NAPWA), for instance, echoed Mbeki's recurrent ideas. He asserted that the nature of the epidemic in South Africa was different from the rest of the continent because of the unique legacies of apartheid, forced labor migrations, and the stifled discussions of sexuality.[81] NAPWA, along with the government, sought to resist the derogatory and disempowering stigmatization of African people living with AIDS as "sufferers" and "victims."[82] Similarly, Thanduxolo Doro, another leader of this organization, insisted that fighting poverty along with improving nutrition and ending discrimination were necessary preconditions for mitigating the impact of the epidemic.[83] As Mbeki's determination to defend his reappraisal of the epidemic waned, Nxesi still insisted that traditional medicines and holistic healing were more important than conventional medicines. He defended Manto Tshabalala-Msimang's statements about the importance of nutrition and food security as part of the comprehensive strategy to respond to the looming health crisis. And even after the remarkable change in the course of health governance under the new president, Jacob Zuma, NAPWA's leaders were still more concerned with food security and proper nutrition than with the sustainable expansion of treatment to all who are ready for it.[84]

The reappraisal of the South African epidemic fell on the rich soil of conspiratorial suspicions that in the 1990s and early 2000s were in broad circulation. These collective articulations included beliefs that global pharmaceutical firms exported junk medicines to Africa and that Westerners artificially created the human immunodeficiency virus to undermine African population growth.[85] Some deciphered the acronym AIDS to read "American (or on occasion Afrikaner) Invention to Discourage Sex." Other conspiratorial notions ranged from the belief that the U.S. CIA propagated the idea that HIV causes AIDS to the reinvented imageries of witchcraft performed by white doctors, treatment activists, and representatives of the Western pharmaceutical sector.[86]

In summary, South African elites questioned the similarity of HIV/AIDS's epidemiological circumstances in South Africa compared to the rest of the world. Elites framed the domestic epidemic as a local developmental problem and presented lifestyle issues and the massive consumption of various toxic drugs, antiretrovirals included, as the causes of the plague in the West. This reasoning came out of the African Renaissance and resulted in important governance consequences. Political attention to complementary, alternative, and traditional medicines was the direct result of countervailing external guidelines and promoting indigenousness as the core goals of the state. This orientation cannot be reduced to a mere policy blunder or an unfortunate outcome of Mbeki's idiosyncratic mistakes. The following subsection provides details regarding alternative and traditional treatments in South Africa.

Complementary and Traditional Medicines

The South African Ministry of Health promised to uphold alternative and traditional medicines as the cornerstone of its comprehensive health care program. Government officials often scoffed at the results of domestic and international trials that proved the efficiency of antiretrovirals.[87] In contrast, health officials blew out of proportion the concerns about conventional drugs' safety and efficiency while suppressing similar concerns in regard to a snowballing variety of unorthodox products with unproven medicinal effects. Local remedies, be they vitamin supplements or complementary or traditional medications, were envisioned as having important health benefits. Despite all the official backing, attempts to promote subpar medicines did not go unchallenged.

How did it all start? Infamous dissident Anthony Brink claimed that Mbeki's awareness of azidothymidine's toxicity was triggered by Brink's self-published book manuscript "Debating the AZT: Questions of Safety and Utility."[88] It is possible that Mbeki read the manuscript early in his first presidential term. No matter what his original impulse had been, Mbeki jumped on the opportunity to accuse multiple international actors of concealing the scientific evidence about azidothymidine. In a similar vein, Nkosazana Dlamini-Zuma (minister of health, 1994–99, minister of foreign affairs, 1999–2009) insisted that AZT was not helpful because it treated people who were already sick. Both agreed that antiretrovirals could not alleviate poverty and malnutrition and therefore were futile in fighting the root causes of the health crisis in the country. This convoluted reasoning was more than mere rhetoric. Questioning conventional medical science and Western pharmaceutical products signaled the desire to suspend the domestic distribution of the internationally approved medicines and replace them with domestic substitutes.

Given the fearful and unreasonable state of top politicians' minds, it is not surprising that between 2000 and 2004 the Cabinet chose to promote various "immune-boosting" concoctions and nutritional supplements as the major alternatives to the certified medicines. In 2003 Tshabalala-Msimang expressed her enthusiasm for the so-called nutritional recovery regimen and the "Mediterranean diet," which consisted of garlic, ginger, beetroot, and olive oil. Her outlandish claims that complementary micronutrients and dietary supplements could prevent the development of opportunistic diseases won her a number of sarcastic nicknames among treatment activists and the public. The health minister also became famous for promoting those sketchy characters who seemingly shared her biomedical convictions.

One of them, Roberto Giraldo, the health minister's official nutrition advisor and a strong advocate of unorthodox treatment programs, gained notoriety for his blunt disregard of evidence-based science. Giraldo claimed that his alternative medicinal products were nothing short of miraculous. Addressing the Southern African Development Community's (SADC) meeting on nutrition and HIV/AIDS in Johannesburg in November 2002, he averred that certain alternative remedies reverse the effects of AIDS, slow down the progression of HIV to the full-blown AIDS, prevent transmission of HIV, and lessen the presence of viremia. On top of all these health benefits, he was willing to sell his products for the modest sum of U.S.$7.00 per month per patient. Another shady person, the former nurse Tine van der Maas, received the health minister's permission to conduct trials of her "African solution" in public hospitals and clinics.[89]

The controversial cases of Giraldo and van der Maas were not that atypical. Throughout the years of Mbeki's presidency, people from different walks of life but with highly questionable medical qualifications jumped on the opportunity to sell a variety of herbal mixtures as genuine alternatives to ARVs. The purveyors of these medicines failed to label their products and avoided any explanation as to how they worked, but they surely did not fail to advertise their remedial powers. The media typically described these products as brown liquids of suspicious origin having no benefits for the health of their consumers. Yet no governmental action was taken to stop the spread of all these questionable concoctions. On the contrary, according to multiple press reports, some of these proprietors enjoyed the usually unstated and sometimes very tangible support of the national and provincial governments. Any criticism of unconventional medicines was met with hostility that spotlighted the alleged "colonialist" attitudes hindering the rebirth of the country.

The number of complementary medicines in South Africa began to multiply. In 2000 a local *inyanga* (healer), Lulu Ngubane, claimed to be able to treat and reverse HIV with a recipe that came to him in a dream. In 2001 Phyto Nova, a South African company, produced the immune-boosting Sutherlandia, potentially useful for HIV-positive individuals. That same year, Siphiwe Hadebe, a medical technologist turned healer, amassed a fortune by treating about six hundred patients with *umbimbi*, yet another nostrum remedium to enter the market. Among his high-powered patients was Mbeki loyalist Peter Mokaba, who soon died from an infection that was rumored to be AIDS related.[90] In 2007 Freddie Isaacs, a codirector of Comforter's Healing Gift, produced yet another untested product to cure AIDS.[91]

A former truck driver, Zeblon Gwala, deserves a special mention in this context. In 2005 he presented uBhejane—a mixture of various herbs—to complement antiretroviral medicines. His nostrum would increase the CD4 cell count and eliminate the viral load in the blood, as the advertisement asserted. Gwala also claimed that his product cured cancer, sore feet, kidneys, pneumonia, and skin problems. Over a number of years, he extensively marketed and sold this panacea against that curious combination of maladies while enjoying the support of various provincial and national health officials. In May 2005 Gwala was invited to address the official HIV information workshop sponsored by the KwaZulu-Natal government, thereby effectively joining the chorus of other loud opponents of antiretroviral therapy. Later on, Gwala was invited to address Parliament's Health Portfolio Committee. In 2006 Obed Mlaba, the mayor of eThekwini municipality, which includes Durban, sponsored uBhejane for local patients. Although the information about the gross conditions under which Gwala's medicines were produced had become public, Tshabalala-Msimang would have none of it. Once again, she chose to defend a subpar product and lash out against its critics. So did Thami Mseleku, in 2005–9 one of the key functionaries in the Ministry of Health who was no less fond of unproven remedies against immune deficiency (as long as they represented African traditional medicine) than he was of vitamins. According to him, any criticism of uBhejane was flatly colonialist. Only years after Gwala's profitable career had begun, the Advertising Standards Authority ordered the immediate withdrawal of an advertisement for uBhejane. But his activities still were not terminated completely.

To put this state of affairs in historical context, a hypothetical nineteenth-century American observer would have found herself at home with all these proprietary medicines, or *nostra remedia*, which since then have been replaced in America with evidence-based drugs. Although at some point politicians refrained from challenging conventional medicines in public, Pretoria continued emphasizing indigenous knowledge and traditional medical practices. The stated objective of reviving indigenous knowledge systems was to demonopolize neocolonial science and show that South Africans were fit to produce original science. The Ministry of Health averred that "essential and irreplaceable" traditional health practitioners "utilise scientific methodologies that stretch back thousands of years."[92] While profiteering Westerners promoted the false dichotomy between traditional and conventional medicine, studying and applying indigenous knowledge, according to Tshabalala-Msimang, provided "an opportunity to reclaim our scientific and socio-cultural heritage which was stigmatised and discredited as primitive rituals and witchcraft during many years of colonialism and apartheid."[93]

There are certainly important preconditions that might warrant incorporating traditional medicines into the system of conventional health care. The estimated number of healers in South Africa is somewhere between 200,000 and 350,000 people; 70 to 80 percent of people allegedly use their services. The ubiquity of traditional healers in southern Africa warrants their involvement in the process of health governance. Traditional healers of South Africa can be roughly divided into four categories: herbalists (*izinyanga*), diviners in illnesses caused by witchcraft (*izangoma*), traditional birth attendants (*abathandazi*), and the purveyors of homemade folk medicines (*muthi*). Many domestic observers have claimed that traditional healers have been effective in providing grief counseling and psychological support. Their role is essential when other avenues of escaping blame and stigma for the virus carriers are not available. But as important as psychological counseling may be, traditional healers can also provide potentially harmful herbal concoctions based on folk wisdom.

The major problem is that many remedies in the guise of traditional medicines were suspiciously similar to the fake cures described above. This is not surprising, given the porous conceptual borders between traditional and alternative medicines. At the very least, the production of these substances requires thorough regulation and the strict application of good manufacturing standards. Although a flurry of organizational innovation has ensued (most notably, the government established the Directorate of Traditional Medicine within the Ministry of Health in 2006, the National Indigenous Knowledge Systems Office within the Department of Science and Technology in 2007, and the Interim Traditional Health Practitioners Council, which was not operational until 2013), consumers' health has been barely protected.

In the middle of Mbeki's rule, the government set forth legislation regarding traditional healing practices and the institutions sustaining them. The Traditional Health Practitioners Act (No. 35 of 2004) was a step toward systematic regulation of traditional medicines and licensing of healers and thus was welcomed by many observers of health governance.[94] But two years later the actual overseeing of those tasks was delegated to the presidential task team that included none other than Herbert Vilakazi, a person with financial interests in uBhejane whose dubious credentials were scoffed at by treatment activists, and a controversial lawyer, Christine Qunta, implicated in the spread of fake cures.[95] Not surprisingly, the way Neliswa "Peggy" Nkonyeni, a prominent health official, saw it, there still was nothing wrong with opposing antiretroviral therapy and introducing herbal remedies for treating HIV/AIDS patients at public hospitals in KwaZulu-Natal.[96] Nor did the new legislation restrain Nhlavana Maseko, head of the Traditional Healers Organization, from publicly condemning antiretroviral medication. Healers kept persuading patients to stop taking antiretrovirals while asserting that their own treatment would reverse the course of the disease or eliminate immunodeficiency syndrome altogether.

With the help of American funding, in 2005 South Africa started examination of local medicinal plants used by traditional healers and their impact on slowing down the virus. Although these studies were not intended to offer recommendations on how to replace conventional medicines with local nostra remedia, the proponents of indigenous medicines clearly used these trials to their advantage. For instance, Nkonyeni, Mlaba, and Vilakazi have promoted uBhejane's use, asserting that it improved patients' health, although that assertion bluntly misrepresented preliminary research findings. Nor was any attention paid to the statements of Dr. Nceba Gqaleni of the Nelson Mandela School, who refused to endorse uBhejane's health benefits.[97] To add to the confusion of ordinary patients, press reports have described that concoction as a possible cure for the immunodeficiency virus. In addition, officials ignored grave warrants that both African potato and Sutherlandia inhibited metabolism of antiretrovirals. Further, Tshabalala-Msimang fought to exclude traditional medicines from the rigorous process of testing designed for contemporary Western biomedical products.[98] She also defended the questionable study of an herbal remedy, Secomet V, conducted by Girish Kotwaal, a principal biotechnological investigator at the University of Cape Town, on the grounds of the inherent and anticolonialist value of natural products.[99]

That building a national policy, an appropriate legal framework for the institutionalization of African traditional medicines in the country's health-care system, and protecting consumers are prerequisites for the quality of health governance is obvious. Questions about how, why, and to what extent to incorporate traditional healers into the system of local health governance and whether and to what degree complementary treatments are desirable should be part of a sensible policy discussion. But that discussion should not discourage the rollout of conventional drugs. It appears that the post-Mbeki Cabinet has slowly moved in this direction. First, training traditional healers to increase their knowledge of HIV/AIDS and giving them legal authorization to distribute condoms, for instance, is a step in the right direction. Second, new health minister Aaron Motsoaledi has proposed tighter safety standards and an efficacy review of complementary medicines under the authority of the revitalized Medicines Control Council (MCC), the South African agency with regulatory functions somewhat similar to those of the U.S. Food and Drug Administration.[100] Given the backlog of 150,000 items, the trials will take some time if the officials perform the task properly. By February 2014 the MCC was not able to force manufacturers of complementary medicines to introduce "new labels warning consumers that the products had not been evaluated for safety and efficacy."[101] Not surprisingly, the representatives of Clicks Group and Adcock Ingram, two large South African firms whose production includes complementary medicines, did not welcome the tightening regulation.

In short, local knowledge can be helpful to increase bottom-up participation and reduce the costs for health care in resource-poor settings. In the 1980s and the early 1990s, when ARVs were not yet available, traditional medicines might be the only treatments available. During Mbeki's rule, traditional medicines, infused with political significance, became something more than a desperate attempt to grapple with the consequences of the contagion. Now, with continuing economic growth across Africa and burgeoning international assistance in procuring necessary medicines, traditional healing practices no longer remain the only accessible and affordable option for the overwhelming majority of the local population. There seems to be a fine line between the productive engagement of a massive body of traditional healers for the purposes of giving care, lending support, and spreading education, on the one hand, and searching for an ethnomedicine that could be a silver bullet, on the other. Mbeki and his political entourage crossed that line for the sake of the African Renaissance while allowing *muthi* traders to undermine adherence to the standard medical regimen.

Resisting Pharmaceutical Colonialism

When governments face the contagion as a public health crisis they are likely to focus on securing a stable supply of essential medicines and high-quality generics for the public sector. Making use of various legal mechanisms, such as compulsory licensing, and bolstering production of generics at home are practical solutions for countries with fairly advanced pharmaceutical industries. In these areas, the South African government's behavior was quite complex. The Cabinet endeavored to stimulate domestic production, empower domestic pharmaceutical companies, and countervail the powerful lobby representing foreign drug firms. At the same time, Pretoria defended its preoccupation with medical pluralism while granting too many licenses at the expense of the essential priorities of public health.

The attempt to develop local drugs was a clear attempt to bolster domestic pharmaceutical research and development. There is a clear parallel here with the Russian case in terms of the state's desire to become a powerful producer of original molecular entities and thereby acquire a position as an influential global player. The controversial but genuine passion for Virodene (Virodene P058) started in 1997, when three physicians from the University of Pretoria announced the invention of a cheap and effective drug based on an industrial solvent used in cryopreservation. From the outset, this claim was suspicious, because the sensationalistic study had been neither peer reviewed nor published in any respected scientific journal, while its inventors possessed no relevant medical qualifications. Not surprisingly, the MCC banned the drug and stopped its testing.[102] However, the inventors skillfully deployed an argument against Western pharmaceutical neocolonialism and thus were able to secure the necessary political and financial support. Eventually, "the Virodene affair" generated too much political heat, and the deal was passed first to Namibia Medical Investments, which marketed the drug under the brand name Imunoxx, and later to some Congolese entrepreneurs.[103] However, the Virodene affair was not an isolated incident of a policy blunder.

In the late 1990s and early 2000s, global activists sought to influence the intellectual property arrangements regarding HIV medicines through vigorous protests, mobilization campaigns, and litigation. When South Africa adopted the Medicines and Related Substances Control Amendment Act (No. 90 of 1997), a law designed to make drugs affordable at low cost, it was a sign that the country was following a conventional way of protecting its public health interests. Domestic activists welcomed the act as "a step towards ending apartheid in health care." But global pharmaceutical companies interpreted it as a law dodging patents protection and sued the government. This was not that surprising, given that one of the provisions of the act required doctors to use generics unless patients asked otherwise.[104] In defending the act, the government resisted Vice President Al Gore's and the U.S. trade representative's pressures to accept the rules for pharmaceutical production as formulated by the international pharmaceutical sector. Although the pharmaceutical companies withdrew their lawsuit over the Medicines Act in 2001, the ostensible success of the South African government in protecting public health interests was undermined by the fact that Pretoria did not follow up on its original intentions. Instead, Pretoria decided to focus on research and development of alternatives to ARVs. South African opinion leaders nailed the purchase of ARVs from foreign pharmaceutical giants as the strategy that reinforced the predatory power of "pharmaceutical colonialism" and brought far more problems than solutions to South Africans. Pretoria refused to accept Boehringer Ingelheim's offer of free nevirapine for pregnant women in mid-2001 and declined Glaxo's offer to buy AZT at a 70 percent discount.[105]

In 2002–3 the South African government did not conceal its fury when it heard about health activists' scheme to smuggle generics into the country and even tried to prosecute the smugglers. Some policy analysts noted that advocates of the generics, such as the Clinton Foundation, found themselves outside the sphere of the Cabinet's interest. It seemed that the Ministry of Health stalled the tenders for generics to heed the concerns of Randall Tobias, who at the time was head of PEPFAR, about using generics to supply antiretroviral drugs to state hospitals.[106] Still, according to one report, "Many generic companies complained of being shut out of the process—which mostly seemed tailored to favour the Western pharmaceutical industry and/or possibly, the development of South African sources."[107] The local production of antiretrovirals began as Aspen Pharmacare, a large multinational company based in Durban, secured multiple voluntary licenses from major pharmaceutical firms to produce generics in sub-Saharan Africa. Clearly, there was more to Pretoria's seemingly erratic behavior than a simple desire to boost indigenous knowledge, described in the foregoing subsection. Many observers surmised that part of the reason for halting the process of procuring generics was to make Aspen the main beneficiary of the Health Ministry's tenders and thus the main recipient of the globally funded projects.[108]

The description of Pretoria's AIDS governance would be incomplete without drawing attention to the government's failures to strike an appropriate balance between intellectual property protection and the needs of public health. For an extended period of time, the authorities were granting patents to nearly any applicant, including those who filed for patents for altered (and so not entirely original) medications. At the dawn of Mbeki's rule, only two out of fifteen antiretroviral drugs were not granted patents in the country. During the last year of Mbeki's presidency, South Africa granted 2,442 pharmaceutical patents, but domestic applicants registered only 10 of these.[109] According to a researcher with the Treatment Action Campaign, the decisive factor for obtaining patents in South Africa was simply an accurate submission of the required paperwork.[110] This review system increased the number of low-quality patents, emboldened patent holders to file for interdicts against the firms manufacturing generics, stifled market competition, and, as a result, sustained the high prices for generic pharmaceuticals. The consideration of the substantive merits of disputed patents was left to the courts to decide. But in the absence of straightforward intellectual property legislation, the courts' judgments, while heeding considerations of the public interest, were not delivered exclusively on the grounds of scientific evidence of each drug's originality.[111]

Pretoria's indecisiveness in devising intellectual property legislation, adjusted to the needs of the public health, left the country far behind best international practices. In contrast to India, which amended its intellectual property legislation in 2005, the process of drafting and enacting the improved national legislation in South Africa remained exceptionally slow. Only by 2014 was the Department of Trade and Industry able to come up with significant revisions to the national rules of patent review in order to address public health needs and take full advantage of the Declaration on TRIPS and Public Health. Pretoria's long-standing aversion to issuing compulsory licenses certainly benefited Aspen, which since 2001 has been able to secure exclusive voluntary licenses from six major originators. Then again, the Mbeki era's relaxed stance on granting patents has had significant implications for the future of AIDS governance in the country. Most germane, the consequence that plagued post-Mbeki health governance was that the government found itself unable to procure antiretrovirals at internationally competitive prices. Further, the increasing number of patients whose health depends on taking the second-line medications and the necessity to devise optimal regimens in order to prevent treatment failures require expanding access to a variety of cheaper second-line versions in the public sector. However, the failure to incorporate the appropriate public health safeguards in the national legislation could undermine the availability of second-line drugs and their variety in the future, despite the overall decline in the prices of second-line regimens.[112] For instance, secondary patents on ritonavir (RTV), a key drug needed to boost a number of protease inhibitors, can hinder the availability of the fixed-dose combination of atazanavir/ritonavir (atazanavir/r).

Paradoxically, the excessive patent protection went hand in hand with vilifying transnational pharmaceutical firms. Instead of deploying tangible legal instruments, Pretoria chose to rely on elaborate but vacuous and ultimately incon-sequential tongue-lashing. In 2000 the presidential spokesperson, Phakamile "Parks" Mankahlana, averred that the pharmaceutical sector had exaggerated the positive effects of their medicines. The main reason for their claims was simple—enrichment at the expense of Africans.[113] One member of the govern-ment argued that "price reductions negotiated with manufacturers were neither substantive nor a permanent solution."[114]

An infamous pill salesperson, Matthias Rath, courted by the government, di-rected his vitriol against the industrialized world and the pharmaceutical drug cartel, which promoted toxic ARV drugs across Africa. He classified antiretro-viral medicines as chemical weaponry that subverted the economic prosper-ity and political independence of African nations. The Group of Eight (G8), in his view, clearly had a genocidal plan for Africa. Further, Rath sponsored *End AIDS! Break the Chains of Pharmaceutical Colonialism*, a perfervid, book-long accusation "exposing" the role of multinational pharmaceutical industries in re-colonizing the continent. According to his diatribe, global pharmaceutical neo-colonialism was infiltrating the country via civil society, which had castigated Mbeki's take on the multinationals only to promote the multibillion-dollar ARV business in South Africa.[115] In Rath's view, civil society simply detracted Mbeki from opposing the mass import of toxic ARV drugs.[116] Later on, Rath was joined by Mbeki's semiofficial biographer, R. S. Roberts, who also linked the interna-tional AIDS drug promotion conspiracy to domestic treatment activists. Using defamatory language, Roberts lashed out against "the elite media and its anti-ANC AIDS-drug agitation," as well as "the AIDS-drug lobby lore" of protreatment activists, politicians, scientists, and writers. David Cameron, Tony Leon, Zackie Achmat, Mark Heywood, Kerry Cullinan, Nicoli Nattrass, and Nadine Gordi-mer were dubbed "celebrity colonialists."[117] In general, Mbeki-friendly opinion leaders claimed that the advocates of generics had concocted a plot to under-mine President Mbeki's and the ANC's authority, threatened black lives, and as-pired to turn the country into a banana republic.

In short, all these anticolonial claims "revealed" the Western conspiracy to cram toxic drugs into African nations. All things considered, rhetorical action against the pharmaceutical industry is self-serving and weak. No perfervid rhet-oric can offset the material power of drug companies. Such rhetoric does not offer any tangible mechanisms for keeping tabs on the global pharmaceutical sector and does not secure cheap medicines. But it surely fits the third core pos-tulation of the African Renaissance vision of the renovated postapartheid state as a moral leader of continental proportions that countervails the global power structure.

Although upholding indigenous values is no longer an official strategy of South African transformation after Mbeki's demise, South Africa's ongoing focus on market-based empowerment sustains its ambitions of producing local antiretroviral medicines.[118] Quite strikingly, the South African government seemed to protect the interests of the private sector. In contrast to Brazil and Thailand, where governments run pharmaceutical companies, South Africa has kept its commitment to buy ARVs exclusively from private and primarily local companies.[119]

Summary

Thabo Mbeki yearned for a comprehensive public discussion about the African condition and did not want a simple evidence-based answer about the etiology of the virus. Mbeki asserted that external actors misrepresented the nature of the epidemic in South Africa, and he simultaneously challenged the life-saving value of the antiretrovirals. Not surprisingly, given the immediate threat of a grave HIV crisis, international observers, medical professionals, and health organizations were not interested in taking part in an unproductive exchange. Pretoria was left alone with its normative ideas about the liberating power of indigenous knowledge. As a result, the Cabinet promoted the mixture of complementary medicines and bogus cures and later institutionalized African traditional healing. Mbeki's Pretoria resisted Western medical colonialism and enabled international health dissidents. But after the ANC ousted Mbeki, Pretoria's longing to promote nonconventional methods of health governance all but vanished.

As Mbeki's administration waned, localized ideas about health and healing were no longer preferred as an institutional solution to the domestic health crisis. Nevertheless, this should not be taken as evidence that the whole AIDS debacle occurred solely because of Mbeki. This only shows that the constitutive ideas failed to gain strong social traction. Having whipped up these attitudes, Mbeki unwillingly yet officially withdrew from the HIV/AIDS debate. Suffice it to say that his silence did not mean that he had learned anything genuine.

CONCLUSION

This chapter has started tracing how, why, and to what degree social purposes shape governmental responses to internationally agreed-upon principles of good AIDS governance. Despite the obvious empirical dissimilarities between the two cases, in both countries a dedication to unique social purposes pushed governments to understand matters of HIV and public health differently from the global mainstream. While not operating outside of the conventional paradigm of public health, both governments sanctioned social practices that were wrought to solve problems beyond the realm of public health.

First, while international actors define the nature of HIV/AIDS as a massive public health crisis, both South Africa and Russia decided to interpret the meaning of the contagion in unique localized fashions. For Putin's entourage, the continuing spread of the infection was one of the many faces of the demographic menace to the state. For Mbeki's associates, the epidemic was a local developmental problem to be resolved by local solutions. The second core theme discussed in this chapter pertains to the selection of biomedical tools and the implementation of the standardized regimen in health governance. The South African case is especially illustrative in this regard because Pretoria failed to accept the universally agreed-upon principle of evidence-based medicine and picked a fight against the conventional understanding of AIDS and pharmaceutical products. The third theme touched upon in this chapter concerns the standardized practices states use to secure the supply of generic medicines and branded products at discounted prices. Instead of monitoring the activities of the global pharmaceutical firms and using the available legal mechanisms, South Africa chose to defend its preoccupation with medical pluralism by rhetorically countervailing the powerful pharmaceutical lobby. Moscow's preoccupation with bolstering development and production of essential medicines was all about attaining import substitution and climbing to a position of influence in the international power hierarchy.

At this point, many additional questions persist. Most importantly, what is the core set of activities that governments undertake in order to solve the issue at stake, and to what extent does it match international recommendations? Is it conceivable that the core goals of the state influence how governments decide to deal with issues of prevention? Is it plausible that leaders suppress harm-reduction services not because of the social stigma attached to "demon users" or for reasons of political expediency but because of an internalized understanding of the goals of the state and intentional efforts to attain those goals? Is it probable that social purposes affect the processes of scaling up treatment, underwriting HIV-related programs, and funding health care in general? Because expanding access to treatment and removing barriers to prevention are important components of good AIDS governance, the next chapter inquires into them.

CHAPTER 4

Expanding Access

Approaches to Prevention and Treatment

INTENSIFYING EFFORTS TO achieve universal access to treatment and striving to offer adequate prevention services tailored to local epidemiological circumstances are now two intertwined standardized practices of AIDS governance that governments should enact in order to solve the looming health crisis. While the debate about how to strike an appropriate balance between access to treatment and prevention has been long, both are needed to curb the epidemic. Access to prevention services and medications as a broad, standardized practice is not only a matter of economic calculations but also a step to fulfill everyone's right to health.[1]

Issues of sex education, public discussion of sexual behavior, alternative lifestyles, and drug consumption have been controversial and are likely to remain politically sensitive. But these complications do not exonerate governments from the responsibility to provide extensive access to basic prevention services. When prevention services are available, governments will save much-needed resources and diminish public health spending in the long run. As the number and quality of realistic preventive measures increase, domestic opportunities to embrace prevention increase as well. Even the predictably divisive idea of harm reduction, although it goes against the global punitive prohibition ideology, has gained many pragmatic supporters.

Equally necessary is to mobilize the requisite amount of resources to put on medication all infected individuals who qualify for the therapy from the medical standpoint. Providing universal access to treatment is about underwriting HIV-related programs and interventions. Although providing drugs to everybody is costly, when prices on brand-name medicines fall and their cheap generic versions enter markets, policy makers, even those in countries with limited resources, can realistically increase the number of people on treatment. With the generous help of global donors, low- and middle-income countries have access to truly unprecedented resources.

That international actors have agreed on these health practices is, no doubt, a hallmark of the level of sophistication global AIDS governance has achieved. Notwithstanding this consensus, domestic ideas about the legitimate goals of the state can interfere with the global spread of the standardized approaches to prevention and treatment. Public officials can intentionally thwart access to prevention services and protect legal and cultural barriers that obstruct effective HIV governance. They can also deliberately freeze spending for health and decrease budgetary allocations for HIV-related programs.

The people who were responsible for making policy calls in Russia cultivated their own intolerance of human rights as a subversive antistatist ideology associated with Western liberalism. As a result, they intentionally rejected harm reduction, needle exchanges, and opioid substitutes, interpreting select preventive practices as illegitimate methods of health governance. On the other hand, increases in domestic health spending and generous investments in health systems were fully compatible with Putin's devotion to the developmental state. Public officials, health administrators, and activists welcomed spending money on HIV. In South Africa, on the contrary, state officials challenged the principles of resource allocation but not the principles of human rights. The focus on market-centered empowerment and self-reliance prompted the Cabinet to protect private actors and keep the public sector small. At the same time, Mbeki was hardly motivated to challenge the principles of human rights as hostile to the core goals of the African Renaissance. South Africans worked hard to identify and remove legal barriers to effective HIV prevention, although the health outcomes of their efforts were not always exemplary.

The chapter proceeds as follows. The first section explores a baseline approach to the universality of access to prevention services and treatment to make that approach operative for the further analysis of my cases. The second and the third sections consecutively inquire how Russian and South African ideational commitments have selectively affected the ultimate governance goal of scaling up universality.

INTERNATIONAL APPROACHES TO
PREVENTION AND TREATMENT

This section discusses how the idea of universality became an international norm.

The first subsection addresses the fact that although important prevention services that mitigate the spread of the epidemic are evidence based, they rest on a recognition of human rights as well. In this respect, the universality of access to prevention, treatment, and care, especially when vulnerable populations are involved, is about the principled ideas and values regarding human rights. UNAIDS leaders argue that increasing access to essential medicines and prevention directly relates to "expanded political space for affected people and the utilization of human rights discourse in demanding not only access to HIV-related services but to confront broader issues of social justice."[2] Human rights as an organizing principle of AIDS governance is distinct from the notion of the human right to health, understood as the broad socioeconomic right to enjoy the highest standard of health regardless of one's ability to pay.[3] It is important to keep this distinction in mind.

The second subsection discusses scaling up as a proxy for universality of treatment. Since the invention of ARVs, many international actors—scholars, activists, and advocacy groups—have struggled to promote treatment as a public, not private, good. Because at the dawn of this century fewer than half a million people were able to receive treatment, it should not be surprising that activists chose to spread awareness about governmental failures to ensure adequate access to life-saving medicines. After serious entrepreneurial efforts, the notion of "scaling up" made it onto the list of standard recommendations to curb the contagion. Scaling up basically means that governments must increase treatment coverage proportionately to the number of people who qualify for it. In recent years, the number of people on treatment has increased dramatically, rising from fewer than half a million individuals in 2003 to almost ten million people in 2012. Although I do not delve into details of political economy of HIV pharmaceuticals or the issues of the long-term financial sustainability of the currently achieved level of treatment, the presented evidence indicates that scaling-up treatment and mobilization of resources are crucial international recommendations for curbing AIDS. That in 2006 and 2011 the UN General Assembly adopted two political declarations on HIV/AIDS is a reliable indication of the firmly established international commitment to implement comprehensive, evidence-based prevention approaches and to accelerate efforts to achieve the goal of universal access to antiretroviral treatment.[4]

"Prevention Must Be the Mainstay of Our Response"

The first core set of activities that governments should undertake in order to solve the issue at stake is to either expand access to prevention services or remove barriers to them. Because putting people on treatment alone is not enough to address the challenge of HIV/AIDS effectively, it is indispensable to emphasize prevention as a key for eliminating the contagion. Early preventive interventions are likely to be cost efficient, as they will lower the rates of virus transmission to the general population. In the end, this will likely diminish public health spending and free resources for additional HIV-related needs.

In 2002 the Global HIV Prevention Working Group, an international panel of leading public health experts, listed only three "proven" prevention strategies: prevention of sexual, parenteral, and mother-to-child transmissions. Later on, everybody agreed that prevention is also about strengthening health systems, supporting behavior change programs, promoting abstinence, institutionalizing access to contraception and family planning services, providing sex education, providing routine HIV testing, securing the safety of the blood supply, and so on.[5] In recent years, research has shown that male circumcision, the use of antiretroviral-based microbicides, and pre-exposure antiretroviral prophylaxis are also valuable tools of prevention. In 2012 a Food and Drug Administration (FDA) panel recommended the fixed-dose combination Truvada (tenofovir [TDF], originally approved in 2001, and emtricitabine) for pre-exposure prophylaxis of HIV to prevent the risk of contracting the virus.[6]

Although treatment and prevention seem to imply different strategies of health intervention, in reality they are closely intertwined. In 2009 Robert Gallo and Luc Montagnier, the famous codiscoverers of the human immunodeficiency virus, called for universal testing and widespread treatment as the most reliable methods of prevention. Universal HIV testing turned out to be somewhat controversial, as activists became afraid that such a strategy would undermine human rights. The idea of treatment as prevention turned out to be more successful. Recent international randomized trials, known as the HIV Prevention Trials Network (HPTN) 052, have demonstrated that taking antiretrovirals substantially reduces the risk of the sexual transmission of HIV.[7] Thus, providing treatment to people with HIV significantly reduces the risk of transmission to their HIV-negative partners. The discussion below goes as follows.

Striking a balance between treatment and prevention, as well as adjudicating among different tactical strategies that might be devised on the basis of the wide range of currently available preventive measures, remains difficult. In theory, prioritizing prevention at the expense of treatment may signal a warped policy process and possibly will result in falling back on the underprovision of treatment as a public good. That is why global activists took personally Randall

Tobias's comments about AIDS being a fully preventable disease to be curbed primarily by abstinence. Equally critical (and not always reasonable) was their response to George W. Bush's conservative approach to the epidemic. But the so-called ABC principle (abstinence, be faithful, use condoms) is not prioritized at the expense of other prevention services and hardly ever hinders the collective effort in mitigating AIDS.

What influential global players count as appropriate prevention strategies might cause controversies as well. Suffice it to say that conservative and liberal political groups have conflicting ideas about the appropriate methods of health governance.[8]

Governmental commitments to observe human rights and provide necessary health services to vulnerable groups are central to sustaining effective preventive efforts. Because high-risk subpopulations do not live in airtight conditions isolated from the rest of the population, aiming at universal treatment at a country level is the most reliable way to curb the pandemic. Depending on a country's epidemiological circumstances, the category of vulnerable individuals includes intravenous drug users (IDUs), commercial sex workers, prisoners, men who have sex with men, HIV-positive mothers, women and girls, youths, people living in poverty, migrants, refugees, and orphans. The sign of bad health governance is when governments choose to either deploy severe restrictive measures or criminalize high-risk populations while denying them treatment and necessary health services.

The international community traveled a long way before accepting the importance of access to preventive services among vulnerable and negatively constructed populations. At the onset of the pandemic, it was easy to associate the disease with deviant and promiscuous minorities with an almost 100 percent mortality rate. In the 1980s many policy makers understood AIDS as "gay cancer." The short-lived nomenclatures (the pejorative GRID [gay-related immune deficiency] and the informal "four H disease") capture these early attitudes.[9] At that time, the U.S. administration believed that the epidemic should be contained through severe regulative measures, including quarantine.[10] One of the most high-profile restrictive measures was barring the entry of affected foreign nationals into the United States.[11] Yet even much later, compulsory surveillance and criminalization were used as methods of AIDS governance.[12]

Many activists and practitioners still pessimistically talk about the many complexities of overcoming the stigma of the disease that negatively influence governments' efforts to launch a broad-based response to AIDS. In many cases, high-risk groups have to endure discrimination, resentment, and hatred. Nevertheless, consensus that excluding certain groups is a significant breach of the standardized policy that puts the general population at risk has strengthened. At the forefront of the movement that linked the issues of HIV and human rights was Jonathan Mann. He understood that the devotion to human rights enhances the commitment to expand the universality of access to prevention as a key component of fighting AIDS. In the early 1990s, internal politics and fights at the World Health Organization undermined his activity and aborted the slowly emerging international regime; his plea to use a human rights framework against HIV/AIDS went unheeded. In the long run, but regrettably after his tragic death, Mann's proposition that "promotion and protection of human rights and promotion and protection of health are fundamentally linked" became a foundational principle in AIDS governance.[13]

In 2004 the World Health Organization prepared the Dublin Declaration on Partnership to Fight HIV/AIDS in Europe and Central Asia, which in large part stressed action against local-level stigma and discrimination against vulnerable populations. The declaration noted that "the respect, protection and promotion of human rights is fundamental to preventing transmission of HIV, reducing vulnerability to infection and dealing with the impact of HIV/AIDS."[14] In essence, its signatories affirmed that observing human rights had become crucial for preventing HIV/AIDS from moving into the general population. The European Centre for Disease Prevention and Control (ECDC) monitors the Eurasian countries' progress in the implementation of the principles and commitments expressed in this declaration.[15]

Although the present-day approach to good AIDS governance explicitly acknowledges that excluding high-risk populations not only makes the elimination of the disease difficult but is also morally wrong, the battle for prevention is not over. Threatening the global spread of the norm of prevention is the state propensity to fall back on coercive methods, since it vindicates a state's intolerance for highly controversial but evidence-based interventions. Only leaving punitive ideology behind allows states to embrace harm reduction, a controversial but effective method of prevention, as legitimate. Initial support for punitive methods of health governance can come from many sources, but with principled rejection of human rights as an organizing principle of AIDS governance that support can become permanently settled. The remainder of this subsection talks about harm reduction as the cornerstone of an effective method of AIDS governance. The discussion that follows is relevant mostly for the subsequent analysis of my Russian case.

Harm reduction is intended primarily to reduce negative health consequences for individuals who cannot stop using drugs intravenously. Harm-reduction programs include opioid substitute treatment, needle and syringe exchanges, and drug consumption rooms. Benefits are numerous. In general, needle exchanges reduce the risks of the spread of HIV, hepatitis, and other bacterial infections; substitute treatment can help intravenous users reduce injecting drugs and prevent symptoms of withdrawal; administered in a controlled environment, methadone treatment prevents addicts from pursuing illicit narcotics through criminal networks.

The methadone maintenance treatment uses synthetic opioids, chemicals that mimic the action of natural substances derived from the opium poppy plant. First-line synthetic substitutes for opioids include buprenorphine and methadone products. In October 2002 the FDA approved Suboxone and Subutex, two buprenorphine products, as sublingual tablets. Similarly, other methadone products (Dolophine, originally approved on August 13, 1947) treat pain that is not responsive to nonnarcotic analgesics, provide detoxification, and maintain treatment of opioid addiction.[16] Although methadone has been known to cause serious side effects, it is not life threatening. In the United States, the Controlled Substances Act (CSA) classifies methadone as a Schedule II drug and buprenorphine as a Schedule III drug.

There are clear distinctions between harm reduction and use reduction: "Use reduction may be a strategy to achieve harm reduction, but when use reduction becomes a goal in its own right the policy or programme should not be described as harm reduction. Harm reduction is not in conflict with abstinence as a possible strategy for reducing drug-related harm, even in the long term, but it gives priority to the more immediate and practical goal of reducing harm for users who cannot be expected to stop using at the present time."[17]

The broad understanding of harm reduction contains ideas and values associated with respect for human rights. This issue framing implies the necessity to provide services for drug users and stop the institutionalized prosecution and harassment of those addicted to controlled substances. Despite attempts to define harm reduction in value-neutral and evidence-based terms, in various societal and political contexts, policy makers who do not explicitly commit themselves to eliminating the supply of narcotics and reducing their overall consumption might lose electoral support. Part of the problem is the widespread fear that needle exchanges and opioid substitute programs excuse and legitimize the consumption of illicit drugs. Because of this and other reasons, governments' degree and pace of accepting the harm-reduction approach to the threat of HIV has varied. Only in December 2009 did the U.S. government, for instance, partially lift the 1988 ban on the use of federal funds for syringe exchange programs for drug users. Prevention, in other words, is not safe from political concerns. Often, agencies implementing harm reduction proceed without enthusiasm and at a slow pace.

I am far from claiming that there is complete consistency in how harm reduction is being interpreted and implemented across the globe. Even the term itself remains somewhat controversial. But the overall direction of health governance is set by those countries that include explicit and supportive references to harm reduction in national policy documents, institutionalize operational needle exchange programs, sponsor operational opioid substitute programs, and allow drug consumption rooms.[18] Canada, Australia, Germany, Luxembourg, Norway, Spain, and Switzerland lead by offering stellar examples of good AIDS governance. The majority of states, except Russia, use some combination of the aforementioned policy components, excluding drug consumption rooms. Recently, the Global Fund has started sponsoring harm-reduction programs.[19] Such luminaries as Michel Sidibé, executive director of UNAIDS, Michel Kazatchkine, former executive director of the Global Fund, and Eliot Ross Albers, executive director of the International Network of People Who Use Drugs (INPUD), endorse the efforts of Harm Reduction International. This organization describes its mission as "to reduce drug related harms by promoting evidence based public health policy and practices and human rights based approaches to drug policy through an integrated programme of research, analysis, advocacy and civil society strengthening."[20]

For those countries where injecting drug users are the main vector of the epidemic, harm reduction is critically important to protect public health. Russian HIV prevalence among people who inject drugs is around 37 percent. This number is slightly lower than that of Brazil, Thailand, Indonesia, and Ukraine.[21] But given that there are almost twice as many IDUs living with HIV in Russia as there are in Brazil, opioid substitute therapy is not available in Russia, and needle exchanges cover only 7 percent of the Russian IDUs, health professionals have even more reason to worry about the next wave of the national health crisis. So should top Russian leaders, who instead exude overconfidence in their health governance methods. Recently, Russia failed to supply relevant data on injecting drug users to the UNAIDS world report, which might indicate a further desocialization from international norms and a Russian attempt to conceal a looming crisis.[22] Learning about national harm-reduction programs would have been a smart decision, but, for the reasons explained below, that education is not likely to happen.

In short, governments that are accustomed to the organizing principles of human rights are well attuned to best-evidence-based practices. At the same time, the countries that display a disdain for human rights most likely will reject the best practices and will try to guard their societies against utilizing them and even strengthen legal barriers to doing so.

Mobilizing Resources to Scale Up Treatment

According to one important report, "in the highest prevalence countries, only urgent expansion of treatment will forestall continued catastrophic rates of illness and death and the attendant social and economic devastation."[23] In a few words, this statement captured the second core set of activities that governments must undertake in order to deal with a public health crisis effectively: expand access to treatment, which requires mobilizing sufficient financial resources adequate to putting people on medications.

Only treatment prolongs the lives of the forty million people who already carry the human immunodeficiency virus and, by preventing the progression of the virus to AIDS, allows them to return to productive work. The invention of highly active antiretroviral therapy unburdened state budgets and made treatment economically feasible. Because prices of antiretroviral treatment are currently low, governments can put on therapy an increasingly large number of HIV-infected individuals. Treating AIDS-defining illnesses is costlier than hitting the virus hard at the early stage. Introducing treatment is most efficient at the outset of the epidemic, when the absence of drug resistance warrants the disbursement of the cheapest first-line regimen. But it is clear at the same time that covering everybody is nearly impossible. For this reason, the relevant international guidelines talk about scaling up as a proxy of the universality of treatment, while the ultimate goal, of course, is still to provide access to antiretrovirals for all those who need them.[24]

Since the invention of triple antiretroviral treatment, intergovernmental organizations, global activists, and policy entrepreneurs have pushed for global access to life-saving ARVs and stimulated domestic awareness about the importance of scaling up. The agreement on scaling up can be found in many international declarations and commitments. The United Nations Millennium Declaration, which was adopted at the Millennium Summit in September 2000, was central among these. It clearly expressed its support for the notion of universality of treatment.[25] The Millennium Summit set forth the goal to "halt and begin to reverse the spread of HIV/AIDS and the incidence of malaria and other major diseases."[26] In 2002 the Policy Project and Merck sponsored a special conference on AIDS and economics whose participants came to the conclusion that the adverse economic impact of HIV/AIDS outweighed the costs of treatment. In 2003, commissioned by UNAIDS, an international panel of the leading AIDS advocates composed a report titled *Access to HIV Prevention: Closing the Gap*. The report called for filling the estimated 3.8-billion-dollar HIV funding gap by 2005. The World Health Organization offered a conceptual platform to accelerate the delivery of ARV treatment to three million people by the end of 2005 within thirty-four priority countries.[27] Although that "3 by 5" initiative fell short of its declared targets, it nevertheless contributed to spreading scaling up as a feasible approach to be adopted by governments across the globe.[28] Other advocates of scaling up include the Accelerating Access Initiative (AAI), a partnership between United Nations agencies and five pharmaceutical companies, and the World Bank's Regional Treatment Acceleration Project.[29]

Scaling up depends upon the mobilization of national resources and an interpretation of antiretroviral treatment as a public good. Today, international financial institutions confirm the necessity to increase public investment in health. The World Bank promotes treatment and advocates governmental responsibility to provide drugs in the public health sector. Its seminal report *Confronting AIDS: Public Priorities in a Global Epidemic* frames AIDS as a public health problem and stresses national governments' responsibility to provide antiretroviral therapy, palliative care, and treatment of opportunistic infections. In the most straightforward formulation, the report states that "governments should ensure that HIV-infected patients benefit from the same access to health care as other patients with comparable illnesses and a similar ability to pay."[30] In 2004 the World Bank joined the GFATM, UNICEF, and the Clinton Foundation to assist developing countries in buying high-quality AIDS drugs at reduced prices. In 2005 the World Bank called for comprehensive programs to include "an increased number of interventions targeted to virtually all groups in society" and to "address gender and other dimensions of equity such as access for poor and marginalized groups and in rural areas."[31] It framed the provision of treatment as a precondition to sustainable development, realizing that health programs require significant financing. Subsequently, the World Bank became one of the largest international funders in the fight against the pandemic. Private foundations and philanthropic initiatives have joined influential intergovernmental organizations. The wave of global generosity has alleviated many earlier problems, such as the necessity to conduct permanent fund-raising campaigns, overcome donor fatigue, and rise above the squabbles about the appropriate amount of donations as related to a country's GDP in the developed states.

Given the failure of the norm of universal primary health care, the emergent norm of widespread access to treatment is remarkable. It materialized because of the efforts of health policy leaders and AIDS entrepreneurs who campaigned and turned the universality of access into an issue of social rights. They also convinced many global actors that treatment was a public, not private, good.[32] Mobilization of resources to scale up treatment featured prominently in PEPFAR's funding strategy. According to the Kaiser Family Foundation's data, in FY 2004–5 PEPFAR allocated $34 million for antiretroviral therapy, which surpassed the funding for prevention and abstinence. The next year, approximately $819 million were spent to purchase ARVs, while the number of people receiving treatment increased from fewer than fifty thousand to more than one million people as of May 2007.

Much as the advent of this principle was not predestined, its future is not set in stone either. For many reasons, a long-term commitment to the universality of treatment is a daunting task. Keen observers indicate that the scope of national treatment programs should reflect the capabilities of a given country, including the health-care infrastructure, the percentage of the infected population, the country's GDP, and the general state of the economy.[33] Pushing this argument to the extreme, some commentators insist that distributing antiretrovirals hinders states' performance in health care in the long haul. While AIDS activists and policy entrepreneurs are likely to continue to fight for universal access to antiretroviral drugs, the demand for treatment constantly rises. Facing hard economic times, donors might wish to reconsider the extent of their foreign assistance. At the same time, the tensions associated with a new global sense of entitlement to the U.S.-funded AIDS treatment might jeopardize a donor's generosity and desire to be actively involved in health governance.[34]

At the very least, the expansion of global financial commitments becomes vulnerable. But the number of people eligible for treatment does not abate: the World Health Organization suggests that a stupefying number of almost thirty million people are ready to be on treatment. It is likely that in 2030 more than 55 million people will need these life-saving medicines. The issue of affordability looms large for everyone. Governments will have to keep pace with changing epidemiological conditions and increases in drug resistance and eventually will have to purchase increasingly expensive lines of pharmaceuticals.[35] At the same time, the generic industry will have to adjust to match its supply to the increasing demand, but whether markets will remain open to generics is not yet clear.[36] All this adds up to a challenging new trend that governments will have to grapple with in the near future. Right now, however, freezing spending on health and scaling down treatment are not viable options.

In summary, the decreasing prices of life-saving medications made possible an unprecedented wave of global financial generosity and generated optimistic expectations among international bodies that governments will be able to foot the bill without going bankrupt. That and the dwindling costs of triple treatment therapy temporarily disable the arguments of those who question the economic feasibility of rolling out treatment anywhere except in the wealthiest countries. Governments, therefore, should not skimp on providing treatment and scaling up their response. They should not suspend treatment for any reason other than a patient's death.

Summary

Prevention services are complementary, not antithetical, to the global orientation to expand treatment coverage. Various strategies of health promotion, including education and prevention campaigns, should join campaigns that focus solely on the access to medicines. Until the vaccine against HIV/AIDS is found, widespread access to essential medicines is indispensable. But as treatment costs increase and the need for second- and third-line regimens intensifies, the importance of access to prevention services becomes paramount.[37]

The second and third sections of this chapter consecutively explore how Russians and South Africans undermined expansion of prevention and treatment as standardized practices of AIDS governance. In a nutshell, for Moscow the uncomfortable choices were about human rights and prevention, while for Pretoria those choices were about underwriting conventional medicines and treating their provision as a public good.

PREVENTION AND TREATMENT IN PUTIN'S RUSSIA

The Kremlin mobilized substantial finances to underwrite various HIV-related activities. While it did not challenge the growing consensus on prevention services in general, it surely frowned upon harm reduction because it was associated with human rights norms. The first subsection provides details about the intentional roadblocks to institutionalizing adequate national harm-reduction programs in Russia. *Siloviki*, conservative opinion leaders, church functionaries, and a sizeable fraction of the professional medical community converged on the conclusion that harm reduction undermines the mores and goals of the Russian state. Central to the goals of the government were a significant reduction in the use of illicit substances and increasingly punitive laws rather than protecting the health of intravenous drug users. The second subsection demonstrates that the Kremlin scaled up access to treatment, poured money into various healthcare projects, and built new AIDS centers. Generous spending on health projects at the federal level was consistent with the elite's commitment to restore a powerful centralized authority, to fulfill its social obligations, and shore up its public image of the developmental state. The combination of the Kremlin's financial generosity and normative rigidity in its approach to health governance makes an AIDS-free future in Russia precarious.

Obstacles to Prevention in Russia

Although Russian public officials increasingly understand prevention and health promotion as the means to improve public health, the future of HIV prevention in the country remains highly uncertain. I start this subsection by indicating that Russian politicians have recently begun grasping the vital importance of health promotion in health governance. I then discuss how and why Russian actors involved in health governance deliberately paralyzed internationally agreed-upon preventive measures and thus failed to bridge the gap in HIV prevention among drug users.

Until recently, the Russian government failed to challenge the inherited Communist emphasis on curative medicine and to promote preventive medicine as the core component of public health. Health professionals tend to emphasize treatment as the best approach to health. Dimitriy Medvedev took a special pride in the specialized curative centers and boasted about the high-end technological equipment provided for citizens in the framework of the National Priority

Projects. At the same time, he signaled a clear understanding of the necessity for disease prevention and health promotion.[38] In an interview for the official newspaper *Rossiyskaya gazeta*, Ol'ga Borzova, chair of the State Duma Committee for Health from 2007 to 2011, praised the ongoing transition from curative medicine to health promotion as the core component of public health.[39] Notwithstanding these promising developments, the hostility to health promotion and evidence-based prevention among many health-care professionals endures.[40]

In Russia, a key high-risk population includes approximately 1,825,000 intravenous drug users, although some estimates give a much higher number. Intravenous drug users and heroin addicts are the main bridge population that transmits the disease to other social groups. Incidences of HIV among women and the heterosexual population have increased rapidly. Thus, heeding international recommendations to devise methods of reducing the spread of HIV among drug users is of critical importance for good AIDS governance in Russia. The remainder of this subsection focuses on the governmental action toward intravenous drug users.

By the end of the 1990s, many policy participants across the globe had grasped the benefits of harm-reduction services for improving the standards of health governance. Many Westernized Russian health-care professionals, as well as domestic and international civil society organizations, clearly saw the value of harm reduction and tried to promote it. But many others did not.[41] As mentioned in the previous section, internalizing harm reduction is hardly possible without at least minimal devotion to the principles of human rights. But many Russians, including Putin, came to envision human rights as the pernicious implementation of external forces that had been conspiring to undermine Russia's sovereignty.[42] That is why Russian politicians and opinion leaders decided that punitive measures were more appropriate than rehabilitative ones.

The Moscow government continuously promoted prevention, sometimes mixing it with criminalizing measures. Lyudmila Stebenkova, chair of the Committee for Health Care and Protection of Public Health at Moscow City Duma, correctly claimed that promoting healthy lifestyles and moral sexual behavior would curb the epidemic. But she also erroneously insisted that "under the guise of prophylaxis the Western foundations advertise pedophilia, prostitution and immoral behavior."[43] In 2006 she petitioned President Putin to restrict the outreach of the nonstate sex education campaigns in Russia. Nikolay Kaklyugin, professional psychiatrist, a specialist in addiction medicine, and head of a faith-based social charity, displayed a similar attitude. He claimed that the U.S.

government covertly supported these organizations' subversive activities to turn Russia into a liberal democracy. He went as far as claiming that transnational HIV/AIDS programs aim to "create and consolidate elements socially harmful and dangerous for the rest of the population—homosexuals, prostitutes, narcotics users."[44] The removal of barriers to prevention services, sex education, and implementing harm-reduction programs proved to be daunting.

Key Russian public officials hardly bother to conceal their contempt for Western norms. In his 2005 interview on the proliberal radio station Ekho Moskvy, Aleksandr Mikhailov, deputy head of the Federal Drug Control Service (FSKN), argued against harm-reduction measures because they reproduced "incomprehensible reflections related to human rights."[45] Similarly, Viktor Ivanov, head of the State Antinarcotics Committee (GAK) and the new director of FSKN, on many occasions tried to persuade his listeners that harm reduction, as well as human rights, implied tolerance of social sins and were incompatible with the common good.[46] Moscow mayor Yuriy Luzhkov claimed that the Russian approach to drug users and homosexuals should differ from that of the Western democracies.[47] Some health-care professionals and medical doctors surmised that harm-reduction programs aggravated contemporary demographic problems in the Russian Federation.

Conservative opinion leaders fanned the flames of societal uncertainty about harm reduction and spread the disdain for human rights. They claimed that harm reduction weakened the state and exposed it to the mercy of aggressive alien ideologies. They portrayed the liberal proponents of harm-reduction programs and the human rights watchers (*pravozashchitniki*) as dangerous agents of foreign governments. Some accused liberals of building societal tolerance to social sins and sneaking onto Russian soil destructive ideas that jeopardize many lives. Similarly, Alexey Nadezhdin, in 2005 the chief of the Division of Adolescent Narcology of the National Scientific Center at the Ministry of Health, claimed that only repressive medical practices could protect the healthy majority against the abnormal deviants and their advocates. He lashed out against foreign-sponsored subversion: "*Pravozashchitniki* and 'humanists' shift the vector of public perception from the interest of the majority . . . to the pathological minority. And, supporting this minority, [they] crudely impinge on the interests of the healthy majority, threatening the security of the state."[48] Some conservative commentators interpreted repressive policy choices—without appropriate evidence—as an effective approach to eradicate the consumption of narcotics and mitigate the epidemic of HIV/AIDS.[49]

That the Russian society en masse does not favor internationally agreed-upon prevention strategies such as the substitute treatment and syringe exchange is obvious. These attitudes, however, are poor excuses for the Russian government. Although the Kremlin can influence and change popular opinions, it has chosen not to promote professional claims and not to overturn the self-serving feelings of intolerance to social vices. On the contrary, both federal and regional policy makers have bluntly rejected any major findings regarding the benefits of de-criminalizing health governance.

Assorted *siloviki* and governmental officials scoffed at the validity of the conclusions offered in the June 2011 report of the Global Commission on Drug Policy, the central drug policy–making body within the United Nations system. Radical voices claimed that the UN Office on Drugs and Crime was promoting narcotics instead of putting up a fight against them. Given this profound skepticism about international health organizations and policy guidelines, the deeply seated Russian perception that humanitarian rhetoric disguised a furtive subversive agenda becomes less surprising.[50]

These official statements insisted that the domestic epidemic was mostly a result of the swelling domestic abuse of narcotic substances related to the increased harvest of opiates in Afghanistan that followed the U.S. invasion. During the State Duma's hearings for the Russian Federation on the causes and consequences of the Afghan narco-traffic, its speaker, Boris Gryzlov, claimed that Russia had entered into a state of war with those who spread opiates from Afghanistan in a deliberate strategy to destroy the Russian gene pool. The head of the Federal Drug Control Service, Viktor Cherkesov, joined the strengthening domestic chorus. He averred that a transnational lobby had gone all out to undermine the strength and sovereignty of the Russian state by promoting decriminalization of drug use and advocating harm reduction.[51] The widespread view stated that to control the spread of HIV/AIDS the state should become less lenient toward intravenous drug users and stop the production of opiates right at their source, in Afghanistan.[52]

Russian policy makers tried to camouflage their ideological resistance to harm reduction on technical grounds as well. Dr. Gennadiy Onishchenko, the chief public health official, went on record claiming that opiate substitute treatment and needle exchange programs were never effective.[53] In 2009 he averred that drug users simply walked away from treatment, thereby obliterating the benefits of treatment and increasing drug resistance. Onishchenko is certainly correct in some respects, since "past data shows that only 16% of IDU receiving substance abuse treatment completed the course without relapse, and only 40% of IDU on ART remained on treatment at 6 months."[54] Under a different set of circumstances, adherence concerns could have been the starting point for a pragmatic public policy debate, one that could be resolved by the compelling medical research showing the outcomes of large-scale harm-reduction programs. But Russian health officials defended inefficient and punitive withdrawal programs and kept on blaming their victims.[55] To justify a punitive criminal justice approach to drug policy, Russian opinion leaders invoked the questionable evidence of allegedly small HIV/AIDS infection rates in China and its arguably successful fight against narcotics. Although China surely can be seen as an example of a state that does not heed Western recommendations and does not fully observe human rights standards, the Chinese embrace of methadone therapy and its pragmatic recognition of the effectiveness of harm reduction should have been acknowledged nonetheless.

In practice, the Russian government failed to provide harm-reduction services within the state health-care infrastructure. The federal authorities replenished various antidrug initiatives and law enforcement needs but depleted harm-reduction programs. Heroin addicts remained a low priority on the treatment waiting lists. Sometimes, local AIDS centers denied HIV treatment to active drug users. The involuntary withdrawal programs are the new game in town.[56] Numerous newspaper articles and advocacy reports indicate that state officials harassed substitute treatment and harm-reduction programs offered by nonstate actors.[57] At the same time, high-powered officials looked the other way when lower-level bureaucrats and police harassed addicts instead of punishing such behavior. It is worth highlighting that these prevailing attitudes toward IDUS among Russian officials create a self-fulfilling prophesy and perhaps weaken drug users' desire to undergo treatment in the public sector in the first place.[58] Further, without governmental support, only small-scale nongovernmental harm-reduction programs are likely to remain operational in the country.

Arguably, legislation on controlled substances and prevention strategies could have evolved in any direction. In the late 1980s, the stress on eliminating traffic and supply did not portend the unavoidable resistance to evidence-based prevention. Federal Law No. 3, "On Narcotic Means and Psychotropic Substances" (1998), an initial legal framework, was written before officials had grasped the significance of injecting drug use for the spread of HIV infections. Further, at the dawn of the new millennium, some decisions, including that of the Duma to decriminalize personal possession of controlled substances, could have paved the road to legalizing substitution treatment and embracing harm reduction. However, law enforcement agencies became a prominent force in health governance, and human rights ideology all but crumbled. The resistance to harm reduction in Putin's Russia therefore reflected intentionality stipulated by the core tasks of the state.

It would not be a conceptual stretch to say that the looming failure in controlling the spread of the contagion in Russia in large part stems from Moscow's commitment to hard-nosed ideational predilections despite the unambiguous recommendations of multiple behavioral and biological studies. That the *siloviki* stressed punitive measures was not surprising. That they failed to acknowledge the limitations of the supply-control drug policy was not so striking either. Astounding was the intersubjective tendency to equate harm reduction with an ontological threat to the Russian state as an autonomous political organization. This unusual interpretation materialized because the underlying normative context in Russia became antithetical to human rights. Politicians failed to internalize harm reduction as a useful health-oriented intervention, but they surely interpreted it as a licentious and anti-Russian tool. In short, the metaphor of "sovereign narcology" might adequately capture the gist of the Russian government's policy toward vulnerable populations. Part of the reason that the professional medical community failed to expostulate was because the policy debate on AIDS governance and especially on harm reduction was in the hands of *siloviki*. I discuss this issue in chapter 5.

Mobilization of Finances in Russia

The federal government committed to an extensive treatment coverage and, therefore, complied with international guidelines and best practices. In principle, the federal laws guarantee free and universal access to ARV therapy. Russia's first comprehensive legislation concerning HIV/AIDS directly called for extensive access to HIV medication and comprehensive public education.[59] Subsequently, in November 2001 the federal government approved a program on preventing and combating "socially significant" diseases. It covered HIV/AIDS and specified provisions for purchasing and disbursing the "most effective" antiretrovirals.

In September 2005 Vladimir Starodubov, the deputy minister of health and social development, claimed that the budget would cover all mothers to prevent transmission of the virus to children (6,253 people), as well as all those who needed treatment (up to 15,000 people).[60] By 2008 most regions covered more than 70 percent of people who needed treatment. Several years later, more than seventy thousand patients received therapy in regional AIDS centers. Compared to 2002, when antiretrovirals were available for fewer than two thousand patients, the progress is truly staggering. The country progress reports boasted a very high number—from 80 to 96 percent—of adults and children with advanced HIV infection receiving treatment.[61] Undeniable progress notwithstanding, there is a discrepancy between the numbers that appeared in congratulatory domestic reports and the numbers estimated by independent observers. According to Michel D. Kazatchkine, executive director of GFATM, by the end of 2009 only 23 percent of the HIV-infected population received treatment. Compared to the average of 40 percent among other nations, this was a plain underachievement. The ambiguity might arise from the fact that the number of HIV-positive Russians might be significantly higher than official statistics recognize. In addition, the Russian government accepted the model of treatment that recommends providing highly active antiretroviral therapy (HAART) after the viral load has increased to a certain point and not when the infection has been detected.

I would like to conclude this subsection by discussing the overall level of health spending in Russia. Prior to 2006, the government spent only about $5 million per year to fight AIDS, had no streamlined national policy, and was vague on the implications of the virus spread for the strength and development of the state. In 2005 the Kremlin announced its decision to create a new form of governance under the direct patronage of the president: the Council for the Implementation of National Priority Projects and Demographic Politics. The council's mission was to reverse adverse demographic tendencies and "smartly" invest money in several critical areas, including health. In 2007 Dimitriy Medvedev asserted that National Priority Projects would be the most effective way to solve domestic problems.[62] The decision to use NPPs as the organizational form to invest in health matched Putin's normative commitment to the developmental state. In 2008 Putin stated that his government had designed and implemented national projects in order to fulfill the goals of the developmental state (or "modern social politics," in his parlance).[63] This gives an observer necessary rhetorical evidence on the links between the devotion to attain the core goals of the state and the process of governance. There is no doubt that the skyrocketing prices of hydrocarbon products made possible the initial expansion of the state health-care sector. But the Kremlin continues to increase its spending on health care despite intensifying budgetary constraints.

The majority of Putin's liberal opponents simply did not recognize the NPPs as meaningful vehicles of economic transformation. Many commentators thought that the sole purpose of the NPPs was either to redistribute the revenues generated from the oil sector or to ensure the political survival of Putin's entourage after his second presidential term expired in 2008. Putin's detractors thought of National Priority Projects as public relations exploits and the springboard for Medvedev to kick-start his presidency, for which he allegedly had been previously short-listed. As if anticipating the liberals' criticism and incredulity of this initiative, Medvedev determinedly noted that National Priority Projects were not public relations exploits but genuine tools to uphold social justice and promote economic growth. Putin and Medvedev alike contrasted their generous investment in health to Yeltsin's 1990s, when the government allegedly shied away from any social obligations. Despite the independent expert community's continuing skepticism about all this, the NPPs continued to pump money into public health.

Despite the Russian tendency to overestimate its success in AIDS governance, the commitment to extensive coverage is evident. How much money did the government spend on AIDS governance? The numbers in table 3 and table 4 give a snapshot of governmental spending on AIDS.

The government thus became a generous spender and supported a whole range of research and development activities. In addition, in 2008 the federal budget allocated about $5.7 million to the State Centre of Virology and Biotechnology, about $614,000 to the Ivanovsky Institute of Virology, about $1.2 million to Saint Petersburg State University, and about $8.7 million to the Federal Medico-Biological Agency.[64] In 2008–10 the federal budget allocated $41 million for HIV/AIDS vaccine research and improvement of the HIV/AIDS monitoring and control centers.

The Kremlin decided to pour money from windfall mineral rents into the problem, scrapping further reform plans. Despite the dramatic increase in state funding for public health, government spending in most cases lagged behind urgent needs. Old infrastructure, outdated medical equipment, and poor quality of health care continue to frustrate ordinary Russians. More recently, many domestic public health-care experts have identified the lack of strategic vision and a clear road map of reforms in the Health-Care Development Concept (the first draft of which was published in 2009) and the ensuing State Program of Health-Care Development as the core impediments for the successful transformation of public health.[65]

On balance, the lack of state efficiency and capacity plagued this massive spending, significantly undermining the urgent need to upgrade public health

Table 3   HIV/AIDS Funding from the National Health Project, National Priority
           Projects (millions of rubles)*

	Diagnosis	Prevention	Treatment	Research	Construction	Total
2006	1,200.00	200.00	1,700.00	0.00	0.00	3,100.00
2007	2,277.50	200.00	5,322.50	0.00	0.00	7,800.00
2008	2,799.32	200.00	4,800.00	0.00	0.00	7,799.32
2009	3,400.00	400.00	5,500.00	0.00	0.00	9,300.00
2010	3,404.74	400.00	8,143.30	0.00	0.00	11,948.04
Total	13,081.56	1,400.00	25,465.80	0.00	0.00	39,947.36
% of total	32.75	3.50	63.75	0.00	0.00	

Source: Data available at http://hivpolicy.ru/publications/index.php?id=469.
*$1.00 = 27 rubles

Table 4   HIV/AIDS Funding from the Department of State Targeted Programs
           and Capital Investments, Ministry of Economic Development of the
           Russian Federation (Minekonomrazvitiya) (millions of rubles)*

	Construction	Research	Various	Prevention	Treatment	Total
2006	107.90	16.10	0.00	56.80	13.70	194.50
2007	249.40	25.59	95.20			370.19
2008	372.29	27.50	63.73			463.52
2009	221.76	0.00	75.28			297.04
2010	415.34	3.62	8.86			427.82
Total	1,366.68	72.82	243.07	56.80	13.70	1,753.07
% of total	77.96	4.15	13.87	3.24	0.78	

Source: Federal target program "Prevention and Treatment of the Socially Important Diseases,"
subprogram HIV, data available at http://fcp.vpk.ru/cgi-bin/cis/fcp.cgi/Fcp/ViewFcp/View/2010/218/.
*$1.00 = 27 rubles

care. The real benefits of all that spending for health improvement are far from
certain, too. Putin himself acknowledged that overall only 33 percent of patients enjoyed good-quality services despite the overall increase of invested resources.[66] Commitment to state-led development suggests that the Kremlin will
continue to allocate money for public health and will cover the costs of antiretroviral treatment. The spending spree continues, even though material conditions
have become unfavorable.

Summary

In Russia, the Putin administration set forth legal provisions and law enforcement practices that limited the availability of substitute treatment and syringe

exchanges for intravenous drug users. This practice was a result of the government's unwillingness to accept human rights as an organizing principle of health governance on which the success of access to prevention in part depended. Although many Russians abhor drug users, the available evidence does not lend much support to the proposition that society is unanimously against harm reduction. According to the findings of Knowledge for Action in HIV/AIDS in the Russian Federation, a program funded by the UK Department for International Development from 2003 to 2007, while harm reduction was controversial and difficult to scale up, "the overall societal resistance to these strategies seems to be more of a widely believed myth than a fact. Harm reduction is supported and opposed by approximately the same proportion of decision-makers and the population with about a third taking neither side."[67]

The government, of course, could have either misunderstood the social cues or deliberately acted on conventional misperceptions in this regard, but there is no rhetorical proof that the Kremlin ever based its health-related decisions on public opinion. Nor do we have clear evidence of any political benefits for erecting legal obstacles to harm reduction. Instead, another interpretation seems more feasible. Russian policy makers fostered hostile attitudes to harm reduction as a tool for defending the country from the liberal ideals and policy proposals that contravened the Russian raison d'être. In this regard, Moscow's method of AIDS governance is self-defeating. Neglecting the vital needs of the most-at-risk population has morphed into huge inequalities in who gets adequate HIV-related services in Russia today. In addition, some deep-seated cultural factors will no doubt play a significant role in resisting additional international recommendations on the appropriate preventive practices. For instance, although scientific trials have provided compelling evidence that adult male circumcision can significantly reduce men's risks of becoming infected with HIV, this practice, despite its public health benefits, is not likely to spread in Russia. Currently, less than 20 percent of men who are circumcised in Russia belong to the country's Muslim population. It is likely that this state of affairs will not change in the near future.

At the same time, the Kremlin embraced the notions of universal HIV testing and extensive access to treatment. While favorable material conditions supported expanding investments in health, an internalized obligation to manage the economy for the sake of development was the reason behind the strategy of the country's leaders. Even after finding himself overwhelmed with mounting social obligations, Putin has refused to trim his spending. In the near future, the importance of access to prevention in Russia will grow precisely because the government scaled up access to life-saving treatment so successfully and because it failed to expand prevention.

PREVENTION AND TREATMENT IN MBEKI'S SOUTH AFRICA

In South Africa, the virus has spread to the general population. One of the most vulnerable groups and at the same time the driver of the spread of the disease has been HIV-positive mothers who pass the virus to their children during child-birth or while breast-feeding. Although nevirapine was effective for minimizing the risks of vertical transmission, for a while the Cabinet argued against mother-to-child prevention programs as too expensive and unsafe. Both Pretoria and provincial health officials neglected and even stalled national programs (see the first subsection below). The Cabinet ignored voices advocating a more state-centric approach to health than the market-centered empowerment would allow. Further evidence suggests that Pretoria chose to protect the private sector and did not employ it to improve the dismal health-care conditions in the public sector (see the second subsection below). Mocking the delivery state as the false god of his detractors, Mbeki assaulted the principle of universal access to health-care in the public sector. I qualify the common view that the level of treatment coverage is best explained by economic constraints. In a fledgling economy, the government is forced to keep expenditures in the public sector low. Ironically, with the advent of the global financial troubles, Pretoria's recalcitrance to external models of good health governance now seems like a sensible policy choice.

Access to Prevention in South Africa

International recommendations commonly underscore that treating most-at-risk groups is of critical importance. In South Africa, prevention efforts should focus on three large-scale interventions to stop predominantly heterosexual transmission of the human immunodeficiency virus.

First, individuals with multiple sexual partners, such as sex workers, should be empowered to engage in safe sex practices and should have good access to a variety of preventive and protective methods. The most effective way to prevent the spread of the virus among commercial sex workers is perhaps to decriminal-ize sex work and to regulate it thoroughly while improving access to condoms, reproductive health care, and HIV services. Another factor complicating HIV prevention among this at-risk population is that a significant number of commercial sex workers use various drugs during sexual transactions.[68] Some advocacy groups (such as the Cape Town–based Sex Worker Education and Advocacy Taskforce), politicians (Gauteng's current premier, Nomvula Mokonyane), and the African National Congress Women's League and the Commission for Gender Equality argue in favor of these goals. Although removing socioeconomic and gender barriers remains a daunting task, as early as 2000 the Cabinet understood that efforts to develop an appropriate social and legal environment for people living with HIV/AIDS, sex workers, and rape victims, as well as the urgent need to address gender-based violence, were crucial in fighting the contagion.[69] The High Court's ruling that the police were guilty of harassing sex workers on one occasion is also a promising sign that removing legal barriers to prevention and putting an end to organized harassment can be realistic policy goals. Without these incremental developments, the recent national strategic plan for sex workers that integrates public health and a human rights approach would not have been possible.[70]

Needless to say, the issue of sex work is also a part of the larger problem of gender inequality and the disproportionately higher prevalence of HIV among females. Despite the wide expression of conventional concerns for women's health and the rhetorical embrace of the Westernized organizing principles that underlie prevention strategies, evidence tentatively suggests that the continuing positive appraisal of traditional leadership structures keeps diminishing the power of otherwise effective messages on prevention and gender equality.[71] In other words, although myriad official documents and strategies follow internationally agreed-upon sensibilities, perpetuated structural factors still undermine the desired outcomes of health governance. Some seemingly time-honored and culturally appropriate social practices might appear to complement modern prevention strategies, but in reality, they only reinforce gender inequality and jeopardize human rights.[72] Thus, in order to stipulate the avenues for lifting the burden of AIDS in South Africa, the government should tackle the structural factors and address the complicated links between gender inequalities, patriarchal culture, and market-based means of socioeconomic empowerment.

Second, health education, awareness campaigns, and risk-reduction strategies should target youth. South Africa's largest ongoing HIV communication projects include Khomanani, Soul City, Soul Buddyz, and loveLife. While Soul Buddyz focuses on children age eight through twelve, it also reaches out to two-thirds of young adult females. LoveLife promotes sexual health education and awareness among adolescents and young adults age fifteen to twenty-four through the use of popular culture.[73] Sex education, which became an integral part of the South African Life Orientation curriculum after the Department of Education introduced it in 2002, now complements these large-scale awareness initiatives. As a result, there is modest encouraging evidence that by 2008 prevention strategies targeting adolescents and young adults had helped lower the prevalence and incidence of HIV within these two groups. Condom use among South African adults has been increasing as well. Although all these initiatives deserve positive mention, by and large they have failed to improve knowledge about various aspects of HIV/AIDS, including how the virus is transmitted. The persistent negative influences of various structural factors impede the rates of progress toward an AIDS-free generation. For instance, observers often note that shortages of highly trained educators and the soaring rates of school dropouts impede the effectiveness of the Life Orientation curriculum and undermine the influence of mass media campaigns and social marketing projects.[74]

Third, mother-to-child transmission must be prevented. South African children acquire the virus because their infected mothers transmit HIV to them during pregnancy, childbirth, or breast-feeding. To minimize the chances of HIV transmission to children, seropositive mothers should take preventive drugs during prenatal care. Preventive nevirapine has been at the center of domestic contestation regarding the appropriate methods of curbing the epidemic. It is surprising that potentially the least controversial dimension of the prevention strategies discussed above—reducing the rate of HIV transmission from infected mothers to their children in a medical setting—has generated the most domestic contention. The remainder of this subsection delves deeper into this issue.

In South Africa, the provision of antiretrovirals to mothers is a high priority because mothers constitute the key target vulnerable population in which the transmission of HIV is highly preventable. According to the South African Department of Health, by 2002 the level of seroprevalence in prenatal clinics had reached 25 percent, which was significantly higher than the incidence of HIV in the overall population (estimated at 10 percent). Despite the decreasing prices and increasing efficiency and safety of the drugs, the Cabinet was reluctant to offer antiretrovirals in the framework of mother-to-child transmission prevention programs. The central controversy was over nevirapine—the essential drug that significantly reduces the chances of HIV transmission to infants and that would notably alleviate the burden of palliative and pediatric care in the public health sector. In order not to offer the drug in the public sector, the South African government embarked on a course of contorted reasoning that attempted to demonstrate nevirapine's economic inefficiency and medical harm to patients. In practice, the course of reasoning described below meant that the Cabinet ignored the urgent health needs of the most vulnerable population.

The road to prevention by medicines could not have been rockier. In October 1998 the health minister, Nkosazana Dlamini-Zuma, decided to make nevirapine unavailable to mother-to-child programs any longer and to discontinue the pilot projects.[75] In 2000 Parks Mankahlana indicated that the fully implemented mother-to-child prevention programs would result in a dramatic increase in orphans and vulnerable children, which would deplete state resources in the future. Doubtless, in his capacity as presidential spokesman, Mankahlana expressed official ideas. In a cruel twist of fate, he was rumored to have died of an AIDS-related illness, although loyalists claimed that he died because he took the ARVs.[76]

In 1998, just at the time when Glaxo Wellcome drastically cut the price of azidothymidine, the drug that significantly reduced transmission during pregnancy and labor, the Health Ministry stopped trials of the drug, claiming that it was too expensive and that the ministry would focus on other prevention campaigns. In 2001 Boehringer Ingelheim offered to provide nevirapine free for use in the public sector in developing countries, but the government refused the offer. Dr. Ayanda Ntsaluba and Dr. Nono Simelela, chief director for HIV, AIDS, and STDs in the national Department of Health, repeatedly exaggerated the scientific and public health impact of nevirapine-resistant virus. The Cabinet insisted that the logistical costs of providing free treatment would be too high. That same year, however, the government offered preventive drugs to eliminate the chance of mother-to-child transmission on a trial basis at selected sites. While the provinces of Gauteng, KwaZulu-Natal, and the Western Cape were able to start decent mother-to-child programs, provincial officials obstructed the logistical support and planning of these programs in the other provinces.[77]

Over a period of several years, Treatment Action Campaign (TAC) activists argued that treatment was indispensable for prevention strategies and that it should be provided within the public health-care system. The organization initiated legal action against the government to offer nevirapine at all public hospitals. As a result, the High Court ordered expanded access to nevirapine in all provinces. Then again, in 2003, the Medicines Control Council (MCC) withdrew the license for the use of nevirapine. It rejected both the domestic studies at the Chris Hani Baragwanath Hospital in Johannesburg, the largest hospital in the country, and the Ugandan study that declared the drug safe and effective in preventing mother-to-child transmission.[78] Thus, the Cabinet attempted to stay its course, although the practical repercussions of doing so turned out to be disastrous.

In 2005, according to UNAIDS, less than 15 percent of pregnant women with HIV received preventive treatment. Because of that foot-dragging, in 2006 half a million babies were estimated to be infected with HIV during birth or breastfeeding in Africa, and many of the babies infected in the previous years of resistance to nevirapine survived only to puberty.[79] In November 2007 Deputy President Phumzile Mlambo-Ngcuka chaired a meeting with the South African National AIDS Council (SANAC) and announced a new mother-to-child treatment protocol consistent with global prescriptions.[80] Only in 2008 did pregnant women start receiving zidovudine (AZT). Many precious years that could have been devoted to prevention had been lost.

Policy was turned around eventually, but the change did not occur because of the calculations offered by prominent domestic health economists. There are reasons to believe that they had no impact on the position of the Department of Health, "despite medical and economic research showing that the costs of MTCTP [mother-to-child transmission prevention] were more than offset by the cost-savings associated with reduced numbers of HIV-related paediatric cases."[81] More consequential was the impact of prominent political figures, including Nelson Mandela, Desmond Tutu, and Mbhazima Shilowa, whom Mbeki and the Cabinet could not ignore. According to Patrick Furlong and Karen Ball, "State response to criticism from traditional supporters was the cabinet's dramatic recommitment on 17 April 2002 to fighting AIDS. . . . The cabinet also asserted that universal rollout of PMTCT [prevention of mother-to-child transmission] drugs and supportive programs for rape survivors were on track."[82] Over a period of several years, TAC activists argued that treatment was indispensable for prevention strategies and that it should be provided within the public health-care system. The final change in the policy occurred because of generous financial aid from international sources. The availability of international funding placated the Cabinet's financial concerns. The president's emergency plan made the following disbursements: 3,045,400 pregnant women received HIV counseling and testing services; 462,400 HIV-positive pregnant women received antiretroviral prophylaxis; and 528,100 orphans and vulnerable children benefited from the program in FY 2008 alone.[83]

In short, Mbeki's concerns about the alleged toxicity of Western medicines combined with the focus on restraining spending in the public health sector pushed the Cabinet to cancel nevirapine programs, despite their absolute necessity. Only several years after Mbeki's downfall did domestic prevention guidelines finally fall in line with the WHO strategy.[84] The results of the change are telling: according to the summary provided by the international charity AVERT, "Since 2009 South Africa has had one of the sharpest declines in new infections among children. In 2011, more than 95 percent of pregnant women with HIV received treatment to prevent the infection of their child. Yearly infections in children have dropped from 56,500 in 2009 to 29,100 in 2011."[85]

Mobilization of Finances in South Africa

Much has been said about the pernicious impact of neoliberal ideology on South African health governance. The most important aspects of that impact include the slowness of transformation in the health sector in the 1990s; the reduction of state resources spent on AIDS programs; the expansion of the finance ministry's power over other health departments' policies and programs; and the narrowness of the public debate on health, which has been limited primarily to issues of financial affordability.[86] The major point that bears emphasis here is that marketization as the core component of the African Renaissance impelled the government to reduce spending on public health in general. In 2003 health-care spending in the country was almost 5 percent lower in real terms than in 1996, while some provinces spent little more than a dollar per person per year. The devotion to market-centered empowerment also urged the Cabinet to shrink from strong spending commitments for HIV treatment. South African leaders argued that the government could not have afforded treatment in the public sector, despite the abundant external evidence that the rapid improvement of biomedical technology, the fast-growing industry of generics in India, Brazil, and Thailand, and the decreasing prices of medicines made antiretrovirals affordable at least in principle.

Protreatment coalitions and the critics of neoliberal economic predilections contributed to the public outcry against the Cabinet's ideas and policies. At the dawn of the century, a variety of high-profile activities, civil disobedience and litigation campaigns, and negotiations and talks at key "consensus-seeking institutions," such as the National Economic Development and Labour Council (NEDLAC), characterized the domestic policy environment. As a result of various pressures, the Cabinet gave in and on November 19, 2003, announced the new Operational Plan for Comprehensive HIV and Aids Care, Management and Treatment for South Africa. This plan stipulated the extensive provision of treatment in the framework of the public health-care system, arranged for a significant increase in AIDS-related funding, and suggested the appropriate number of patients to receive antiretrovirals.[87] Promises looked good on paper, but in reality, Pretoria stayed its course. The Cabinet did not hurry to mobilize the resources necessary to fulfill its promises. Although the number of treated patients in the public sector increased, Pretoria continued to hinder the scale-up efforts.

Between 2003 and 2005 such prominent think tanks as the South African Health System Trust (HST), the International Treatment Preparedness Coalition (ITPC), and the Institute for Democracy in South Africa (IDASA) were raising serious concerns about the implementation of the Operational Plan and the degree of financial commitments to it.[88] Their reports indicated several major flaws in South African health governance. First, the government had designated much less money for the full implementation of the announced targets than was required in reality. Second, provincial authorities that were directly responsible for social services in South Africa either delayed the procurement of drugs or failed to use the significant portion of resources allocated for the fight against the epidemic. For instance, in 2003 Gauteng and Mpumalanga failed to spend even half of the money allocated to them in conditional grants to fight the pandemic. According to press reports, provincial treatment numbers were either hard to obtain or not reliable. Provincial authorities evaded scrutiny because the Treasury and the Health Ministry failed to set up adequate monitoring and evaluation mechanisms that would have alleviated the persistent problem of underspending allocated resources. Third, although in fiscal year 2005–6 total HIV and AIDS budgets increased by 36 percent, the government failed to acknowledge the extent of the epidemic in the country. Thus, by 2005, although there were 192 public health facilities providing antiretrovirals in the country, only 18 percent of all individuals in need of treatment in the public sector were getting them.[89] Increased spending notwithstanding, in 2006 the provision of treatment did not reach approximately six hundred thousand patients who were in need of antiretrovirals.[90]

Needless to say, the hostility to antiretrovirals that was displayed by all too many provincial authorities was not crushed. Between 2006 and 2008, Peggy Nkonyeni, a member of the Executive Council who had forged strong connections with local organizations, invited thirty prominent antitreatment advocates to take part in an official information workshop. She also courted such outspoken opponents of conventional medicines as Dr. Cyril Khanyile of Medunsa University and Nhlavana Maseko, president of the Traditional Healers Organisation of South Africa (THO). Khanyile and Maseko condemned antiretrovirals and criticized spending money on biomedical research. Similarly, Mpumalanga health official Sibongile Manana frequently ordered doctors not to prescribe antiretrovirals.[91] Not surprisingly, in the province of KwaZulu-Natal, problems with the provision of ARVs persisted until 2009. In the Free State, the Department of Health imposed a moratorium on treatment therapy that lasted longer than the originally promised four months.[92]

Underperformance in health governance is commonly related to multiple logistical challenges and limited capacity and efficiency of the state and its bureaucracies. But it was intentional shirking that aggravated actual challenges. For instance, the government's focus on deficit reduction limited the public resources that otherwise could have been devoted to alleviating the often-lamented staff shortages in the public health sector.[93] There is enough rhetorical evidence to suggest that the Cabinet simply did not want to put all individuals who needed it on treatment. Besides considerations of affordability and sustainability, which at least were legitimate from the economic standpoint, Pretoria evoked the all-too-familiar images of the overbearing West pushing Africans to do things they did not want to do. Very illustrative was the episode when the health minister picked a fight against the WHO's "3 by 5" initiative. Tshabalala-Msimang offered that Pretoria did not "want to be pushed or pressurised by a target of three million people on antiretrovirals by 2005. WHO set that target themselves; they didn't consult us. I don't see why South Africa today must be the scapegoat for not reaching the target."[94]

Although both Pretoria and provincial health officials consistently stalled the implementation of national programs as a way to prevent overspending and block the spread of conventional medicines, they were losing social support. Even the Congress of South African Trade Unions (COSATU), part of the longstanding alliance with the African National Congress, joined TAC's quest for the universality of treatment. It is important to note here that these two organizations joined forces not because of COSATU's principled commitment to Western evidence-based medicine but rather because of the perceived failure of the Cabinet to improve the public health system and provide basic services to the poor. During the TAC Congress in September 2005, COSATU's general secretary, Zwelinzima Vavi, made it abundantly clear that Pretoria's inability to reach the poor in its consumerist-oriented prevention and education campaigns and its persistent underfunding and poor management of the public health sector impelled him to act.[95]

Finally, in October 2006 the new Strategic Plan for South Africa set clear and highly ambitious targets for scaling up treatment with the goal of putting 80 percent of all HIV-positive individuals on medicine. But the plan was developed under the leadership of new Deputy President Phumzile Mlambo-Ngcuka and at the moment when crumbling support for Mbeki coincided with a significant influx of external resources. South African activists were predictably impressed both by the process of consultations that culminated in the final document and the strategic plan itself.[96] The estimated costs of the new plan turned out to be quite staggering. Mlambo-Ngcuka projected that providing antiretroviral drugs for the duration of the plan's term would cost around 5.6 billion rand (roughly U.S.$750 million). Not surprisingly, implementation lagged way behind ambitions. National expenditures became adequate only by 2009.

Summary

The South African case illustrates the implications of social purposes for adopting international health governance standards. The increasing international commitment to treatment as a common good went against the internalized dedication to market-oriented economic empowerment and development. Neoliberal implications for mobilization of finances are not that hard to see and explain. At the same time, because human rights ideology was far from controversial for the proponents of the African Renaissance, issues of human rights and access to justice featured heavily in all South African national HIV/AIDS strategies. South African policy makers understood well that minimizing human rights violations, focusing on the rights of women and girls, and promoting gender and sexual equality to address gender-based violence were crucial for good AIDS governance. However, any further progress toward an AIDS-free generation in the country remains complicated, as it involves both correcting the recurring problems of policy implementation and lessening the multifaceted influence of various social and structural factors.

CONCLUSION

The evidence presented in this chapter supports the proposition that social purposes were the main obstacles on the course of adopting some components of the broad norm of universality of access to prevention and treatment. In Russia, the government equated harm reduction with the outright legalization of illicit substances, which would play into the hands of the subversive Westerners and undermine the ontological security of the Russian state. In South Africa, both Pretoria and provincial health officials consistently stalled the public introduction of national prevention and treatment programs and continuously sounded off about the critical importance of keeping the levels of expenditures low. The government's unwillingness to recognize essential medicines as a public good was a result of Pretoria's dedication to a market-centered empowerment that limited spending on social goals.

Given the stress on IDUs in this chapter, putting Russian public health strategies in various comparative contexts is necessary. Consider the South African context first. (Because drug use is not the main vector of the contagion in South Africa, the limited attention to harm reduction in this chapter seems reasonable.) Because intravenous drug use in South Africa has been relatively low (estimated at about 0.2 percent of the population), there are still very few official and operative sites that support harm-reduction strategies. There is only one site for the exchange of needles and syringes and six operational methadone and buprenorphine programs. While drug addiction treatment has been accessible mostly to white IDUs who co-pay or pay out of pocket for clinical services, almost half of South African intravenous drug users reported that hospitals and pharmacies refused to give them needles. At the same time, to rectify the impact of socioeconomic inequalities, Pretoria integrated public funding for drug treatment into primary health-care networks.[97] Thus, although South African decision makers have not yet adequately promoted harm-reduction programs, the core difference from Russia is that the South African Cabinet has not dismissed harm reduction as a legitimate method of public health governance. On the other hand, putting Russia in the post-Soviet regional context is illustrative as well. Ukraine, a country that apparently carries similar sociopolitical baggage, since 2004 has developed a vast harm-reduction program that includes 1,323 operational sites for needle and syringe exchanges and operational programs that dispense both methadone and buprenorphine.[98] When Russia annexed the Crimea in 2014, it immediately stopped all opioid substitute treatment programs, leaving eight hundred patients without necessary maintenance treatment. Clearly, then, the constraining influences of the past (including the often-mentioned inertia of Russian health administrators) are not the main or sole reasons for the current deficiencies in Russian health governance.

While this chapter delineated the impact of social purposes on the universality of prevention and treatment, it did not fully touch upon the complexity of relationships between various domestic actors in health governance. Many questions remain unanswered thus far. It behooves me to reflect on the interaction between governments and nonstate actors in more detail. In the next chapter I focus on the following questions. First, did policy debates in either country reflect the widening competency of health bureaucracies or the parochial goals of the state? Were health agencies able to exercise their functions to the extent that was warranted by the scope of their organizational missions and competencies? Second, how did social purposes affect the partnership arrangements between governments and private actors? Did the Russian devotion to the autonomous state as the core goal of the state predispose the government against some individuals and groups in health governance? Did South African leaders engage some of the country's nonstate organizations as respected partners because these organizations shared Pretoria's ideational preoccupations? And third, how did Putin's Russia and Mbeki's South Africa try to alter the global health landscape? The next chapter is an inquiry into the underlying tendencies that shaped the patterns of AIDS partnership in Russia and South Africa.

CHAPTER 5

Selecting Partners

The State and Key Stakeholders

TRANSBOUNDARY COOPERATION IN response to AIDS and domestic collaboration between the state and all relevant stakeholders improve the quality of health governance. Governments, bilateral and multilateral donors, the private sector, civil society organizations, affected communities, faith-based organizations, academic institutions, and people living with HIV should join forces to fight AIDS. The state, of course, remains highly relevant for mobilizing individuals and groups against the contagion, but to restrain partnerships and exclude key stakeholders is to create an environment that inhibits good health governance.

To embrace external and domestic nonstate actors as equals, the state has to accept the notion of nonhierarchical relations as an organizing principle of governance. Some governments cannot accept this principle without much effort, because nonstate actors make novel claims of justice and set new standards of appropriate behavior that might be uncomfortable to the state's modus operandi. Certain normative obligations, expressed in legitimate social purposes, might also undermine the state's willingness to cooperate with those actors that do not share the elite's normative predilections.

The structure of this chapter follows the blueprint established in the preceding chapters. The discussion of international approaches to partnership sets the stage for examining my empirical cases. Russian and South African stories reveal how committed elites chose to deal with nonstate health actors in order to fulfill their ideational commitments. First, Russian law enforcement and government-friendly opinion leaders captured the policy debate and dominated it; the top tier of South African politicians continuously tried to reshuffle and dominate the AIDS bureaucracy. Second, Russian government brusquely reined in civil society and the private sector; South Africans pursued a selective engagement with those individuals and groups that shared Pretoria's devotion to alternative and traditional medicines. Third, governments of either country tried to act as norm givers and endeavored to secure an authoritative position in the global health landscape, although material prerequisites for doing so were not in place.

In general, while from the empirical standpoint the patterns of partnerships in Russia and South Africa were quite different, in both countries committed elites developed expectations about the appropriate role of domestic groups; elites then based their management of social groups involved in health governance on those expectations.

INTERNATIONAL APPROACHES TO PARTNERSHIP

To make sure that health governance systems operate properly, governments must be open to collaborate with all relevant stakeholders. At the beginning of this century, a clearly identifiable norm of diffuse partnership was entrenched in numerous health institutions.[1] This section operationalizes this best practice: first, it looks at public-private partnerships, then discusses the indispensable role of civil society, and concludes with international AIDS organizations.

Public-Private Partnership

The partnership between the government and the private sector in health governance is a relatively recent phenomenon.[2] The National Council for Public-Private Partnerships defines a partnership as "a contractual agreement between a public agency (federal, state or local) and a private sector entity. Through this agreement, the skills and assets of each sector (public and private) are shared in delivering a service or facility for the use of the public. In addition to the sharing of resources, each party shares in the risks and rewards potential in the delivery of the service and/or facility."[3] Christer Jönsson highlighted the significance of diffuse partnerships to combat HIV/AIDS and underscored the absence of any lead agency in such an arrangement.[4]

Since HIV/AIDS presents an enormous challenge for everyone, governments should invite the private sector to fight the epidemic with them. The opposite of this standardized practice is either trying to safeguard the private sector by excluding it from solving problems of common action or purposefully overcommitting to fight the pandemic exclusively within the framework of the domestic public health sector. Both choices can generate detrimental consequences, especially in countries operating in resource-poor settings.[5]

In 2001 Richard Holbrooke turned a small group named the Global Business Coalition on HIV/AIDS, Tuberculosis and Malaria (GBC) into a major international health actor. This consortium of organizations mobilizes businesses to sponsor public health emergencies and advocates a broader involvement of business in HIV/AIDS as a matter of national and human security. Merck, for instance, joins and sponsors different global and regional partnerships, as well.[6] In sum, the emphasis on public-private partnerships is part of the consensus on the appropriate methods of good AIDS governance.

Partnership with Civil Society

Civil society organizations often act as innovators in AIDS governance and simultaneously challenge the inert structures of the state's authority. Nonstate stakeholders often embrace new ideas, implement innovative health interventions, and excel at dealing with complex and sensitive public health issues. Partnerships with relevant domestic stakeholders, both private and public, allow governments to tailor domestic policy responses to the conditions on the ground, diversify services, and improve outreach.[7] For these and other practical reasons, the state must support the work of volunteers, health service organizations, and noncommercial entities, both domestic and transboundary. At the very least, governments should not erect insurmountable bureaucratic barriers, exclude social groups from the policy formulation and implementation process, and choke them financially. Solely relying on governmental programs is not likely to sustain good AIDS governance.

One of the first prominent efforts to spread the norm of partnership belonged to WHO's Global AIDS Programme (GAP, 1986–1995). GAP focused on improving surveillance, encouraged governments to develop national AIDS plans, promoted human rights, and facilitated fund raising. The literature praising GAP's contribution to the international efforts against AIDS sees GAP as a successful agency that helped connect governments to other subnational actors and the civil society sector. GAP was also able to link international donor organizations, including the United States Agency for International Development (USAID), to domestic recipients.[8] Despite all these achievements, the absence of effective and affordable HIV therapies triggered donor fatigue and undermined interest in developing a strong partnership with civil society organizations.

The invention of the highly active triple therapy empowered AIDS activists and health advocacy organizations. Instead of building partnerships and networks based exclusively on human rights principles, civil society can do so using professional claims and evidence-based solutions. Today, various stakeholders across the globe can receive financial support from many sources. Launched in January 2001, the Global Fund to Fight AIDS, Tuberculosis and Malaria (GFATM) is a major financing mechanism that ensures sustainable funding for numerous local projects and leverages additional financial resources from a variety of governmental and private sources. In 2007 alone, the total of disbursed resources amounted to almost $4 billion. The Framework Document of GFATM indicates that this organization supports simplified, rapid, and bottom-up disbursement mechanisms that "reflect national ownership and respect country-led formulation and implementation processes."[9]

Nonstate actors apply to the state for approval and funding of their proposals for necessary programs. Further funding depends on the performance of these programs. An important mechanism to foster civil society's and service organizations' engagement with the fight against AIDS at the country level is the country coordinating mechanism, which promotes multistakeholder partnerships, local ownership, and participatory decision making. Although there is valid criticism that these mechanisms are vulnerable to state capture, a state should understand that such behavior is not desirable and not condoned. These mechanisms indeed bring together state officials and the representatives of a wide range of nonstate actors that fight AIDS on the ground.

In addition to the spread of the general understanding that nongovernmental organizations are indispensable for fighting AIDS, there are many think tanks that offer specific recommendations on how to engage domestic civil society for good health governance and that tailor their messages to specific governments. For instance, in 2003 the experts from the Center for Strategic and International Studies and the Brookings Institution specified the principles that the Kremlin should have embraced in order to involve domestic civil society effectively. They suggested that the Russian government promote policies that not only tolerate the existence of the nongovernmental organizations but also encourage their growth and robustness. Generous tax incentives, training programs for the leaders of NGOs, financial influxes, and predictable rules of interaction could have mended the relationships between state officials and NGOs.[10] These goals were extensive and ambitious, but at the dawn of Putin's rule, they were reasonably attainable. But, as will be shown below, that permissive environment did not last very long. Putin's Russia took an entirely different route.

Partnership with International AIDS Organizations

The global landscape of health-related organizations is immensely complex.[11] It is impossible to give here full justice to all significant initiatives and programs. The discussion that follows simply sets the stage for the ensuing analysis of governance choices in the two countries under investigation. The bottom line is that, in the early twenty-first century, governments have been encouraged to work in tandem with multiple global and transnational organizations and discouraged from obstructing their activities.

For resource-limited countries, the success in curbing the epidemic is often directly dependent on the quality of partnership with international AIDS organizations. Invaluable is access to modern epidemiological expertise, an uninterrupted supply of effective medications, and the availability of various grants and funding. Working with international organizations is especially important for the governments that either lack the requisite financial and infrastructural capacities to curb the epidemic on their own or require assistance to increase the capacity of the public health-care sector, institutionalize financial flows, or improve service quality and outreach. In certain cases, countries shirk from strong spending commitments and decide to rely on foreign-sponsored programs. Overreliance on external help leads to outright donor dependency, which might generate negative externalities and diminish domestic incentives to develop a strong public health-care system. Among the countries fighting HIV/AIDS, Russia and South Africa occupy a unique place. These two countries are neither fully dependent on international donors nor fully able to rely on their own resources.

Today, multilateral health organizations have converted some of the generic political pledges of developed nations to fight HIV/AIDS into an institutionalized routine that is not easily reversible. The new generation of AIDS organizations sponsors HIV-related programs and therefore provides strong incentives for governments to follow the global consensus of methods for good AIDS governance. GFATM and President's Emergency Plan for AIDS Relief (PEPFAR) have helped overcome the problem of the erratic supply of drugs, a problem that undermines the benefits of treatment and triggers drug resistance. Those two organizations recently became the most important global instruments for stimulating the improvement of public health in nations constrained by limited resources. For the developing nations, gaining external resources and receiving transfers from the Global Fund is contingent on following international norms and best practices.

Many practitioners and activists have habitually lamented the insufficient level of funding from the major international donors. But this concern does not imply that broad financial commitments on behalf of the international health organizations and the donor community are nonexistent. Rather, activists are pushing donors to allocate the extremely high and often unrealistic amount of resources.

There is a clear understanding now that international health organizations pursue exclusively humanitarian goals. Unfounded are realist-like suspicions that the industrialized world uses these organizations as a hypocritical implement to pursue its parochial goals. Further, less-developed states have found out that international health assistance does not really give organizations' wealthy donors any political leverage to influence domestic affairs in the countries that accept such assistance. Quite the contrary—the recipients of health assistance have gained leverage over the sponsors of health programs.[12] When governments claim otherwise, it means that they either have misinterpreted the nature of global health governance or are chasing an internal political agenda that has other motivations than improving public health.

Serious reservations about the impact of the World Trade Organization and the World Bank on domestic health might be warranted. Concerns about GFATM and PEPFAR might be justified too, but only to the degree that these concerns help enhance their transparency and increase the effectiveness of these institutions. It does not mean, however, that these organizations are devoid of any internal problems. A sober analysis identifies both strong and weak aspects of their performance.[13] Indeed, international health organizations in general have to rectify many potentially debilitating shortcomings, such as the crisis of credibility, the emergent corruption, uneven allocation of resources, and prioritizing the fight against some "fashionable" and "exceptional" diseases while ignoring other grave health challenges.

PEPFAR is the biggest global program dealing with the HIV/AIDS pandemic. In his 2003 State of the Union Address, President George W. Bush announced the generous commitment of $15 billion over five years to fight AIDS globally by providing antiretroviral treatment for two million people, preventing seven million AIDS deaths, providing care to ten million people in the focus countries, and building a self-sustaining health infrastructure. Besides increasing treatment coverage and treatment promotion, on a larger scale, PEPFAR promotes country ownership and helps developing local infrastructures to establish self-sustainable local health programs. Judged by its general design, this infrastructure-building plan looks valuable for fostering good health governance across the globe. Targeted countries include twelve African, two Caribbean, and one Asian states.[14] The selected countries account for approximately 50 percent of the world's HIV/AIDS infections. Among these countries, Uganda, Kenya, and South Africa are receiving the lion's share of contributions. Although the Russian Federation is not technically PEPFAR's focus country, in 2006 it was put on the second tier of five additional countries of interest that receive additional bilateral funding. In 2008 Congress reauthorized the Emergency Plan and approved up to $48 billion over the next five years to combat global HIV/AIDS, tuberculosis, and malaria. PEPFAR is also the cornerstone of the American vision for an "AIDS-free generation."

PEPFAR works with key South African departments at the national level and all provincial governments, thereby promoting the multisector governance of AIDS in the country. During Mbeki's presidency, PEPFAR's bilateral funding amounted to approximately $1.44 billion. PEPFAR put South Africa in a somewhat unique and privileged position among the other recipient countries, as the program directly underwrote a sizable share of the expenditures intended for treatment, prevention, and clinical care in the country. According to the official data, during the first six years of PEPFAR's operation in the country, more than nine hundred thousand individuals were put on antiretroviral treatment, almost seven hundred thousand HIV-positive pregnant women received necessary services to prevent mother-to-child transmission of HIV, and about two hundred thousand of them obtained antiretroviral prophylaxis. South Africa's Emergency Plan Small Grants Program empowered community-based organizations and grassroots groups (e.g., the Maboloka HIV/AIDS Awareness Organization and the Lighthouse Foundation) to engage in various small-scale activities. In 2007 PEPFAR supported technical training and improved capacity to manage treatment regimes in Eastern Cape's Frere Hospital. The program's portfolio also included the support of domestic initiatives that promoted behavioral changes and spread messages about the critical role of abstention, faithfulness, and the use of condoms in order to prevent sexual transmission of the virus. During South Africa's transition phase, PEPFAR has continued its efforts to strengthen South African health systems and maintain financial support totaling half a billion dollars a year.[15]

For Russia, the prerequisites for engaging transnational civil society in the fight against HIV were all in place. Many international NGOs have distinguished themselves by doing excellent health-related work. The list of the most known and renowned organizations includes American International Health Alliance,

Doctors without Borders, GBC, International Medical Corps, Aide Médico Sociale Russie, International Union against Tuberculosis and Lung Disease, Partners in Health, Project HOPE, People to People International, Center for Human Services–University Research Company, and AIDS Foundation East-West. Transatlantic Partners against AIDS (TPAA) galvanized interorganizational alliances, raised awareness about the social implications of HIV, engaged in advocacy, and provided treatment and various services for people living with AIDS in Russia. TPAA has broad public outreach via the Online Policy Resource Center on HIV/AIDS and high-level policy conferences that feature prominent politicians and famous TV personalities. TPAA's annual policy reports, policy briefs, analysis of regional health programs, and advocacy efforts remain an independent international source of information on the epidemic and governmental policies.

The point that bears emphasis here is that concerns about the performance of international health organizations are legitimate, but these concerns should not turn into motivations to either disrupt these organizations' work or reject their recommendations and guidelines. To sabotage the work of international AIDS organizations or to try to insulate a state from their activities is counterproductive in terms of mitigating the continuing spread of the virus.

Summary

Despite many actual and potential roadblocks to cooperation between governments on the one side and all relevant stakeholders on the other, international agreement on the utility of building partnerships is hard to ignore or dismiss as irrelevant. In the following two large empirical sections, I demonstrate how and why Russia and South Africa responded to the principle of nonstate and nonhierarchical governance. Under certain conditions, accepting the principle of nonhierarchical and nonstate cooperation with multiple individuals and groups is painful. Some states refuse to suffer this pain and instead make deliberate choices that are likely to create a frustrating policy environment. The first sign that a state is likely to resist that organizing principle is when some high-powered elite groups hijack the policy debate and undermine the routine tasks of health bureaucracies. Although AIDS bureaucracy, of course, is part of the government, the state should not intrude into the specialized sphere of that bureaucracy's professional competencies and expertise. I deal with this issue in the opening subsections of my Russian and South African cases. First, I trace how ruling groups limited the discretion of policy participants to decide a policy course and constrained their actions. Second, for the purposes of the subsequent discussion, I divide the group of relevant partners into three broad categories: the private sector, domestic civil society, and international health organizations.

HEALTH PARTNERSHIP IN PUTIN'S RUSSIA

Liberal principles of partnership threatened the Russian devotion to hierarchical and state-centered governance as substantiated in the ideas of sovereign democracy. In Putin's Russia, the *siloviki* captured the policy debate on HIV/AIDS and framed it according to their ideas and organizational mission. The first subsection locates the Federal Drug Control Service (FSKN) as an especially important policy actor whose power to shape the public discussion on AIDS exceeded that of the Ministry of Health and the members of the organized medical community combined. FSKN's officials linked the crisis to the threatening growth of narcotics consumption and downplayed the image of the epidemic as a public health crisis in its own right. The second subsection substantiates the proposition that the Kremlin designed the National Priority Projects (NPPs)—the framework for disbursing resources and transforming the health-care sector—in order to deliver on the government's social obligations and crowd out the private sector as an independent force in public health. The third subsection traces the increasingly belligerent attitudes that many state officials no longer feel obligated to conceal when they have to engage with civil society. This negativity bordering on overt disdain is not very surprising, given that civil society is surely a threat to the goal of hierarchical and state-centered governance. As long as the current social purpose dominates, the independent role of Russian civil society in health governance will remain limited. Finally, I discuss Moscow's ambitions to put its stamp on the international health landscape and insulate its civil society from any sources of external nourishment.

Capturing the Policy Debate in Putin's Russia

In October 2006 the government created a special governmental committee on HIV/AIDS, which, at least in theory, was intended to foster a multisector dialogue and streamline the consolidated national strategy to respond to HIV/AIDS as a broad public health crisis.[16] Unfortunately, this special multisector committee has remained largely defunct since its inception and has not convened even once since 2009. After several years of initial recognition of AIDS as a potential threat, it became obvious the Russian government did not want to formulate a comprehensive strategy against AIDS. This seems counterintuitive, especially since the Kremlin used the epidemic as a public relations tool in its attempt to lionize its own efforts to eradicate the epidemic. Satisfied with the direction of HIV/AIDS policy, top leaders did not stop the efforts of law enforcement agencies, most notably the FSKN, to dominate the debate on AIDS.

As explained in chapter 3, the *siloviki* in general acted as the main champions of the common good. The dramatis personae includes the head of FSKN, Viktor Cherkesov; the deputy head of FSKN, Aleksandr Mikhailov; the head of the State Antinarcotics Committee (GAK) and the new director of FSKN, Victor Ivanov; and the deputy prime minister, Igor Sechin, who is believed to be the informal leader of the *siloviki* "clan." It is not by chance that when the Kremlin set up the Council for the Development of the Pharmaceutical and Medical Industry, Sechin became its supervisor.[17] The State Duma deputy Mikhail Grishankov, one of the most highly visible political leaders involved in the fight against HIV/AIDS, has a KGB background as well. Together, all these individuals were able to capture the policy debate on HIV/AIDS and tweak it to match their ideas and tastes. They spread their views via multiple newspaper interviews, radio appearances, and policy publications. In his April 2006 interview for radio station Radio Rossii, Grishankov stated that the outbreak of the epidemic of HIV was secondary to the scourge of heroin consumption. Grishankov explained that he had been deeply alarmed about the skyrocketing numbers of addicts in his native province. Accordingly, that concern motivated him to join the fight against HIV. In essence, his outlook succinctly expressed the *siloviki*'s failure to address the spread of the virus as a public health problem.

The *siloviki* had enough power to act as energetic policy entrepreneurs. They also sought to engage the conservative wing of the Russian Orthodox Church as their tacit ally. To do so, in 2007 FSKN distributed to all of its regional branches a book penned by Anatoliy Berestov, a Russian Orthodox monk and the founder of the Charitable Center of Saint John of Kronstadt in Moscow. In a nutshell, that book was a lengthy diatribe against Western human rights–based approaches to health governance. It also dwelled on the seemingly irreconcilable differences between the righteous war on drugs and the moral shakiness of harm reduction. The book also implied that drug addicts should be treated with prayer and religion.[18] Recently, that tacit alliance seems to have become explicit. In February 2010 Viktor Ivanov opened a conference entitled "Spiritual and Medicinal Help in Overcoming the Sins of Narcotics Addiction, Alcoholism, and Tobacco Smoking."[19] In January 2011 the deputy director of FSKN, Nikolay Tsvetkov, took part in the antinarcotics section of a faith-based educational conference. Tsvetkov talked mostly about forging a partnership between the church and the law enforcement agencies. In 2012 the agency and the faith-based radio station Radonezh recorded and aired an educational series entitled "To Save Children from Narcotics."

FSKN became a major player in Russian health governance by means of expanding its organizational mission way beyond its original law enforcement mandate. Although the director of FSKN, Viktor Ivanov, never concealed this expansionist ambition, only in 2013 did he openly claim a mandate to suspend any questionable substance on the market without any formal consultation with the Ministry of Health or the professional medical community. FSKN is also in the process of creating its own system of rehabilitative centers for illicit drug users. The *siloviki*'s understandable preference for the punitive approach to vulnerable populations is likely to trump the solid statistical evidence that such measures as syringe exchange programs are extremely helpful to mitigate the impact of intravenous drug use as one of the primary driving forces of the epidemic in the country.

According to a renowned antialcohol and antinarcotics social entrepreneur, Oleg Zykov, the de facto expansion of the FSKN has routinely jeopardized the use of conventional painkillers in Russian hospitals. With an expanded and loose definition of narcotics and psychotropic-like substances, FSKN will be able to interfere with any firm that legally uses products such as industrial solvents and poppy seeds. Less amusing than that, FSKN also wishes to expand its organizational mandate to supervise both the structure and finances of all extant government antidrug and HIV-related programs.

The steadily growing allocation of federal resources to fight the consumption of illicit substances and to supervise all narcotics-related programs means the *siloviki* have acquired an immense power to dispense and channel financial resources. The government allocated 212 billion rubles for the federal program against drug trafficking for 2013–20, which marked an incredible seventyfold increase compared to the moneys allocated for similar a program from 2005 to 2009. But that bid for organizational expansion did not go as smoothly as Ivanov hoped. In December 2013 the members of the Public Chamber contested his aspiration to regulate the core aspects of narcotics policy and interfere with the activities of social actors and other health-related agencies that did not fall in the official sphere of law enforcement oversight. In addition, the Russian liberal-minded expert community resisted FSKN's bid to acquire leverage on both business and nonprofits and even called for its disbandment.[20]

As the strength of the *siloviki* and conservative voices in the policy debate has increased, the role of health professionals in both Cabinet-level positions and more modest midlevel bureaucratic roles has dwindled. The Ministry of Health was especially unlucky since it was not able to exercise policy-making power independently of the *siloviki*. While its head officials often took the blame for the failures of AIDS policy design and implementation, in reality, neither Mikhail Zurabov nor his successor, Tat'yana Golikova, were able to act as independent policy makers. Russia's chief medical officer, Dr. Gennadiy Onishchenko, until his retirement in 2013 seemed to toe the *siloviki* line as well. While not tied to law enforcement via any prior or current organizational affiliation or his own personal background, on many occasions he derided the vital importance of harm reduction.

Above, I discussed how the *siloviki* captured the policy dialogue on HIV and turned it into a monologue emphasizing the issues of narcotics consumption in the country. This policy capture would hardly have been possible were it not for the prior framing of HIV not just as a public health crisis but rather as an artificially provoked demographic menace to the Russian state to be resolved by active state intervention. In general, this evidence also complements one of my core observations that the state bureaucracy, with all its top decision makers, insulated themselves from key domestic stakeholders and the professional medical community.

The Government and the Private Sector

Purposeful government efforts to implement public-private interaction mechanisms and contract the private sector for public needs are pivotal to increase the capacity of the public health-care sector.

On balance, although throughout Putin's presidency, many roundtables, discussions, and public panels were attended by the representatives of both business and government, these initiatives can hardly be classified as meaningful and consequential. In March 2003 the representatives of high-powered business circles of the Russian Union of Industrialists and Entrepreneurs (RSPP) lamented that they could not meaningfully participate in the fight against HIV/AIDS because the government failed to formulate a clear strategy for how the private sector could contribute to the eradication of HIV/AIDS.[21] In 2007 GBC and TPAA organized a conference entitled "Leaders Forum on Public-Private Partnerships" that engaged more than 180 leaders from around the world. The following year, Moscow hosted a roundtable entitled "Training of Employees in the Health Sector" that involved more than twenty Russian and international corporations as the roundtable participants. They shared the experiences of HIV, alcoholism, and other socially significant diseases among their employees and discussed plans to improve health in the workplace. Paying lip service to the necessity of involving business as an equal partner in AIDS governance, the Kremlin simply poured more and more money into upgrading the public sector, while the private sector was never involved in the fight against AIDS to its full capacity.

Most importantly, Russian officials designed the NPPS as a state-centric tool in initiating and implementing national economic improvement. In essence, the NPPS provided funding to upgrade the public health sector. By Russian standards, the amount spent turned out to be truly colossal and historically unprecedented, especially compared to the cash-strapped 1990s. In general, state funding for HIV/AIDS-related programs grew exponentially from 2005. In 2007 alone, the government spent $444.8 million to fight HIV, and an additional $105 million went to the Global Fund. In 2009 Russia pledged about $392 million for various HIV/AIDS initiatives.

Total funding through the NPPS between 2006 and 2010 amounted to more than $1 billion. The funding for HIV/AIDS went primarily through NPPS and far surpassed other sources of funding for AIDS, including the Federal Targeted Program, World Bank project, Globus program, and GFATM disbursements. Between 2006 and 2010, overall health-related spending in the framework of the NPPS reached 400 billion rubles (approximately U.S.$13.5 billion). In April 2010 Putin, then in his temporarily humble role as prime minister, announced an additional 460 billion rubles (approximately U.S.$15 billion) to be invested to modernize the health-care infrastructure and increase its capacity within the next several years.[22] The Council primarily directed NPP Health to rebuild the public health-care infrastructure, to raise the salaries of doctors and nurses, and to increase the number of broadly trained health-care practitioners as opposed to narrow specialists. According to analyses done by TPAA and GBC, the government channeled as much as 86 percent of the committed resources to construction, while the provision for treatment and palliative care received only 14 percent.[23]

The 2006 collective report compiled by well-known domestic liberal economists and health-care practitioners positively evaluated the general NPP approach to reforms in the health sector.[24] At the same time, this report indicated that the Kremlin had committed itself to too many social obligations. For this reason, insightful observers came to view the NPPs as a return to a quasi-socialist system of health governance.[25] Backpedaling on the market mechanisms surely had become a hallmark of the Putin health administration. Consider additional evidence.

While the government rapidly expanded the public sector, its partnerships with the private sector deteriorated. To pay for public health, the Kremlin chose to burden the private sector with more taxes. In the spring of 2010, Putin announced that the private sector would be taxed an additional 2 percent to cover the anticipated shortages in public health care in 2011–12.[26] He proposed to allocate the money—460 billion rubles—to reconstruct hospital buildings and clinics, increase the quality of health-care services, and include some unspecified additional help for pensioners. This decision effectively disregarded the multiple pleas made by members of the RSPP and representatives of business circles. The liberals noted that, while ignoring the private sector, the government perpetuated the flaws in the public health-care sector.

In the 1990s the Russian government liberalized domestic pharmaceutical markets. Russian consumers were no longer victims of prescription drug shortages and enjoyed access to a wider variety of brands.[27] Yet the idea of the developmental state galvanizing economic growth and domestic markets supported policy reversal.[28] In 2007 the Ministry of Health and Social Development intervened to regulate the prices on pharmaceutical products. In doing so, the ministry neglected to consult with experts from the Formulary Committee of the Russian Academy of Medical Sciences. Paved with good intentions, the road to price control led to administrative restrictions, shortages of cheaper drugs and disincentives to produce them, and the growing anxiety of the drug firms and medical professionals. The price control stabilized prices, but only negligibly so.[29]

In summary, the purpose for becoming a developmental state contributed to a rapid expansion of the state-managed and state-financed sector of health care and gave the government reasons to control pharmaceutical markets via noneconomic means. The money available from the sale of hydrocarbons mattered because that income supported a permissive financial environment, but intentional devotion to state-led development was the chief reason for the government's actions. The evidence presented in this section suggests that the Kremlin overcommitted to act as the sole provider of funds for the health sector while shying away from meaningful engagement with the private sector. Throughout this period, the government remained willing to cover the costs of treatment exclusively from its budget.[30]

Restraining Civil Society

During the early stages of the domestic fight against HIV/AIDS, Putin's administration accepted nongovernmental organizations (NGOs) as partners in improving public health but gradually became hostile to most of them. Why did that happen? After all, the openness of Russia's external borders suggests that learning about the importance of nonhierarchical and nonstate principles of governance was possible. In general, the idea that civil society acts on the liberal conception of the common good and sustains decentralized spheres of authority that menace the self-contained state shaped Putin's orientation toward the nonstate sector.

There are many domestic nonstate actors with distinguished records of fighting AIDS. Healthy Russia Foundation, Open Health Institute, Russian Harm Reduction Network, Russian Health Care Foundation, ESVERO, AIDS-Infoshare, and FOCUS-MEDIA have spearheaded health promotion efforts and implemented many successful programs across the country. If nothing else, for the Russian government, fostering partnerships with these organizations is a rational governance course that allows diversifying the ways of providing treatment and prevention services and reaching out to places not currently covered by government programs. But these organizations embody the principle of nonhierarchical governance insofar as they are not co-opted into the domestic top-down power hierarchy, to the degree that they are legally able to receive global funding, and as long as they are able to implement programs that they deem important.

As explained in chapter 2, the Kremlin detested the idea of an autonomous civil society but tolerated those noncommercial entities if their missions, styles, and strategies were compatible with Moscow's goals. For instance, the Health and Development Foundation, a Russian NGO that develops and implements health communication and improves maternal health in Russia, acquired massive sponsorship from USAID. This sponsorship did not incur the state's animosity because the foundation's cardinal mission matched the government's focus on demographic security and increased fertility.[31]

To be fair, during the early stages of the domestic battle against the epidemic, many elected politicians demonstrated a willingness to work closely with HIV-related organizations. Tat'yana Yakovleva, the chair of the State Duma Committee for Health from 2004 to 2007, for instance, on multiple occasions underscored the essential role of civil society in educating wider audiences on prevention and increasing trust in the domestic health-care sector. In order to prevent the large-scale spread of the epidemic in Russia, Artur Chilingarov, Ol'ga Borzova, Vladimir Ryzhkov, Valeriy Zubov, and Nadezhda Gerasimova joined an interfactional deputies working group on prevention and treatment of HIV/AIDS and other socially significant infectious diseases. But over time that willingness dissipated.

As the country became increasingly wealthy, the Kremlin pledged to fund charities and "socially valuable" organizations. According to different estimates, there are between one hundred and three hundred smaller nongovernmental AIDS service organizations working as subcontractors for the bigger NGOs and the regional governments.[32] In 2011 the government simply retracted its previously generous pledges to sponsor domestic nonstate service organizations and returned to the treasury a significant portion of the money that had been officially earmarked for prevention programs.[33] In 2012 no presidential grants were awarded to any mainstream nonprofits with a good performance record of helping people living with HIV and AIDS. As a result, health NGOs that are now devoid of any source of funding have to either let their personnel go or simply shut down. The massive flow of the workforce from nongovernmental AIDS organizations to the state-run AIDS medical facilities is a telltale sign of the organizational depletion of the nonstate sector.

Further complications paralyzing health partnerships between the government and key domestic stakeholders arise from the fact that politicians and the general public have gradually embraced the idea that the independent NGOs were subversive agents of external influence. This intersubjective understanding impels Russian health policy analysts to take a scunner against transnational nonstate actors and their activities.

A study recently published by the Russian Institute for Strategic Studies, a prominent think tank headed by a retired foreign intelligence general, featured many barely concealed accusations against transboundary actors but skated over any rigorous evaluation of their work. The authors exposed the pernicious effects of the evidence-based methods of prevention and were dismayed to admit the influence of those methods on youths. The study's main conclusion, in just one paragraph, tied together a great variety of Russian insecurities:

Despite the fact that "medical" NGOs usually claim that their activities are free from politics and ideology, the results of their ten-year-long work in Russia nevertheless show that their programs had a marked impact on the Russian mentality, behavior, and system of interpersonal relationships. In particular, during numerous long-term projects on Russian soil, foreign NGOs managed to impose the "Westernized," mainly American, model of resisting HIV/AIDS on the Russian youth. . . . [D]istribution of syringes "legitimized" addiction, and "safe" sex among youth increased their disposition to an unconstrained freedom of choice and hedonism. And it's safe to say that the Western fight against HIV/AIDS has contributed to the spread of these diseases in the Russian Federation.[34]

Insofar as the *siloviki* and conservative opinion leaders have taken umbrage at an autonomous civil society that espouses liberal values, their friendliness toward conservative domestic charities that operate under state guidance has increased. It is not surprising, then, that the ultraconservative rehabilitative centers of Saint John of Kronstadt received governmental accolades and became a priority for government funding, while mainstream nongovernmental health organizations that had previously received assistance from independent international sources were snubbed.[35] There is mounting evidence to suggest that the church's role in health governance is on the rise. For instance, Berestov's charity centers emphasize the rehabilitation of drug addicts, alcoholics, and gamblers and promote a heavily conservative and faith-based approach to HIV/AIDS eradication. In July 2009 the Russian Orthodox Church presented its own comprehensive reappraisal of the meanings and implications of the HIV epidemic in the country. The document stated that the root cause of the rapid spread of the epidemic was the loss of fundamental spiritual values and religious guidelines in Russian society. The HIV epidemic, in short, was the direct consequence of the sinful lifestyles of ordinary Russians and their misguided lapses from virtue. No one should have expected any other phrasing coming out of a conservative faith-based organization, but since Putin's interpretation of the core goals of the state has progressively engaged conservative and antisecular values, this document might indicate which methods of AIDS governance the Kremlin will likely sanction as the most appropriate in the foreseeable future.

In summary, throughout Putin's and Medvedev's presidential tenures, frequent changes in legislation created confusion among internal and external observers about the baseline relations between the Kremlin and civil society. On the one hand, the Russian government was reluctant to nourish civil society's independence. On the other hand, the Kremlin encouraged the service work performed by members of society. The overall governmental strategy was to exercise surveillance and strict control over any independent NGO.[36] Because few Russian NGOs have true financial security, possess necessary advocacy competencies, and enjoy the requisite capacity to implement health services independently from the state, the Kremlin purposely amplifies the fledgling civil society's inherent vulnerabilities. At the dawn of Putin's third presidential term, it became clear that dependence on the state has impeded civil society's fight against the pandemic. The next subsection analyzes Russia's efforts to assert itself as an international leader and donor.

Chasing Leadership in International Health

The Kremlin has collaborated with various global and transnational health organizations but gradually decided to put its own stamp on the global health landscape. The role of a humble recipient fits neither Putin's self-serving largesse nor the dearly held collective images of Russia's great power status. Once windfall mineral rents made Russian financial circumstances more comfortable, the Kremlin immediately jumped on the opportunity to offer international health assistance. This behavior would not have been possible without improved material circumstances, but it was the pride of becoming a contributor to global health that motivated the Kremlin to act. The Kremlin's fixation on sovereignty and internal state autonomy prompted its assault on those transnational agents who embodied different conceptions of the common good and allegedly challenged sovereignty as an inviolable principle of governance. As the imagery of great power crystallizes, so does the government's intolerance of external influences. That is why the Russian government recently set at international humanitarian organizations and expelled some of them.

Since the early 2000s, the Russian government has maintained normal connections with various international organizations, including the World Bank, the Global Fund, UNAIDS, and the United Nations' specialized agencies. The United States Embassy in Moscow reported that several people in key Russian policy positions, despite Putin's swelling anti-Western rhetoric, had expressed an interest in further partnership with foreign governments.[37] Indeed, initially, Russia collaborated with various international health organizations, often living up to the best expectations of fruitful cooperation and adoption of external recommendations.[38] But even at the dawn of Putin's rule, the Kremlin displayed clear signs that it wanted to move away from being a recipient of international assistance and advice, despite the fact that its health spending had not yet reached levels matching international assistance. The early examples of such behavior are as follows. In 2002 Moscow was spending just 1.5 rubles per person per year for HIV treatment and prevention while generously giving more than $20 million to international charities. In 2003 Russia rejected $150 million offered by the World Bank. After protracted negotiations, Russia signed a forty-eight-million-dollar loan with the World Bank to improve regional HIV/AIDS services, including treatment. For a while, international donations surpassed the amount of resources the government was able to spend domestically. In 2004, for instance, the international grants for prevention were three times more than the funding coming from the federal budget.

In the late 2000s the Kremlin became more assertive in chasing its desires for external grandeur. That is why the Russian government decided to reimburse most of the Global Fund's contributions for HIV-related programs in Russia. Once Russia decided to become exclusively a contributor to the Global Fund, it officially refused supplies of AIDS drugs from the Global Fund and chose to phase out all international assistance. In December 2013 the Russian government pledged to give the fund $60 million, hoping that such generous support will enhance Russia's status as one of the leading international actors in addressing public health problems. Perhaps that behavior would have been justified if global AIDS organizations were no longer willing to provide financial assistance to an increasingly wealthy Russia. But that is definitely not the case with the Global Fund's vision. The fund's executive director, Michel Kazatchkine, proposed to continue such funding and possibly to employ loans as a new mechanism in the fund's work.[39] Because Putin and Medvedev were willing to part with a lot of money in order to buy their way into the global health club, Kazatchkine's arguments went unheeded.

Furthermore, the Kremlin's ascension to donorship allowed it to cut domestic nonstate AIDS organizations from independent sources of support previously available via the Global Fund. For more than a decade, merit-based external funding had given domestic civil society some degree of autonomy from the Russian state. A notable example is the Globus program, which has received numerous international accolades. For eight years, from 2004 to 2011, this collaborative program, which was implemented by a consortium of five leading nongovernmental organizations, received more than $110 million in external funding.

According to the official description, the program developed an integrated approach to improve knowledge about the epidemic among the general population, implemented prevention programs among specific vulnerable groups, and campaigned to improve the effectiveness of government counterparts' participation in AIDS policy. As external funding dried up, the Kremlin acquired the freedom to ignore one of the core principles of the Global Fund, that is, competitive and transparent funding driven by local needs. Today, there is no formalized mechanism left to prevent Moscow from closing any program that does not fit its heavily idiosyncratic policy course, which in the future is likely to be premised on the newly designed conservative values.

The changes in how prominent politicians view the role of transnational health actors are palpable as well. In the early years of Putin's rule, the domestic political establishment was relatively sympathetic to the missions and aspirations of the transnational health NGOs. Sergey Mironov, Mikhail Margelov, and Mikhail Grishankov served on the board of directors of TPAA. However, this favorable disposition did not last very long. At the end of Putin's second presidential term, the ideas of state autonomy and the desires to insulate the nation from external influences were taking a firm hold on the officialdom and the public. Official representations of NGOs as puppets of foreign intelligence agencies trapped politicians, who were no longer free to throw their support behind civil society. Domestic politicians who understand the necessity to collaborate with transnational health agents have become highly vulnerable to domestic opprobrium: even moderate support for any innocuous cause can trigger wild allegations that these politicians are subverting the state. Not surprisingly, some of these politicians have chosen to distance themselves from nonstate health charities sponsored from abroad.

Those who were never sympathetic to transnational partners now feel that they no longer have to conceal their intolerance to external health agencies and agents of change. In 2011 Gennadiy Onishchenko accused UNICEF of lobbying in the interests of foreign pharmaceutical companies and thereby undermining Russia's efforts to eradicate polio in Central Asia.[40] At the onset of Putin's third presidential term, Russians expelled USAID and UNICEF from the country, despite their impressive legacy of policy change and prospects of further health improvement. One spokesperson from the Ministry of Foreign Affairs openly acknowledged that driving foreign agencies out was politically motivated.[41]

Externally, the Kremlin tried to establish an extensive and credible reputation as a regional health leader. In 2005, for instance, the Russian government hosted a ministerial meeting, "Urgent Response to the HIV/AIDS Epidemics in the Commonwealth of Independent States," which convened from March 31 to April 1 in the President Hotel in Moscow. It was attended by government officials from the former Soviet republics, representatives of civil society, health-care practitioners from the public and private sectors, and officials from UN specialized agencies. The parties adopted the so-called Moscow Declaration.[42]

The G8 summit held in Strel'na, just outside Saint Petersburg, the former imperial capital of Russia, offered another opportunity for the Kremlin to promote its self-image as an indispensable global player. In July 2006 Russia used its G8 group presidency to put the issue of HIV/AIDS on the agenda of the thirty-second summit. President Putin elevated infectious diseases and global health issues as core priorities. Putin's formal address to visitors to the official site of Russia's G8 presidency articulated his vision for international health regulation: "The spread of all kinds of epidemics in the world emphasizes the need to step up the fight against infectious diseases. We are convinced that the creation of a global system to monitor dangerous diseases, the development of regular interaction between experts from different countries, and broader exchange of research information about dangerous viruses will have a major positive influence on the solution of these serious problems."[43]

The image of restored great power status required Russia to act like an active builder of the organizational health landscape while reinventing its integrative role in the post-Soviet space. To achieve these goals, Moscow pursued an assertive leadership role by sponsoring and managing a series of regional initiatives against HIV/AIDS. Since 2006 the Federal Surveillance Service for Consumer Rights Protection and Human Well-Being (Rospotrebnadzor) has hosted four regional Eastern Europe and Central Asia AIDS Conferences (EECAAC). Officially, the first conference's "main objective was to strengthen and consolidate the region's response to HIV through political commitment and leadership and enhanced partnerships with civil society, especially people living with HIV."[44] For a majority of delegates and attendants, this conference provided an invaluable opportunity to develop new professional contacts; improve their knowledge regarding the nature of the epidemic in the region; and develop new or refine existing skills in monitoring programs, evaluating high-risk populations, writing abstracts, and so on. The majority of the attendants were by and large satisfied with the second and third conferences as well.[45]

However, despite the overall positive evaluation of these conferences, the attendees also highlighted the necessity to address issues of prevention and the urgent needs of vulnerable and marginalized groups. Dissatisfaction swelled as the subsequent 2009 conference failed to generate any meaningful strategies to improve the sorry state of affairs concerning human rights in Eurasia and failed to design practical mechanisms to overcome discrimination and reach the most-at-risk target groups.[46] As Moscow failed to rectify these shortcomings, prominent representatives of civil society came to view these conferences as the Kremlin's tool to spread its ineffective and unjust methods of health governance abroad. On the eve of the fourth convention, the leaders of the Andrey Ryl'kov Foundation published an open letter to Michel Sidibe expressing deep concerns in regard to UNAIDS being involved in these conferences.[47] There is little reason to dispute or qualify this highly critical assessment. Moscow surely strengthened regional cooperation, but its initiatives strongly reflected the Kremlin's imbalanced health agenda, which all but ignored issues of human rights and obstructed evidence-based prevention among the most-at-risk target groups, including drug users.

In recent years Russia has groped for the position of international health leader by attempting to develop its own system of international health assistance. In 2007 the Ministry of Finance published a concept paper on Russia's participation in international development assistance that subsequently got the approval of the president. This paper signaled the next step in fulfilling Russia's external health ambitions. While the government was spending money on external assistance (about $220 million in 2008 and about $800 million in 2009), it was also interested in learning from the World Bank and the Organization for Economic Co-operation and Development about the appropriate logistical measures to implement them. Taking the notion of "soft power" seriously, the Kremlin moved to create the Russian version of the United States Agency for International Development.[48] In principle, the desire to implement humanitarian aid programs might increase the Kremlin's multilateral commitments, promote collaborative efforts with Western developmental agencies, and open up the country's leadership to learning about good health governance from experienced donors, as the optimistic argument goes.

Whether Russia's initiatives will improve health abroad and will help mitigate the pandemic in the post-Soviet region remains an open question. It is too early to determine if this agenda will replicate Soviet-style assistance as a foreign policy tool in supporting friendly political regimes, generate some benevolent and productive partnerships in mitigating the consequences of HIV/AIDS, or just fizzle out. That Russia's international ambitions are not fully shored up by the necessary prerequisites should be taken as a serious warning against praising the Kremlin's plan for health assistance. The focus on leadership without modern health-care capabilities and medical professionalism will generate adverse consequences to public health abroad. Before becoming a successful regional health leader, the government should focus on training medical personnel, developing a sophisticated institutional and legal framework, and stamping out corruption in the health-care industry.[49] These are the bare minimum prerequisites for success.

Although there is nothing wrong with taking pride in Russia's status as an international donor and leader of international initiatives, recent actions and statements cannot but warn of negative developments being in full swing. Russia's external ambitions no doubt will affect emerging patterns of transnational health politics in the post-Soviet space as long as Putin and his supporters stay in control. That the growing economic potential of Russia as an emerging power was an essential factor is apparent. Mineral rents will sustain the Russian self-image as a great power and will finance the Kremlin's international endeavors.

Summary

As the *siloviki* strengthened their power position in Putin's Russia, they became a dominant force in the public debate on HIV and health governance. Accordingly, the interests of law enforcement and drug control officers now overshadow the vital needs of improving public health and bringing Russian standards of biomedical ethics and professionalism in sync with international ones. Russian leaders were devoted to the fight against HIV/AIDS but downplayed the desirability of working hand in hand with civil society and the private sector. Many domestic opinion leaders welcomed punishing the liberal segment of Russian civil society for its alleged wrongdoings and its contribution to the worsening of the epidemiological situation at home. At the same time, the readiness of the *siloviki* and church functionaries to forge an explicit alliance might portend the emergence of a new type of hard-line, antiliberal civil society in the near future. Church functionaries and faith leaders might seem to be strange bedfellows for the *siloviki*, but Russian Orthodox aspirations to cultivate citizens' responsibility for morally resurrecting the Russian state match the *siloviki*'s resentment of protecting the autonomy of an individual from the state.[50]

In contrast to Mbeki's South Africa, a legitimate social purpose gained strong social traction in Putin's Russia. That is, one clearly identifiable ruling group (the *siloviki*) came to dominate the domestic normative landscape, while wider audiences shared the prevailing justifications for the state's existence, and the other prominent political groups increasingly conceded to those justifications. It follows that the level of contestation among actors involved in health governance in Russia was low, although liberal-minded groups and individuals detested core elements of the Kremlin's approach to curbing the contagion. Although dissenting voices were heard and respected in narrow professional circles, the overwhelming majority considered the enacted system of health governance to be normal. Thus, societal compliance with the Kremlin's health strategy ensued primarily on voluntary grounds.

HEALTH PARTNERSHIP IN MBEKI'S SOUTH AFRICA

Central to South African approaches to AIDS was expanding the boundaries of medical knowledge for African renewal. Pretoria wanted to make sure that major regulators of medicines and autonomous health institutions operate on principles that are consistent with the goals of indigenous authority and medical pluralism. Thus, the Cabinet tried to undermine the authority of the Medicines Control Council (MCC), tried to rein in the Medical Research Council (MRC), and struggled to weaken the South African National AIDS Council (SANAC). I discuss this course of action in the first subsection. The second and third subsections discuss the complexities of building partnerships with the private sector and nonstate actors. Despite the broad international support behind protreatment activists who promoted Western antiretrovirals and generic medicines, Mbeki's administration favored the nonstate advocates of alternative medicines and complementary diets. The Cabinet forged relations with those organizations whose missions were close to the vision of the African Renaissance and frustrated partnerships with its perceived detractors. Finally, turning to the government's responses to the international health landscape, I suggest that the emergence of the African Renaissance enabled choices that were not legitimate before.

Dominating the AIDS Bureaucracy in Mbeki's South Africa

In the 1990s the South African government cooperated with domestic health organizations in order to formulate and implement an appropriate response to the epidemic. In the early 1990s the National AIDS Coordinating Committee of

South Africa developed a national AIDS strategy, bringing on board a diverse group consisting of NGOS, AIDS service organizations, government officials, business representatives, the private sector, political parties, individual AIDS activists, and trade unions. They all played a major role in drafting the 1994 National AIDS Plan.[51] But Thabo Mbeki's administration pursued a different path in shaping health policy networks.

The story that attracted the attention of the media and scholars started in the early 2000s, when Pretoria turned to AIDS dissidents to help formulate appropriate policies in response to the epidemic. This decision went against the grain of the common biomedical expertise. Most importantly, the denialist movement had hardly been a recognizable and legitimate international force since 1996. In an ironic twist of fate, many AIDS dissidents passed away after too many of them refused to take the available ARV medications. Nevertheless, the Cabinet valued the dissidents' policy input, as the government considered dissidents to be open to African knowledge and not committed to conventional medical science. The latter was true by definition. The former was not really so. As many political observers snidely remarked, the dissident theory was not Afro-centric at all. Be that as it may, sponsoring select biomedical pariahs from across the globe foiled the expertise of mainstream international health organizations and the medical and pharmaceutical establishment of the global North. The Cabinet interpreted public criticism of the dissidents as an orchestrated campaign to use racially skewed science to suppress Africa's independent quest for unique solutions.[52]

In 2000 President Mbeki commissioned the Presidential AIDS Advisory Panel (also known as the Pretoria Panel), of which the dissidents comprised at least half. The Pretoria Panel featured infamous dissidents Peter Duesberg, Sam Mhlongo, Valendar Turner, and David Rasnik. Their recommendations highlighted their beliefs that AIDS was not contagious, although many of the opportunistic infections were; that AIDS was not sexually transmitted; that HIV did not cause AIDS; that the admittedly toxic anti-HIV drugs were more effective in killing than curing people; and that the drug-induced toxic effects caused AIDS-defining conditions and could not be distinguished from AIDS.[53] The summary policy document reads like a counterpoint of two contradictory sets of recommendations. What AIDS denialists recommended, conventional medical experts rejected. Dissidents' call to suspend all HIV testing in the country and abstain from antiretrovirals when treating AIDS patients generated resistance. This counterepistemic community gave President Mbeki and his supporters a quasi-scientific vocabulary to refute the conventional epidemiological wisdom that HIV was the cause of AIDS and reject cost-efficient and safe drugs. As a result, Mbeki created a self-deceptive possibility to select among a large number of legitimate groups and individuals to cooperate with.

Under the strong pressures applied by the transnational protreatment coalition, the Pretoria Panel was disbanded and never reconvened again in the same format. The termination of the Pretoria Panel, however, did not inspire the Cabinet to accept the expertise of the international health organizations or endorse mainstream science. After an enormous international and domestic outcry, Mbeki distanced himself from AIDS dissidents by asking them not to use his name for fund-raising purposes. This distancing, however, remained somewhat duplicitous. In 2007 Mbeki's biographer, Ronald Suresh Roberts, politicized the public criticism of adding dissidents to the panel. He accused critics of being the self-delusional victims of colonial scholarship, racial stereotypes, and beliefs in black incompetence and native unfitness to govern:

> But why, upon mature reflection, would anybody be surprised that a responsible elected official wants to acquaint himself "with all sides" of a science that everybody says is central to a massive health crisis under his watch? It is an elementary intellectual procedure, unless of course the leader is implicitly denied the right to or faculty of intellect. He must just shut up. He must just obey. . . . Mbeki's sin was to reject a drug-based intellectual protectionism in favour of a free exchange of ideas on the proper solution to the AIDS pandemic. . . . Mbeki's methodical inquiry was recast as native stubbornness. . . . Mbeki is cast as a heathen, a non-believer—indeed as the proverbial Kaffir in that rich and resonant word's original sense.[54]

Since the end of the dissident debacle, the general pattern has hardly altered. The Cabinet interfered in the work of its domestic health agencies in order to undermine their conventional medical competencies and promote medical pluralism. The Cabinet's strategy was to circumscribe the independent policy-making power of various health agencies, medical research units, health regulatory bodies, and prominent individuals. For instance, the weakness of SANAC was the result of an intentional strategy to maintain Pretoria-friendly strategies of AIDS governance. In 2001 this newly formed institution replaced the Inter-ministerial Committee on AIDS. As such, it was supposed to consolidate political leadership and increase civil society involvement in the fight against HIV/AIDS. Indeed, SANAC proved instrumental in developing a national integrated plan for children infected and affected by HIV and AIDS and designing a strategic plan for sexually transmitted diseases and HIV for 2000–2005. However, Health Minister Manto Tshabalala-Msimang has dominated the institution from the get-go, thereby ensuring that universality of treatment will not feature in its initiatives. Jacob Zuma, at that time still deputy president, has also been instrumental in turning SANAC into a rubber-stamp institution and worked to undermine its organizational mission. Nevertheless, some domestic policy makers fought for SANAC as an institutional framework that could promote standardized treatment protocols.[55] In 2005–6 the new deputy president, Phumzile Mlambo-Ngcuka, tried to restructure the organizational governance of HIV/AIDS in the country. The new national strategic HIV/AIDS plan (2007–11) intended to return SANAC to its status as a link between the government and civil society. To fulfill these objectives, Mlambo-Ngcuka brought on board a number of civil society representatives, including Mark Heywood of the Treatment Action Campaign (TAC) as the deputy chair. Under her brief leadership, SANAC organized the Third National AIDS Conference in order to resolve the key contentious issues regarding HIV/AIDS.[56] Although these efforts received international recognition, the health minister reinstated things to her liking once she was able to return from a sick leave. Quickly after her recovery, Tshabalala-Msimang tried to restructure SANAC in order to counterbalance the growing influence of the civil society representatives. Although her plan to keep on board only functionaries and loyalists ultimately failed, SANAC remained by and large powerless.

In general, Tshabalala-Msimang applied her administrative power to make midlevel bureaucrats conform to health governance systems predicated on the core tenets of the African Renaissance. In the late 1990s Pretoria intentionally undermined the authority of the MCC by reversing its decision on Virodene as toxic and unsafe and disputed the MCC's approval of nevirapine. The MCC, the main regulator of medicines in the country, however, reaffirmed its independence, as it kept refusing to sanction Virodene's clinical trials.[57] The Cabinet went as far as firing Peter Folb, then director of the MCC and an ANC member. In 2004 the government-backed Dr. Rath Foundation published a petition to disband the MCC, calling it "an agency whose members are directly or indirectly dependent on the international pharmaceutical industry, and whose decisions have consistently served these foreign interests at the cost of the health and lives of the people of South Africa."[58] The idea to terminate "a statutory body that regulates the performance of clinical trials and registration of medicines and medical devices for use in specific diseases," as the Department of Health describes the purpose of the agency, was a bold move. In 2008 Tshabalala-Msimang promoted the legislation to replace "the ineffective and slow" MCC with the Regulatory Authority for Health Products. The proposed body would have closed the "loopholes by covering traditional and complementary medicines" and enjoyed a large staff and vast resources.[59]

No less significant were attacks on Malegapuru Makgoba, president of the MRC, a prominent epidemiologist, and formerly Mbeki's supporter. Their personal partnership ended after Mbeki dismissed Makgoba's objections to the government's stance on ARV treatment policy. The Cabinet put constraints on the MRC's mandate, censured the body's research findings, and accused it of being hostile to the government.

Many midlevel bureaucrats and health officials resisted pressures to promote the value of medical pluralism and separate conventional medical professionals from domestic health agencies. Some were punished for their positions. The episode with sacking Deputy Minister Nozizwe Madlala-Routledge is quite telling. She was fired after she participated in the International AIDS Conference in Barcelona. Officially, she was let go because she had failed to secure direct presidential approval to travel abroad. The media, however, highlighted Madlala-Routledge's independence and conventional beliefs about ARV treatment as the actual reasons for her sacking. The dismissal of Madlala-Routledge backfired and ignited wide criticism of Tshabalala-Msimang's professional and administrative incompetence. In addition, the papers discovered that the minister of health allegedly had a record of stealing hospital property in the past and reported her frequent alcohol abuse. Although bad press did not make Mbeki reconsider his decisions to fire Madlala-Routledge and to retain Tshabalala-Msimang, he was hardly in control of the unfolding challenge to his authority anymore. Many doctors seemed to follow Western, evidence-based medicine and ignored the governmental embrace of medical pluralism. And they could not have been restrained. Independent individuals, prominent medical professionals, and policy entrepreneurs never stopped criticizing the government. In 2006–7, as Mbeki's support was crumbling, calls to dismiss Tshabalala-Msimang intensified.

According to Nicoli Nattrass, the assault on the scientific regulation of medicine and the challenge to the independent power of the MCC were central to Mbeki's legacy in public health.[60] This challenge was far from an irrational hatred toward domestic medical regulators and the scientific establishment: terminating the MCC would have removed institutional obstacles to the further spread of alternative and indigenous medicines. In accordance with the grand vision of the African Renaissance, this erosion of scientific regulation reflected the conscious strategy to resist colonialist science and promote medical pluralism.

In short, while the Cabinet and dedicated Mbekiites worked hard to dominate health policy networks, on balance they failed to erode the independent policy-making power and scientific expertise of the relevant bodies. The ideas of indigenous authority and the African Renaissance were spreading much slower among medical professionals, media commentators, and health experts compared to ordinary South Africans.

The South African Government and the Private Sector

To increase the capacity of the public health-care sector means to develop public-private interaction mechanisms and contract the private sector for public needs. The strength of the private health sector has been a long-standing general trend in South African health care. The trend started with mission hospitals and industry-specific facilities that provided health care for white mine workers. According to Hoosen Coovadia and his coauthors, "By the end of the 1990s, almost three-quarters of generalist doctors worked in the private sector," while "64% of the population are entirely dependent on the public sector" and cannot afford out-of-pocket expenses. Despite these disproportions, the government continued to increase support to private health care while keeping the public sector stagnant.[61] This evidence is consistent with the strategy of marketization (neoliberalism) as the core ideational component of the African Renaissance.

Similarly, in regard to the HIV/AIDS epidemic, the critical evidence suggests that the South African government opted to protect the private sector while keeping expenditures in the public sector as minimal as possible in order to prevent overspending. Prior to 2001, 90 percent of seropositive patients received therapy in the private sector. Overall, this accounted for just a fraction of people who needed treatment at that time. In 2004 only 11,000 HIV-positive people received treatment from the public health system, which was roughly one out of every fifty South African AIDS patients who were medically ready for highly active antiretroviral therapy (HAART).[62] Although after 2004 the government did not resist public-private partnership overtly, it still avoided transferring risks to the private sector in achieving universality of treatment. More specifically, between 2005 and 2008 the annual editions of the *South African Health Review* emphasized the continuing accumulation of resources and expertise in the private sector, the absence of public-private interaction mechanisms, and, with a few exceptions, the government's reluctance to contract with the private sector for public needs.[63] One influential report stated: "The financial disparity in health spending between the two sectors has widened, with the private sector spending approximately seven times more per capita than the public sector, on less than 20% of the population. The public sector serves 84% of the population (mainly the uninsured and poor), spending approximately 41% of total health funding."[64]

Once again, the missed targets indicated that Pretoria did not consider the possibility of sacrificing marketization as the main approach to economic empowerment in order to implement more redistributive, social-oriented programs. In its most outspoken form, the claim that universal access in the public sector was not sustainable lasted from 1998 to 2003. In 2001 Dr. Ayanda Ntsaluba, director-general for policy and planning in the National Department of Health (1998–2003), underscored the logistical and infrastructural challenges behind the extensive access to treatment in the public sector that would hamper its implementation. In 2003 Tshabalala-Msimang argued that the provision of treatment would be sustainable only if the government adequately tackled the problem of improving the domestic health-care infrastructure.[65] These arguments were equally sober comments on the state of health-care systems in the country and a rationalization of why the nationwide expansion of treatment in the public sector was undesirable.

The budgetary constraints were alleviated when external assistance amounted to half the money appropriated for the domestic rollout of drugs. The availability of resources, however, did not change the domestic stress on marketization. Several domestic observers reported that the South African government continued to view the provision of ARVs in the public sector as an "addition to, and not a replacement for, existing ARV access through managed private sector care schemes."[66] That is why the government did not challenge the voluntary licenses granted by multinational pharmaceutical companies. Nicoli Nattrass argued that, although external programs such as the PEPFAR increased the likelihood of HAART coverage, external financial inflows to South Africa also had an adverse effect on the public sector, as they essentially had taken all the pressure off the government to use available domestic resources. In other words, the Cabinet government used the influx of foreign resources not to strengthen its public health programs but rather to protect the private sector.

Another critical dimension of private-public partnerships in a collaborative response to HIV/AIDS is the relationship between domestic business and the state. Some deep-seated structural factors may obstruct this partnership. Long-standing racial boundaries, especially between white managers and low-skilled black workers, factored into the South African government's inability to use or promote the public-private partnerships model among broader constituents, since it would require transcending these boundaries with productive inter-racial cooperation.[67] On the other hand, special interventions by political leaders with broad political and social credibility can generate much-needed social and interracial solidarity and thus foster the required degree of cooperation. But the Cabinet did not stimulate domestic firms to establish treatment and preventive programs and did not intervene to alleviate potentially highly contested and divisive internal issues (such as installing condom dispensers, extending ARV treatment to employee communities, educating the workforce about safe sex behavior, and so on). When the visibility of disease in the workforce had become obvious, South African businesses began acting on their own. At the same time, instead of building health partnerships with the government, firms aligned with the civil society's hostility to the Cabinet in order to promote their narrow business interests and improve their public image.[68]

In short, the critical evidence suggests that Mbeki's Pretoria either consistently chose to protect the country's relatively successful private health sector or simply shied away from stimulating public AIDS programs. The foregoing discussion does not suggest that after Mbeki's fall in 2008 the public sector suddenly improved. On the contrary, the structural and administrative problems of the South African health-care system are likely to last in spite of remarkable breakthroughs in Zuma's and Motsoaledi's approach to health governance. Shortages of trained doctors and essential drugs at the provincial and national levels continue to plague the public health sector. Shortages of ARVs have hit health facilities in Free State and Limpopo especially hard.[69] In some respects, this state of affairs is reminiscent of Russia's problems, which include poor management and corruption exacerbated by overextended social obligations. Newly elected South African leaders, however, seem to recognize these problems and have attempted to alleviate them.

Selective Partnership with Civil Society

During Nelson Mandela's administration, the government worked in tandem with a variety of health-related actors. NACOSA brought on board a diverse

group of NGOS, AIDS service organizations, government officials, business representatives, the private sector, political parties, individual AIDS activists, and
trade unions. All these actors played a significant role in drafting the 1994 national AIDS plan and developing a national AIDS strategy. By the late 1990s,
the broad protreatment coalition included increasingly influential and diverse
groups, such as TAC and the South African National NGO Coalition (SANGOCO),
an umbrella body of South African NGOS. The latter consisted of many provincial affiliates, the Nelson Mandela Foundation, the Congress of South African Trade Unions (COSATU), and the National Economic Development and
Labour Council (NEDLAC). The latter was the peak-level representative and
consensus-seeking body, providing a negotiation arena for business, labor, government, and domestic community-level organizations. The process of policy
formulation, as observers claimed, was faultless. The difficulties of implementation and occasional policy blunders that ensued were another matter.

The general point is that Pretoria acted de facto on the principle of nonhierarchical and nonstate health governance. And yet, at the summit of Mbeki's
popularity and power, his Cabinet distanced itself from those nonstate organizations that did not value medical pluralism. At some point, despite the Cabinet's attempt to ignore domestic criticism, it had no choice but to heed some
basic demands made by the protreatment segment of civil society. But, as will be
explained below, the government acknowledged those demands with great reluctance. The Cabinet sustained its deliberately antagonistic stance against the
protreatment movement while leaning closer to the individuals and organizations that espoused local solutions for the local epidemic. This subsection first
recapitulates the Cabinet's fondness for denialists and traditionalists of varying
provenance and then discusses its tumultuous affair with protreatment activists.

During Mbeki's turn to run the country, the Cabinet began work with those
domestic nonstate actors that adopted unconventional biomedical convictions.
At the dawn of this century, South Africa emboldened a motley crew of domestic antitreatment advocates (Sam Mhlongo, Anthony Brink, Anita Allen), hosted
a number of vitamin salespeople (Matthias Rath, Roberto Giraldo, Patrick Hol-
ford), engaged traditionalists (Nhlavana Maseko, Mlungisi Hlongwane), and,
obviously, did not restrain its own officials (Peggy Nkonyeni, Sibongile Manana,
Thami Mseleku). According to Nathan Geffen's internal sources, the alliance between traditional healers and vitamin peddlers was based on their mutual opposition to pharmaceutical colonialism.[70] This unspoken alliance soon gained the
support of Mbeki's controversial biographer, Robert Suresh Roberts, whom the

media scorned as "Ron the Con."[71] Many examples of such cooperation were discussed in chapter 2.

To reiterate, the Cabinet supported organizations that were hostile to the "AIDS-drug lobby." For instance, Rath's foundation, the South African National Civic Organisation, and Brink's Treatment Information Group were longtime favorites with the Department of Health. Tshabalala-Msimang maintained personal relationships with Rath and treated Roberto Giraldo as her personal nutritionist. The official Operational Plan for Comprehensive HIV and AIDS Care, Management and Treatment for South Africa went as far as incorporating Giraldo's alternative nutrition-related views in its policy recommendations.[72] Giraldo proposed treating HIV/AIDS with his multivitamin supplement Vita-Cell and claimed that the G8 participated in genocide and conspired against Africa. Until 2008, when the Cape High Court ruled multivitamin trials illegal and instructed the government to investigate Rath's activities, Giraldo's positions were quite strong.

There is further systematic evidence that highlights the Cabinet's penchant for those organizations and groups that publicly emphasized poverty and malnutrition as deep structural variables driving the epidemic. Some of these groups and individuals did not flatly reject the life-saving role of the ARVs, but their devotion to traditional medicines was enough to catch the favorable attention of Pretoria's officials. South Africa's National Association of People Living with HIV/AIDS (NAPWA) is one of the groups that deserves some discussion here. Founded at the end of the 1990s, this prominent umbrella organization embraced a sizable number of activists of varying biomedical persuasions. Over the next several years, one of its autonomous groups, TAC, made it its mission to fight governmental denialism, while the association's old guard kept on supporting alternative treatment programs, traditional healing, and nutritional recovery. The formal alliance ended with a bitter debate and mutual animosity. Outshone by its former ally, NAPWA survived, although its organizational weakness, financial troubles, and various allegations of ongoing embezzlement and financial misconduct damaged its reputation and influence.[73] Doubtless, it was the Cabinet's support of NAPWA that ensured its survival. The health minister not only kept Nkululeko Nxesi and Thanduxolo Doro, NAPWA's leaders, close but also became a formal member of the organization herself. In general, NAPWA proved to be invaluable to the Cabinet, as it publicly condemned domestic treatment activists and loudly supported the official course of AIDS governance. After Mbeki's fall, the association failed to address any new problems of AIDS governance that required an immediate response. Instead of helping to solve shortages of essential medicines and fighting for generics, Nxesi seemed to be preoccupied with sharing his legitimate laments about the overwhelming burden of the epidemic, escalating incidents of drug thefts, and the increasingly long lines of people waiting for treatment.[74] In short, NAPWA seemed to follow the charted course and failed to adapt to the changing circumstances and needs of AIDS governance.

As Mbeki commenced his second presidential term, the government turned to individuals and groups advocating alternatives to ARV treatment, despite their limited ability to provide political support and their apparent lack of resources to put together a strong pro-Mbeki coalition. It is true that the estimated number of on-the-ground healers fell somewhere between 200,000 and 350,000 individuals, but healers of varying provenance enjoyed neither a strong organizational structure, nor international support, nor a permanent clientele. Traditional health organizations failed to overcome the differences in their outlooks on the value and appropriate regulation of traditional medicines while being embroiled in organizational rivalries and personal skirmishes. Although the official statistics claimed that up to 80 percent of South Africans used the services of traditional healers, independent studies projected the majority of South Africans to have a decent understanding of ARVs. At the same time, many skeptically minded reporters were not ready to question the value of *muthi*. These journalists referred to genetic medicinal resources and healing practices as "something that has always been there, a familiar belief."[75] Doubtless, a legitimate part of any culture cannot and should not be simply discarded. And yet, these journalists were fully aware of the Cabinet's faults and abhorred the unscrupulous individuals profiteering from desperate people's hope to be cured of AIDS. It is not surprising, then, that wider audiences did not lend Mbeki strong political support, although many groups sought access to the Cabinet even after Mbeki's retreat from the public discussion about AIDS.

In discussing the role of civil society fighting AIDS in South Africa, much of the scholarly literature rightly focuses on the impact of TAC, which elevated itself to the position of the most influential and vocal treatment advocacy group. TAC fully embraced the international consensus on the nature of the pandemic and adopted the norm of ARVs as a biomedical solution. By 2004 it had received many an accolade for its efforts to promote the wide use of antiretrovirals in the country via multiple eye-grabbing campaigns of civil protest, litigation, and shaming. Its members became active participants at international conferences as well. At the XII International AIDS Conference in Durban, TAC and Médecins sans frontières organized a joint satellite conference entitled "Improving Access to HIV/AIDS Drugs in Developing Countries." Two years later, in 2002, TAC tried to create a unified protreatment advocacy network that was supposed to bring together the most visible civil society organizations from all over the continent.[76] At the XVI International AIDS Conference in 2006, TAC co-organized the march for the Global Day of Action in Brazil, Canada, China, and South Africa. TAC's cofounder, Zackie Achmat, and his colleagues toured the United States and appeared in the pages of *Vanity Fair*.[77] In effect, TAC became a link between the domestic and international arenas.[78]

As TAC gained more international recognition and credibility, the members of Mbeki's administration became more hostile to it. Pretoria accused the leaders of this organization of not only holding the government in low esteem and collaborating with neocolonialists but also calculatedly misrepresenting the country's achievements and inflicting undeserved reputational damage. This hostility began in the early years of Mbeki's presidency. According to ANC member Andrew Feinstein, who took notes during Mbeki's speech at the ANC Caucus meeting, Mbeki blamed TAC for lobbying for the special interests of the pharmaceutical sector and acting as an agent of foreign influences.[79] According to TAC's then secretary-general, Sipho Mthathi, government representatives charged the organization with "using international podiums to embarrass the South African government and of not being patriotic."[80] Later on, Pretoria attempted to exclude TAC and its allies from participating in the high-level meeting on AIDS that would take place in New York in 2006.

The most illustrative rhetorical attacks employed wild identity arguments. Activists and protreatment civil society were accused of shifting the blame from the profound consequences of apartheid to black incompetence and callousness. The AIDS debate, then, aimed "to erase apartheid and colonial history from South Africa's present-day self-understanding."[81] Domestic AIDS dissidents who supported Mbeki's AIDS policies were the leading voices in these attacks against Pretoria's "drug-lore" opponents. The independent AIDS dissident Anthony Brink drafted a fifty-nine-page bill of indictment for the prosecution of Zackie Achmat at the International Criminal Court in The Hague "on a charge of genocide for his direct criminal role in the deaths of thousands of South Africans from ARV poisoning."[82] Trying to draw attention to his actions, Brink claimed that the presidency had secretly put him in charge of building an organizational counterweight to TAC and expressing the official viewpoint.[83] These futile attacks peaked at the moment when TAC truly became the leading force of AIDS activism in the country, with more than 16,000 members organized in 250 regional branches at its disposal.[84]

Although the government had to make significant concessions to the mainstream protreatment activists, on balance, activists were not able to persuade or shame the government to change its ideational commitments. Besides the conflict around evidence-based medications that pitted the Cabinet and the civil society against each other, the relations between the Cabinet and the protreatment activists were also strained by another normative clash. Whereas the devotion to neoliberalism prompted the government to think that health issues could be resolved and regulated through market forces, domestic protreatment activists, conversely, viewed health as a political and socioeconomic right.[85] Pretoria remained hostile to those who pushed for universal access to ARVs and accused health activists of disloyalty to the South African transformation process.[86]

To conclude, there is no shortage of academic and journalistic accounts supplying the detailed story of the epic clash between Pretoria and TAC.[87] A standard account of Mbeki's AIDS policy is likely, and quite correctly, to center on his conflict with domestic civil society. Mark Heywood, an active participant in that epic fight, averred that Mbeki's attitudes and actions left "little room for an autonomous civil society, except perhaps as a vehicle to deliver messages and services from the beneficent party/state."[88] But the reality, as evident from the foregoing discussion, was more complex. It is of note that the impartial definition of civil society should not discriminate against nonstate actors based on their political convictions and biomedical beliefs. Civil society does not have to embrace modern, progressive, or Westernized outlooks. Civil society can be illiberal, after all.

In practice, while the Cabinet execrated the advocates of treatment, it also embraced the proponents of alternative and traditional medicines. Although the tangible political benefits of resisting the norm of treatment were far from obvious, the Cabinet preferred to forge connections with organizations that embraced alternative and complementary treatments and did not treat a human right to health as a socioeconomic one. In principle, tapping into the popular sentiment supportive of alternative medications and healing practices seemed like a savvy political move. However, in order to become a force to be reckoned with, most of the aforementioned organizations required strong governmental support themselves. NAPWA, for instance, could not have survived without the government's checks. Ironically, supporting TAC would have improved Mbeki's domestic and even international standing, but forging an alliance with it would have been incongruous with the goals of the African Renaissance.

Challenging International Health Organizations

The evidence suggests that the ideas encompassed by the African Renaissance explain how South African officials chose to deal with the international health architecture. The emergence of this discourse enabled choices and actions that were not legitimate before Mbeki's rule. During the early years of Mandela's presidency, the government explicitly embraced partnerships with international governmental organizations.[89] In the late 1990s, however, the Cabinet started cultivating values of exceptionalism and continental leadership as integral elements of intersubjective social purpose. As the elite's commitment to the African Renaissance crystallized, it had no alternative but to militate against an international arena allegedly astir with colonial legacies and neocolonial sensibilities. These ideational orientations prompted the Cabinet to think that guidelines supplied by international health organizations were ill suited for South Africa, while genuine scientific pluralism had to be asserted. As a result, the Cabinet tried to resist guidelines imposed by major AIDS organizations and countervail the monopoly of the global pharmaceutical sector. At the same time, while the government did not reject external donations, it surely tried to redistribute them as it saw fit.

For a protracted period of time, Pretoria refused to accept the WHO's and UNGASS's recommendations and guidelines. Unnerved by the burden of international scrutiny, the health minister tried to downplay the role of the United Nations' Millennium Development Goals reports. According to the resident coordinator of the UN SA country team, the government chose to make the release of the first South African report a low-key event. The Department of Health failed to adopt an adequate monitoring and evaluation system that would have enabled comparison of South Africa's progress against international guidelines and objectives. In general, the crucial evidence is that the overwhelming majority of the domestic policy documents either did not follow international prescriptions or attempted to reframe them. Consider, for instance, the first official update report, "Progress Report on the Declaration of Commitment on HIV and AIDS," submitted by the Department of Health in 2006. This report received much criticism, as it omitted any tangible data that would have allowed comparing South Africa's internal progress with international thresholds. Evading monitoring and evaluation mechanisms was pervasive on the provincial level as well. By 2006 the provincial health departments had provided neither disaggregated information on HIV/AIDS expenditures nor information about treatment programs for domestic monitoring agencies.[90] According to numerous independent reports, the country had made no progress regarding various international guidelines regarding the universality of treatment as a part of the global consensus on HIV/AIDS. Only in 2007 did the national strategic plan recommend following international prescriptions in establishing a monitoring and evaluation framework.[91]

Another dimension of the story is about Pretoria obstructing the work of GFATM. GFATM's main objective was to empower the AIDS service organizations while circumventing governmental interference and avoiding potential domestic hindrances. Instead of simply disbursing money to the domestic AIDS service organizations on the basis of their prior performance, the Cabinet tried to either control the distribution of the international health-related grants or seize them. In 2002 Mbeki attacked GFATM for "flouting its own rules by funding AIDS programs without proper government approval."[92] The biggest controversy arose when Mbeki announced that the government would seize a grant targeted specifically to the province of KwaZulu-Natal and would add it to the general South African grant. For more than a year, the government stalled the influx of international resources and refused to sign an agreement with GFATM in order to finalize the transfer of funds.[93] In effect, the South African grant portfolio went almost exclusively to the country's Cabinet-level departments. The Cabinet wished to use GFATM's country coordinating mechanism as a means of financial control over AIDS moneys instead of supporting its intended mission.[94] All these problems prompted the International Treatment Preparedness Coalition (ITPC) in 2006 to report that the country coordinating mechanism in South Africa has yet to function properly.[95]

To be fair, Pretoria exhibited not just hostility but also a willingness to collaborate with some external actors. Although the government had picked a fight with those external organizations that could have empowered the "AIDS-drug lobby," it welcomed the support of PEPFAR.[96] The simple explanation for this is that PEPFAR's resources enabled Pretoria to avoid giving any further undesirable financial pledges to fight the epidemic, while those same resources allowed the Cabinet to keep domestic health programs afloat. External financial support took the pressure off the national Department of Health to provide medicines to its public sector. In other words, the government seemed to accept a partnership with international organizations if their assistance lifted the financial burden from the public sector, a stance that was consistent with Pretoria's emphasis on slashing spending. At the same time, the Cabinet's desire to seize PEPFAR's donations was evident. In 2006 Tshabalala Msimang made an argument for stricter governmental control over PEPFAR's 450-million-dollar donation and argued that domestic nongovernmental organizations and international agencies working in the country should not have had direct access to any external funding.[97]

Much like indigenousness and marketization, the stress on benevolent leadership and continental solidarity reflected the strategy to countervail the global power structure and disseminate and promote distinctively African ways to improve public health. An attack on the global pharmaceutical sector was designed to restore continental self-reliance and allow the suppressed dissidents to express their biomedical views on par with conventional scientists.[98] Pretoria galvanized the dissident movement, by then almost extinct, back into existence. Its marginal scientific status, according to Mbeki, was a result of the continuing Western monopoly on science and truth. While the AIDS dissidents in certain circumstances might be able to empower various nonmainstream domestic perceptions of the pandemic and legitimize some obscure local beliefs, for Mbeki they confirmed the righteousness of his quest against the Western monopoly on science. In reality, of course, this move was counterproductive.

Some logical choices never ensued. Developing close partnerships with Brazil, India, and Thailand seemed appropriate, as these nations were rising not only as the principal challengers to the profit-seeking pharmaceutical sector but also as the force countervailing the global hegemony of the West. These countries would have been the natural ally for the South African government in widening its international coalition legitimacy and prestige in the Third World. Pretoria, however, was not ready to commit, since a formal joining of the South-South coalition would have implied the necessity to promote generics at the expense of traditional medicines and enlarge the public sector. Instead, Pretoria promoted traditional medicines in the international arena. For instance, in 2007 the government hosted the Third Ordinary Session of the Conference of African Ministers of Health in the framework of the African Union's decade on African traditional medicine.[99] In addition, the government chose to play no active role in the creation of a new generation of AIDS organizations. Although the relevant literature acknowledges the South African contribution to the foundation of UNGASS and GFATM, this contribution was modest, especially compared to the support provided by other countries.[100]

In conclusion, the argument developed in this subsection links South African behavior toward international organizations and the global health landscape to the aspirations expressed by the African Renaissance. Jacob Zuma's "retrenchment of continental leadership" and his explicit focus on domestic issues characterize the current approaches to AIDS governance in South Africa.[101] This retrenchment is part of shying away from the bold vision of the African Renaissance.

Summary

This section started with some general observations regarding how Pretoria undermined those domestic health institutions that resisted the idea of medical pluralism. It continued by presenting evidence that Pretoria chose to protect the relatively successful private sector by keeping public expenditures small and selectively engage domestic civil society. In chapter 3, I described South African social purpose as power based. That is, although one clearly identifiable ruling group (Mbekiites) dominates the domestic political landscape, not all political groups accept and internalize the elite-friendly justifications for the state's existence. While many ordinary South Africans respect indigenous healing, the notion of indigenous healing authority as a core goal of the state never took on an intersubjective quality.

As social entrepreneurs and treatment activists did not share the government's devotion to the African Renaissance, a conflict around the use of conventional medicines and the desirability of scaling up access to pharmaceutical products ensued. This, of course, did not prevent the government from acting on its ideas. South African elites evoked compliance with their health strategy both on voluntary grounds and by limiting the discretion of dissenting policy participants to decide and act on their own. It follows that societal contestation about HIV/AIDS ensued. The proponents of Western biomedical products and their indigenous opponents clashed.

CONCLUSION

The notion of good governance, broadly conceived, implies that issues of mutual concern are best approached when governments join forces with relevant social groups and individuals. The state also should treat any health stakeholder as an autonomous actor. In both Russia and South Africa, politicians selected health partners in accordance with their understanding of whether or not HIV-related groups and stakeholders enhanced or subverted the cardinal goals of the state. Thus, although it is possible to discern many nuanced characteristics in Russian and South African approaches to building and maintaining health partnerships, adopting the international organizing principle of nonhierarchical and nonstate governance hinged on the elite's obligations to validate their conception of the core goals of the state in practice.

Pretoria engaged civil society and the private sector, taking into account the former's adherence to the national transformation based on indigenous values and the latter's significance for the dearly held market-based economic empowerment. While the Kremlin severely reduced the resources available to mainstream nongovernmental organizations that boasted a decent performance record, it also tested the social waters before allowing ultraconservative social actors to become associated with the government. The Kremlin thought that autonomous civil society, fledgling as it was in Russia, presented an ontological danger to the state insofar as nonstate actors were spreading liberal ideas and facilitating external forces' penetration of the country. Not surprisingly, Orthodox faith-based charities and noncommercial organizations that focused only on delivering social services, both of which were interwoven into the state-centric power structure, were the Kremlin's allies.

Another core theme discussed in this chapter pertains to the external ambitions of the two states. Empirical dissimilarities notwithstanding, the response to the global health landscape depended upon how elites defined their polity's appropriate place in the international power structure and how they stipulated the means of achieving and maintaining that desirable status. With respect to international partners, Russia and South Africa tried to act as regional leaders, although both countries failed to alter the surrounding health landscape. Despite this failure, top Russian leaders still feel obligated to carry on their normative aspirations, while the decline of the African Renaissance as the prevailing discourse after Mbeki's fall made South African leaders cope with their structural limitations in a realistic and humble manner.

The discussion in chapter 2 traced the discursive process in which Russian and South African political elites constructed and communicated their conceptions of the core goals of the state. Chapters 3 and 4 examined how ideational preoccupations with certain goals of the state prompted key decision makers to filter international conventions on good AIDS governance, including the principle of evidence-based medicines and the universality of prevention and treatment. In this chapter, I have explained the reasons why the key political leaders in Russia and South Africa pursued health partnerships with different stakeholders the way they did. The following chapter concludes my investigation. Instead of presenting my results in yet another lengthy narrative, I summarize the implications of my inquiry for three ongoing debates. My concluding thoughts are for practitioners; they clarify the nature and the scope of the underlying difficulties of improving health governance.

Conclusion

Their [externally inspired] reforms were successful only to the extent
that they had been identified as acceptable by the Russian culture. Anything that was incompatible with the life of our culture, anything that
was threatening its foundation, was always painfully rejected. Is it worth
trying [to begin reforms] once more? Is it worth trying to resemble
Dostoevsky's literary character who shot himself, having decided that it
was not worth living as a Russian?

—Vladislav Surkov, "Russkaya politicheskaya kul'tura,"
Strategiya Rossii 7 (2007)

Africa's development and a renaissance cannot be premised on unbri-
dled cultural borrowings from outside. Development in a sustained and
meaningful way can only be achieved on the basis of Africa's own cultural usages in consonance with the history and cultures of the people
of Africa. It is difficult to imagine development taking place along non-
African lines in Africa. . . . [T]his does not mean wholesale return to
cultural practices of the past, or an atavistic revivalism which has no
place in the contemporary world. What we need is a judicious Afrocentric approach which selectively builds on our cultural and historical be-
longings.

—Kwesi Kwaa Prah, "African Renaissance or Warlordism," in *African
Renaissance: The New Struggle*, edited by Malegapuru William Makgoba

THESE STATEMENTS SUMMARIZE the nature of the normative anxieties
that took hold of Russians and South Africans at the dawn of the new millennium. To implement externally inspired reforms in Russia, surmises Putin's
trusted political operator, is to commit ontological suicide. To premise African development on externally validated ideas, speculates a prominent intellectual, is to undercut the rebirth of the continent. These conjectures are harsh in
phraseology and sweeping in implications; they push an observer to ponder why

and to what extent political leaders, prominent intellectuals, and opinion leaders close their hearts and minds to external norms and ideas. This book started with a proposition that the rapidly spreading aversion to external norms in posttransitional Russia and South Africa had something to do with the nature of political authority. Indeed, as shown in chapter 2, Putin's and Mbeki's inward-looking ideas about the cardinal goals of the state sculpted new normative pillars of their authority and suggested the appropriate methods of governance.

Probing heuristic powers of the concept of social purpose gives us usable insights into the reasons that govern official and public views on the benefits of external norms and the suitability of international best practices to address problems at home. Simply put, political leaders' expectations do not always converge around external norms, principles, and conventions. Domestic standards of governance might dovetail with a deep devotion to the contingent goals of the state, goals that are antithetical to the external organizing principles of governance. For committed elites, to accept external recommendations without qualification might mean to threaten their political authority and rescind their ontological security. In the two emergent powers, politicians and key decision makers approached a looming health crisis using social purposes as their conceptual lenses.

Although nonconstructivist scholars often overlook social purposes, their autonomous influence on systems of governance is difficult to overestimate. In certain circumstances, social purposes not only individualize political spaces across the globe but also provide distinct blueprints for collective action and stabilize societal expectations about the appropriate course of policy making. Once accepted at the level of both elites and wider audiences, legitimate social purposes acquire conceptual power, that is, the "capacity to shape patterns and terms of thought and learning."[1] Robbed of attractive and comprehensible social purposes, rulers will not enjoy voluntary compliance and will have to rely on force. While coercive capacity is undeniably important (along with the control of material resources and the power to overrule alternative governance options) to maintain the internal sovereignty of the state, a coherent social and political order is hardly possible without social purposes being internalized by the public.

In the preceding chapters, I examined the systems of AIDS governance in Russia and South Africa. Specifically, I investigated how governments understood the nature of the epidemic, why they removed (or erected) obstacles to the evidence-based prevention services, and to what extent they ensured (or undermined) universal access to proven life-saving medicines. I then probed why states interacted with the other participants in social practice the way they did. As the two governments under investigation embraced different ideas about the core goals of the state, their governing strategies turned out to be different from the empirical standpoint. These obvious differences, however, should not obscure the bigger picture of the conceptual equivalence of the examined cases. Most importantly, domestic responses to AIDS were confluent with the embraced standards and principles of governance that rested on the normative foundation of social purposes. This is why neither the Russian nor the South African elite was ready to adopt external standards of AIDS governance unconditionally and completely. In short, anxieties about normative intrusions from abroad impelled the state to undermine good health governance. There is no need to go over my empirical findings here. Instead, this conclusion first summarizes implications for three important debates. Then, it offers some practical warnings for those practitioners who venture to change the unsatisfying approaches to AIDS governance.

IMPLICATIONS FOR THREE DEBATES

Telling the complex stories of AIDS governance in Russia and South Africa is relevant for three broad debates. The first debate investigates the causal mechanisms that connect international influences with domestic outcomes. Missing from this debate is the broader explanatory strategy that allows highlighting how attempts to construct and maintain political authority at home (with the focus on developing its normative dimension rather than acquiring and dispensing "brute" material power) get in the way of global norm diffusion. To contribute to this debate, I supply such a strategy. The second debate seeks to specify the conditions under which ideational elements play an independent causal role in governance and policy making. The constructivist spin on this debate addresses a long-overdue question about the power of ideas that emerge from the state's justifications for its own existence and rationales for sovereignty. My conceptual elaborations both confirm and advance some of the previous findings that summarize factors contributing to the independence of ideas in policy making. My elaborations also modify constructivist insights in regard to social purposes as one of the most important, but commonly overlooked, types of ideational elements. Instead of painting social purposes with broad strokes and assuming their influence on the systems of governance, I elucidate how social purposes emerge and weigh their influence on systems of governance. Without this theorizing, it is hard to understand how a seemingly random collection of ideas and beliefs becomes coherent and directional. The voices in the third debate call us to come to grips with systems of health governance in a holistic manner. Welcome as they are, previous achievements in investigating the political, social, and cultural determinants of health governments are not without limitations in their explanatory capacity. The time is ripe to probe the analytical potency of the new concepts instead of resuscitating and overstretching the old ones. Using constructivism to parse systems of health governance, as shown empirically, generates nontrivial results. Conceptually, this research confirms the significance of social purpose in adding value to current research strategies.

INTERNATIONAL INFLUENCES AND DOMESTIC OUTCOMES

The first debate for which my inquiry is relevant concerns the causal mechanisms that connect international influences with domestic outcomes. The conventional approach describes policy diffusion as a situation in which change of policies, norms, and ideas in one country increases the chances of their change in others. The dated view on global diffusion centers simply on norm convergence and harmonization of practices across borders. Recently, many constructivist scholars have highlighted conflicts and contestations arising during diffusion processes and stipulated conditions under which norm adoption is likely to occur.[2] Although the focus on norm contestation was a step forward, many new studies seem to satisfy no other analytical purpose than the authorial enjoyment of tweaking the available models to fit any individual case. As the list of cases and models grows, so does the sense of disarray. There is also a clear tendency to misuse constructivist vocabulary, especially in equating norms with policies and norm diffusion with policy transfer. Although there is nothing wrong with using rough synonyms, the inaccurate handling of precise conceptual tools inevitably obfuscates the analytical insights that constructivist perspectives on norms can currently offer. The main theoretical fault is that scholars display a glaring indisposition to disaggregate norms into constitutive norms (such as social purposes), organizing principles, and standardized procedures. But these distinctions, as demonstrated in the relevant empirical chapters, are very important for acquiring an analytical leverage on norm diffusion processes. While my approach does not allow for gathering the available norm diffusion models into a cumulative list or a neat theoretical table, it offers the heuristic power to reason if the collision course is imminent between the state-centric structures of authority, on the one hand, and innovative but not necessarily comfortable organizing principles that spread across the globe, on the other.

This conceptualization sets my analysis apart from those empirically oriented scholars who, without plunging into complex theoretical elaborations, try to grasp what states want from internationally agreed-upon norms and best practices. While they scrutinize complex combinations of constraining domestic circumstances and proximate international contexts in which governments operate, it is worthwhile probing the gap between internationally recognized norms and domestic normative contexts. The concept of the social purpose of the state captures the constitutive notions about the legitimate normative order with which additional regulative norms are suffused. Inquiring into the role of social purposes helps ascertain what constitutes domestic appropriateness, which, depending on its content and the degree of public acceptance, frustrates or facilitates norm diffusion. Domestic commitments to uphold social purposes can interrupt or complicate the process of norm diffusion, which otherwise might propel domestic reforms and pave the way to good governance.

The proposition that seemingly innocuous regulatory standards might challenge domestic authority and legitimacy is enticing, but proving it requires a thoroughgoing inquiry.[3] The practical task of this book was to go back to basics and examine the underlying dynamic—how and why domestic structures of authority make leaders cope with novel international norms and standardized practices. As explained in chapter 3, the dissolution of the intersubjective consensus on the core goals of the state, accompanied by the decline of the state's coercive capacity, unsettles high-powered decision makers and prompts them to rethink their magisterial commitments and the cardinal objectives of the states they lead. Reinvigorating ideas about the appropriate methods of governance and then mainstreaming them are two of the magisterial ways in which governments seek to enhance their ontological security and to exercise their control over the populace. Because these processes are quite palpable in several emergent powers, including Russia and South Africa, we have a good opportunity to inquire into their implications, including their impact on global diffusion. In addition, probing the emerging structures of authority and new normative contexts that stimulate Russian and South African bids for regional prominence can be valuable for the keen observers of the evolving meanings of sovereignty. At the very least, knowing the content of social purposes and the direction of committed elites' ambitions, we will be able to anticipate if the country of interest is moving in a localizing or, conversely, in a globalizing direction.

THE CAUSAL POWER OF IDEAS

The second debate with which this book engages seeks to explore the conditions under which ideational elements generate independent causal effects. Of course, it is tempting to stay away from this question, since the very notion of "idea" tends to provoke conceptual bewilderment, while its uncritical application prompts tautological explanations. Although the heart of the debate is about the explanatory capacity of ideas, additional complications arise from the fact that loose definitions and perplexing taxonomies overwhelm scholars who also have to deal with the reasonable suspicion that each type of ideational element operates through its own unique causal mechanism.[4]

The term "ideas" might refer to a large number of distinct mental constructs. Rationalists commonly argue that ideas (defined as worldviews or principled and causal beliefs) are a substitute for incomplete information, justify how policy actors attain their given interests, and operate as a switch when several paths to the ultimate goal of utility maximization are possible. Cognitivists view ideas as mental shortcuts, biases, analogies, and even psychological responses to confusing data that influence and sometimes distort rational decision making. The standard answer not rooted in rationalism, however, finds the power of ideas in the murky realm of immutable cultures, macroidentities, practices, and deep-seated social values. Any "all the way down" arguments of this sort are excessively bewildering, as they obscure self-conscious and resolute efforts at validating an intersubjective consensus about the core goals of the state and holding on to the state as the ultimate locus of authority. Presumptions that national cultures, histories, and macroidentities tightly fetter decision makers are as untenable as the opposite argument that presents individuals as stern utility maximizers. In contrast to both sides, constructivists do not treat ideas as the property of agency or as oversocializing structures.[5] Instead, they view ideas as socially constructed reasons for actions that emerge out of the systems of representation of meanings about a particular subject matter. But ideas are not always reasons for action. It is the task of a scholar to stipulate the circumstances under which ideas become something more than mere expressions of individual thinking or epiphenomenal collective constructs. Ideas take on their own independent dynamic and become the reasons for action under four conditions.

First, ideas matter when leaders treat them as obligations and thus cannot simply sacrifice them for any parochial goal. Russian and South African ideas about the core goals of the state became much more than rhetorical devices that justified the pursuit of power and wealth. On the one hand, it is hard to argue with Brian Taylor, for instance, who avers that strengthening the state and asserting its autonomy in Russia "has in reality been more about establishing the dominance of the Kremlin than creating the administrative capacity to run a well-functioning 21st century government."[6] However, those who climbed high on the political ladder became deeply committed to these ideas as the preferred solutions for a wide variety of governance issues. It is true that many skeptical observers of South African and Russian politics have commented on the notions of the African Renaissance and sovereign democracy as if these concepts were simply justifications of elites' pursuit of social dominance. Russian liberals averred that sovereign democracy justified Putin's drift toward personalistic rule. Without any doubt, Putin's entourage used ideas about the state and his image as the sole defender of the common good for narrow, self-serving reasons. Similarly, promoting the African Renaissance was a tool in securing Mbeki's status as an anticolonial ruler of continental stature. However, the massive propaganda in the two states does not rule out the independent causal power of the propagated ideas. Further, at some point, the unleashed sensibilities start constraining leaders' freedom of choice; decision makers find themselves defenseless against the ideas they validated and powerless to change the precharted course of governance.

Second, ideas are independently powerful when they operate autonomously from the structural conditions that otherwise constrain leaders' decisions and paralyze the freedom of their choice. Although ideas cannot always break loose from the overpowering weight of material circumstances, the objective conditions quite often allow interpretive flexibility. Once different social actors offer different but equally plausible policy solutions while dealing with the same problem, a consideration that ideas matter becomes warranted.

Third, ideas gain their own force once they are no longer mere intellectual extensions of previously employed governance ideas. Demonstrating the causal power of the nascent domestic conceptions of the common good requires showing that they break with the continuity of some historically durable set of ideational elements that used to characterize a particular political space.[7] Breaking out of the conceptual straitjacket of historically validated norms might depend on leaders' and the public's devotion to self-reflexivity, conceptual complexity, and cultural openness, but in today's world, such factors as skill expansion, information explosion, and proliferation of microidentities are likely to stimulate interpretive flexibility. Individuals and states can and often do break loose from the oversocializing power of prior patterns of cognition.

Moreover, the consideration that muted ideas have a long pedigree and seem to dwell permanently in the public consciousness does not negate the fact that political elites purposefully resuscitate them in order to chase their goals. In other words, the repertoire of available ideas might be limited, but the validation of consciously singled out ideas and fundamental norms is an ongoing process that either shores up intersubjective consensus or impedes it. It is important to bear in mind that norms' validity is not inviolable, even when historical evidence seemingly points to the conclusion that these norms are set in stone. Normative inheritances, as constraining as they might be in certain political and cultural contexts, therefore, do not preordain how elites decide to deal with urgent policy problems. Although perception that the state was the only legitimate locus of authority featured heavily in Russian history, the resurrection of that idea under Putin's rule was deliberate. To illustrate these points, I have presented evidence that Russian and South African elites did not simply inherit the ideas and social purposes of the past but intentionally constructed them.

Fourth, while leaders' premeditated commitments make some ideas prominent, it is the structure of social communication that gives these ideas strong social footing and validates them. Although conventional constructivists might consider such insight fairly ordinary, the prevailing tendency is to focus on the available corpus of books, films, travelogues, and other similar types of fictional representations that, taken in their entirety, constitute the cognitive map of collective articulations. Doubtless, examining fiction is important because it raises socially important themes and communicates politically motivated concerns to the public. In principle, while fiction can serve as one of the vessels of social communication that keeps some ideas alive in the public mind, hasty conclusions that highlight its causal or constitutive impact on the intersubjective consensus about core governance methods are deficient and unsatisfying.

My line of reasoning is different. Elites and opinion leaders promulgate and sustain ideas within the unfolding process of domestic debates and communication. Studying official statements on core ideas helps us discover the formal validity of social purposes; and probing the structure of the discursive communication at home helps us ascertain whether the public confirms these core norms collectively. In this context, identity arguments are of paramount importance. They help sway public opinion and convince wider (initially noncommitted) audiences that any alternative norm undermines the cardinal goals of the state and goes against the accepted conception of the common good. The failure to spell out core ideas and the inability to unfold compelling identity arguments might jeopardize the public's intersubjective consensus on which exact core ideas should be held dear. After all, nobody should follow those who cannot offer reasonable justifications for the existence of a political community and rationales for its sovereignty.

In a nutshell, the central point of contributing to this debate is that ideas acquire their own independent power when they become social goals, that is, when they become confluent with the content of political authority espoused by the ruling group. Although many leaders in many postcolonial countries have mulled over the role of indigenous knowledge, only Mbeki thought to elevate these ideas as the core goal of the state. In other words, the state's justification for its raison d'être makes certain ideas politically meaningful for shaping the systems of governance at home. Surely, ideas about governance can result from rational calculations, but these calculations are likely to be made within the conceptual parameters set forth by the legitimate ideas regarding the cardinal goals of the state.

SOCIAL PURPOSES IN HEALTH GOVERNANCE

Scholars hardly ever complain that the literature on public health fails to examine some important variables and determinants of health governance.[8] This is not very surprising, because concepts of policy tragedy, policy transfer, issue framing, patrimonialism, ethnic boundaries, and social construction of target populations have been fruitfully applied to the study of various aspects of health governance.[9] But time and again health scholars have demurely acknowledged that they are losing their conceptual grip on understanding the system of global health governance as a whole. Quite simply, there are too many actors, institutions, initiatives, and issues in relation to domestic and transboundary politics of AIDS to keep track of. A more important complication arises from the fact that all too many conventional concepts are simply inappropriate for the task.

For instance, concepts from the public policy toolshed might illuminate some aspects of global health governance but hardly ever clarify its deep-seated drivers and underpinnings. It is tempting, for instance, to overuse the comfortable notion of issue framing, despite its limited analytical usefulness.[10] At the very least, scholars should not avoid discussing the extent to which issue framing independently affects health governance. If frames simply reflect rational preferences, material interests, objective epidemiological circumstances, organizational cultures, and deep-seated normative proclivities, then the explanatory power of that concept is overstated. Active drug users, for instance, are often framed as socially untrustworthy and unproductive members of society, but in Russia, as shown in chapter 5, this labeling remains secondary to the master frame of a state-sponsored disdain for human rights. The point that bears emphasis here is that failing to see these distinctions will predictably lead scholars to misinterpret the nature of health governance. Another equally faulty tendency is to employ the notion of practice, currently in vogue with international relation theorists. "Practice" is a new catchall term that describes the patterned nature of meaningful behavior in certain socially organized contexts.[11] That notion impedes our ability to distinguish between independent variables and resultant methods of governance, even though maintaining these distinctions is necessary for doing normal social science.

This book offers a strategy for how to search for coherent but not obvious answers in the midst of the described theoretical disorientation. While internal observers notice unfolding domestic discourses about the appropriate tasks of the state and even take part in them, political scientists often overlook the profound implications of these discussions. As a result of the research presented here, we can assuredly indicate that, at least in Russia and South Africa, systems of AIDS governance have been shaped and defined by the consciously formulated and intersubjectively shared goals of the state. Much as the constructivist study of social purposes sharpens our analysis of norm diffusion, it also enriches the literature on global health governance. Social purposes make possible a range of policy responses that otherwise would have been either less viable or not pursued as the deliberate strategies of health governance. Quite simply, social purposes shape social practices. For instance, the indigenous turn in the South African policy environment as a part of the elite-driven conception of national renewal legitimized and institutionalized traditional medicines. Without the propelling force of the African Renaissance, this kind of action would have been on the margins of health governance rather than in its center. Similarly, in Russia, the harsh restrictions on harm reduction, needle exchange programs, and medically assisted therapy, as well as harassment of their promoters, became possible because of the elite's motivation to impede liberal values and paralyze the value of human rights.

Empirical findings presented here indicate that the effects of social purposes are very important for the adoption of international AIDS guidelines. Evidence suggests that policy makers should evaluate the compatibility of the principles of evidence-based medicines, universality of access to prevention and treatment, and nonhierarchical and nonstate governance on the grounds of their commitments to uphold legitimate social purposes. This finding does not deny the confluent impact of other factors. In the Russian case, low administrative capacity, pervasive corruption, and prejudice against sexual minorities and addicts interfere with tracing the effects of sovereign democracy. In South Africa, weaknesses of the public sector inherited from the apartheid regime and the much-lamented scarcity of health-care professionals and nurses have played an immense role and can be seen as more consequential for the implications of the African Renaissance for health governance systems. I have discussed additional and alternative arguments at length in chapter 1; suffice it to say that no additional factors negate the main conclusions of this research.

LESSONS FOR PRACTITIONERS

Although this study has avoided giving explicit policy advice, practitioners can derive many invaluable insights from academic studies of health governance. For instance, the study of state capacity might be quite relevant to explain some practical challenges to AIDS governance. According to Amy Patterson, the interlocking phenomena of the incapacitating role of traditional patriarchy in Africa, the dependence on international financial resources, the lack of consistency in political and economic commitments, the inability to design and implement long-term treatment and prevention programs, and even the civil society challenging the state's authority undermine the state's capacity.[12] Understanding these challenges and responding to them might increase the efficiency of practitioners' efforts to improve health governance. On the other hand, problems that appear to relate just to implementation or capacity issues might have strong connections to the deep-seated factors whose influence is not that obvious at first sight.

Most importantly, practitioners have to understand that domestic systems of health governance are shaped by factors that originate outside health issue area. For instance, Russian attempts to achieve "pharmaceutical independence" and "food sovereignty," as well as the South African strategy to develop indigenous drugs, were only elements, albeit very important ones, of larger predilections and commitments. In general, loud and sometimes perfervid public commitments to the new social purposes essentially signaled that elites were taking a shot at the sweeping social engineering efforts. Then, attempts to change inefficient and poor health governance, welcome as they are, might not remove the underlying cause of the problem practitioners are trying to deal with.

Practitioners should realize that policy fixes are relatively easy when foundational norms and deeply internalized ideas are not the source of the looming governance crisis. Surely, some methods of prevention of virus transmission are controversial, but practical difficulties on the road to adopting prevention strategies in different countries actually differ greatly in their intensity and complexity. Many governments express deep concerns about harm reduction, but very few muster the strongest possible objection to them, arguing that these methods of health governance go against the very nature of domestic customs and highly valued political orders. Similarly, a devotion to traditional medicines can feature heavily in many political spaces, but rarely do these commitments stem from the perceived pillars of the desired social order. The attachment to traditional medicines does not have to contravene available evidence-based solutions and can peacefully coexist with the deployment of conventional medicines.

In Russia and South Africa, however, the root of the problem was precisely in the emergent normative orders, which turned out to be antithetical to the external principles of governance. These normative orders (which I have referred to as social purposes) determined and narrowed the horizon of the politically suitable approaches to public health. In this context, rectifying policy mistakes would involve more than just correcting separate policy mistakes and shortcomings. In other words, improving AIDS governance in the two cases involves questioning and even subverting the increasingly hidebound goals of the state and self-serving conceptions of the common good that became preponderant in Putin's Russia and Mbeki's South Africa. Although in the latter case the change occurred after the ANC ousted Mbeki in September 2008, the legacy of commitment to and support of traditional medicines is not likely to go away by itself. In the former case, that unlikely change has yet to occur.

For Russia, two additional considerations deserve special attention. First, the prolonged delays in procuring and disbursing antiretroviral treatment were clearly a result of endemic corruption and a lack of state capacity and coordination among various segments of bureaucracy. Multiple scandals have exposed the state's low effectiveness in securing life-saving medications and some elements of corruption in the purchase of medical equipment, even though criminal charges have rarely been brought against any state officials. Graft and ineptitude, which debilitate the best policy intentions and impede good governance efforts, flourish in Putin's Russia precisely because its leaders cannot abolish their devotion to the autonomous state and instead embrace the goals of building modern impersonal administrative machinery. Although the autonomous developmental state is the source of bad governance, a change in the cardinal goals of the state might never materialize. To date, all too many individuals and opinion leaders have accepted the core tenets of sovereign democracy without fully acknowledging it. Even the mass protests that erupted in December 2011 in the country's capital targeted the specific machinations of Putin's lieutenants rather than the normative pillars of the extant political regime. That is why, at the dawn of Putin's second decade in power, general audiences have not linked their swelling dissatisfaction with the Russian health-care system to the desire to abolish the faulty goals of the state.

The second pressing question is under what conditions evidence-based approaches can overpower the climate of hostility to drug users and resistance to harm reduction. Constructivists note that norms, because they are horizons for appropriate behavior, are usually malleable, and, as a consequence, potential adopters enjoy a certain flexibility in how they interpret new norms. That flexibility might facilitate the acceptance of the standardized practices that these norms underpin. But some standardized practices cannot be enacted without difficulty and resistance because their underlying principles go against the prevailing (whether fully legitimate or power-based) social purpose. Politicians and society are likely to consider external principles of governance inappropriate unless these principles match, or do not challenge, the internalized ideas about the core tasks of the state. That is why efforts to promote harm-reduction programs by appealing to human-rights principles are not likely to succeed in present-day Russia. On the contrary, given the elite-fostered suspicion of human rights as a Western-sponsored subversive plot against the autonomy and sovereignty of the Russian state, this might cause a powerful backlash against the agents of change. In other words, pressing for the rights of marginalized and negatively constructed populations will stoke the fire of domestic resistance to what the state already perceives as malignant influences promoting alien norms.

But promoting harm reduction as a value-neutral health policy might slowly depoliticize the internal discourse on prevention and slowly ease the current governmental commitment to punitive criminal justice.[13] Less tactfully put, in addition to arousing public awareness about Putin's stubborn rejection of human-rights principles and his defiance of any external authority, domestic advocates of harm reduction should come to grips with their own failures. Holding the Russian elite responsible for matters in general but trying to make the

Kremlin uphold the rights of intravenous drug users will not suffice. Although the advantages of the value-neutral versus human-rights approach are still under debate in the relevant literature, domestic proponents of harm reduction should definitely explore the value-neutral option.[14] In short, the value-neutral approach might entail a change in policy, while at this juncture the human-rights approach will certainly not be successful.

In South Africa, relevant policy actors, not excluding the president and the health minister, truly believed they were doing the right thing for the rebirth of the country. Despite a rotation in political elites, Thabo Mbeki's focus on indigenousness and disrespect for international prescriptions surely left South Africa with profound legacies that have undermined the implementation of evidence-based strategies at the provincial and local levels in the long haul. That legacy also perpetuates a unique policy-making environment in which even skeptically minded reporters who are sympathetic to conventional policy solutions do not confront *muthi* as an illegitimate option to address the public health crisis. Investigative reporters have exposed multiple unscrupulous entrepreneurs and businesspeople who have tried to turn infected individuals' hopes of a cure for AIDS into a way to make money. But the same reporters have also condoned the high degree of societal acceptance of traditional healers and native medicines. One reporter, otherwise critical of the Cabinet's response to the epidemic, described genetic medicinal resources and healing practices as long-standing and positive components of internal culture.[15] Empowered during Mbeki's presidency, healers and peddlers of myriad cure-alls and nostrums will surely remain the principal part of the domestic policy landscape. Not surprisingly, even several years after his downfall, South African health policies were not fully in sync with international best practices. Undoing the damage of the previous administration can take a long time.

Another predicament is that so far, many policy participants tend not to concern themselves with the bigger picture. A health practitioner, an activist, and someone who works for a health NGO are likely to view epidemiology, prejudice, and stigma as the leading conditions or obstacles that governments face while governing health. In certain circumstances, these variables surely shape governmental behavior. Nevertheless, obligations to fulfill the cardinal goals of the state—understood by elites as a legitimate public good—are not far behind epidemiology and the other usual suspects. Health practitioners and policy entrepreneurs ought to concern themselves with the role of the constitutive ideas, because ideas about the state shape the governance environments in which agents of change operate. Comprehending the nature of social purposes and their significance for the extant systems of health governance will be helpful for those external and internal agents of change who wish to transform domestic contexts. At the very least, understanding the broader picture should help them foresee governmental attitudes toward them.

In summary, although this book deals mostly with analytical concerns, practitioners, policy advocates, and AIDS service organizations can use its detailed empirical descriptions as the basis for changing or correcting the styles and strategies they employ in order to increase the impact of their activities. The degree to which the proponents of reform can realize the complexity of attaining the standards of good health governance and communicate this complexity to the broader public will be the first step in the right direction. Having grasped the role of ideational determinants of norm diffusion, practitioners can apply the lessons from this study to the countries that fall out of the international mainstream because of their changing perception of the nature of political authority. Once again, this book can be relevant inasmuch as it makes clear to any concerned health actor the nature and the scope of the underlying difficulties in improving domestic health. It is also a warning for those political scientists who pay no attention to the deep-seated drivers of governance and thus are likely to give the agents of change misleading or trivial advice on policy improvement.

NOTES

Introduction

1. See, for instance, Audie Klotz, *Norms in International Relations: The Struggle against Apartheid* (Ithaca, NY: Cornell University Press, 1995).

2. Thabo Mbeki, address presented at the Knowledge Management Conference, University of Stellenbosch, January 16, 2012.

3. Thabo Mbeki, response at the debate of the National House of Traditional Leaders, Tshwane Municipal Chambers, April 2, 2008.

4. What counts as a generation and what ideas constitute its conventional wisdom might be subjects of dispute. A plausible interpretation is Jonathan N. Moyo, *Generational Shifts in African Politics: Prospects for a New Africa* (Los Angeles: James S. Coleman African Studies Center, UCLA, 2004).

5. Tom Lodge, *Politics in South Africa: From Mandela to Mbeki*, 2nd ed. (Cape Town: David Philip, 2002), 227–30.

6. I follow the definition of the structure of political authority as formulated in John Gerard Ruggie, "International Regime, Transactions, and Change: Embedded Liberalism in the Postwar Economic Order," *International Organization* 36, no. 2 (1982): 382; and in James N. Rosenau, *Distant Proximities: Dynamics beyond Globalization* (Princeton, NJ: Princeton University Press, 2003), 274–75.

7. My conceptualization of governance builds on the definition supplied by Oran R. Young, *International Governance: Protecting the Environment in a Stateless Society* (Ithaca, NY: Cornell University Press, 1994), 26.

8. For the definition of global liberal governmentality, see, for instance, Iver B. Neumann and Ole Jacob Sending, *Governing the Global Polity: Practice, Mentality, Rationality* (Ann Arbor: University of Michigan Press, 2010), 14–15.

9. For more general discussion of the discourse analysis as a research tool, see Iver B. Neumann, "Discourse Analysis," in *Qualitative Methods in International Relations: A Pluralist Guide*, ed. Audie Klotz and Deepa Prakash (Basingstoke: Palgrave Macmillan, 2008), 61–77.

10. For a similar conceptualization, see Yale H. Ferguson and Richard W. Mansbach, *Remapping Global Politics: History's Revenge and Future Shock* (Cambridge: Cambridge University Press, 2004), esp. chap. 3.

11. Rosenau, *Distant Proximities*, 293–310.

12. For the connections between democratization and health activists in the late 1980s, see, for instance, Amy Nunn, *The Politics and History of AIDS Treatment in Brazil* (New York: Springer, 2009), chaps. 1 and 2.

13. Susanne Choi and Roman David, "Law Enforcement, Public Health, and HIV/AIDS in China," in *The Global Politics of AIDS*, ed. Paul G. Harris and Patricia D. Siplon (Boulder, CO: Lynne Reiner Publishers, 2007), 150.

Chapter 1. Purposeful Choices

1. Steward Patrick, *Weak Links: Fragile States, Global Threats, and International Security* (Oxford: Oxford University Press, 2011), 208–40; Pieter Fourie, "The Relationship between the AIDS Pandemic and State Fragility," *Global Change, Peace & Security* 19, no. 3 (2007): 281–300.

2. Stefan Elbe, *Virus Alert: Security, Governmentality, and the AIDS Pandemic* (New York: Columbia University Press, 2009), 27, 56. For a broader discussion of the evolution of political approaches to AIDS as a security issue, see Colin McInnes and Simon Rushton, "HIV, AIDS and Security: Where Are We Now?," *International Affairs* 86, no. 1 (2010): 225–45.

3. Fred Frohock, *Healing Powers: Alternative Medicine, Spiritual Communities, and the State* (Chicago: University of Chicago Press, 1992), 241–43.

4. James F. Keeley, "Toward a Foucauldian Analysis of International Regimes," *International Organization* 44, no. 1 (1990): 92.

5. For a useful summary of this perspective, see David Roberts, *Global Governance and Biopolitics: Regulating Human Security* (London: Zed Books, 2010), 38–44.

6. For an example of such analysis, in which different independent variables produce essentially similar results, see Didier Fassin, "The Politics of Death: Race War, Bio-power and AIDS in the Post-apartheid," in *Foucault on Politics, Security and War*, ed. Michael Dillon and Andrew W. Neal (Basingstoke: Palgrave Macmillan, 2008), 154–64.

7. Christian Reus-Smit, *The Moral Purpose of the State: Culture, Social Identity, and Institutional Rationality in International Relations* (Princeton, NJ: Princeton University Press, 1999), 127–29.

8. Rawi Abdelal, *National Purpose in the World Economy: Post-Soviet States in Comparative Perspective* (Ithaca, NY: Cornell University Press, 2000), 25–27.

9. The spiral model of norm diffusion is presented in Thomas Risse and Kathryn Sikkink, "The Socialization of International Human Rights Norms into Domestic Practices: Introduction," in *The Power of Human Rights: International Norms and Domestic Change*, ed. Thomas Risse-Kappen, Stephen C. Ropp, and Kathryn Sikkink (Cambridge: Cambridge University Press, 1999), 1–38. For a useful summary of main norm diffusion

models, see Wade Jacoby, "Inspiration, Coalition, and Substitution: A Review Essay on External Influences on Postcommunist Transformations," *World Politics* 58, no. 4 (2006): 623–51; Beth Simmons, Frank Dobbin, and Geoffrey Garret, "Introduction: The International Diffusion of Liberalism," *International Organization* 60, no. 4 (2006): 787–801; Sonia Cardenas, "Norm Collision: Explaining the Effects of International Human Rights Pressure on State Behavior," *International Studies Review* 6 (2004): 215.

10. Peter Haas, ed., "Knowledge, Power, and International Policy Coordination," special issue, *International Organization* 46 (Winter 1992).

11. For a further discussion of these distinctions, see Eric Stern, "Crisis and Learning: A Conceptual Balance Sheet," *Journal of Contingencies and Crisis Management* 5, no. 2 (1997): 82.

12. Wade Jacoby, "Minority Traditions and Postcommunist Politics: How Do IGO's Matter," in *Transnational Actors in Central and East European Transitions*, ed. Mitchel Orenstein, Stephen Bloom, and Nicole Lindstrom (Pittsburgh: University of Pittsburgh Press, 2008), 58.

13. For a detailed discussion of the donor responses to AIDS, see Joshua W. Busby, *Moral Movements and Foreign Policy* (Cambridge: Cambridge University Press, 2010), 151–209.

14. For a detailed discussion of PEPFAR, see chapter 5. Theo Smart, "Is PEPFAR Competing or Cooperating in Treatment Scale-up?," *Health-e News Service*, June 23, 2006.

15. See, for instance, Frank Schimmelfennig, "The Community Trap: Liberal Norms, Rhetorical Action, and the Eastern Enlargement of European Union," *International Organization* 55, no. 1 (2001): 47–80; Jeffrey Checkel, "Why Comply? Social Learning and European Identity Change," *International Organization* 55, no. 3 (2001): 553–88; Michael Zürn and Jeffrey T. Checkel, "Getting Socialized to Build Bridges: Constructivism and Rationalism, Europe and the Nation-State," *International Organization* 59 (2005): 1045–79.

16. See, for instance, Yuriy Luzhkov, "My i zapad," *Strategiya Rossii* 6 (2006); Konstantin Kosachev, "Rossiya i zapad: Nashi raznoglasiya," *Rossiya v global'noy politike* 4 (2007). For a further discussion on the Russian elite's foreign policy discourse, see Petr Kratochvíl, "The Discursive Resistance to EU-Enticement: The Russian Elite and (the Lack of) Europeanisation," *Europe-Asia Studies* 60, no. 3 (2008): 410–11, 415–16.

17. Vladimir Putin, "Demokratiya i kachestvo gosudarstva," *Kommersant*, February 6, 2012.

18. See, for instance, Yanzhong Huang, *Enter the Dragon and the Elephant: China's and India's Participation in Global Health Governance* (New York: Council on Foreign Relations, 2013), 3.

19. For a recent elaboration of this model, see, for instance, Amitav Acharya, "How Ideas Spread: Whose Norms Matter? Norm Localization and Institutional Change in Asian Regionalism," *International Organization* 58, no. 2 (2004): 239–75. See also

Joshua W. Busby, *Moral Movements and Foreign Policy* (Cambridge: Cambridge University Press, 2010), 2.

20. Constructivists seem to understand this point well. See, for instance, Ted Hopf, *Social Construction of International Politics: Identities and Foreign Policies, Moscow, 1955 and 1999* (Ithaca, NY: Cornell University Press, 2002), 13.

21. For a similar approach to disaggregating norms, see, for instance, Antje Wiener, "Normative Baggage in International Encounters: Contestation All the Way," in *On Rules, Politics, and Knowledge: Friedrich Kratochwil, International Relations, and Domestic Affairs*, ed. Oliver Kessler et al. (Basingstoke: Palgrave Macmillan, 2010), 208–10.

22. Patrick Thaddeus Jackson, *Civilizing the Enemy: German Reconstruction and the Invention of the West* (Ann Arbor: University of Michigan Press, 2006), 8.

23. Informative accounts of the history of the epidemic and responses to it include Greg Behrman, *The Invisible People: How the U.S. Has Slept through the Global AIDS Pandemic, the Greatest Humanitarian Catastrophe of Our Time* (New York: Free Press, 2004); Jonathan Engel, *The Epidemic: A Global History of AIDS* (New York: Smithsonian Books/Collins, 2006).

24. Evan S. Lieberman, *Boundaries of Contagion: How Ethnic Politics Have Shaped Government Responses to AIDS* (Princeton, NJ: Princeton University Press, 2009), 115.

25. Jeremy Youde, *AIDS, South Africa, and the Politics of Knowledge of Global Health* (Aldershot: Ashgate Publishing, 2007), 43–57.

26. For an overview of the pre-Mbeki AIDS policy, see Patrick J. Furlong and Karen L. Ball, "The More Things Change: AIDS and the State in South Africa, 1987–2003," in *The African State and the AIDS Crisis*, ed. Amy Patterson (Aldershot: Ashgate Publishing, 2006), 127–53.

27. Alec Russel, *Bring Me My Machine Gun: The Battle for the Soul of South Africa, from Mandela to Zuma* (New York: Public Affairs, 2009), 205–6.

28. Boris Yeltsin, *Ispoved' na zadannuyu temu* (Leningrad: Chas pik, 1990), preface.

29. Leon Aron, *Yeltsin: A Revolutionary Life* (New York: St. Martin's Press, 2000), 322–23.

30. Frank Chikane, "Angel or Demon?," *Star*, July 23, 2010.

31. "Thin-Skinned Mbeki Will Require Deft Handling," Cable 01PRETORIA1173, created February 23, 2001, released August 30, 2011.

32. See Rebecca Cassidy and Melissa Leach, "Science, Politics, and the Presidential Aids 'Cure,'" *African Affairs* 108, no. 433 (2009): 559–80; Ebenezer Obadare and Iruka N. Okeke, "Biomedical Loopholes, Distrusted State, and the Politics of HIV/AIDS 'Cure' in Nigeria," *African Affairs* 110, no. 439 (2011): 191–211.

33. Pregs Govender, *Love and Courage: A Story of Insubordination* (Johannesburg: Jacana Media, 2008), 239.

34. For a broader discussion, see Steven Robins, "Sexual Politics and the Zuma Rape Trial," *Journal of Southern African Studies* 34, no. 2 (2008): 411–27.

35. Tom Parfitt, "Russian Politicians Fight to Legislate against False Science," *Lancet* 366, no. 9,497 (2005): 1597–98.

36. Susanne Wengle and Michael Rasell, "The Monetisation of L'goty: Changing Patterns of Welfare Politics and Provision in Russia," *Europe-Asia Studies* 60, no. 5 (2008): 739–56.

37. Virginia van der Vliet, "South Africa Divided against AIDS: A Crisis of Leadership," in *AIDS and South Africa: The Social Expression of a Pandemic,* ed. Kyle D. Kauffman and David L. Lindauer (Basingstoke: Palgrave Macmillan, 2004), 84–85.

38. For a historical account of traditional healing in South Africa, see, for instance, Karen E. Flint, *Healing Traditions: African Medicine, Cultural Exchange, and Competition in South Africa, 1820–1948* (Athens: Ohio University Press, 2008).

39. For the key events of this story, see Vladimir Voronov, "Tomografiya natsional'noy korruptsii," *Sovershenno sekretno,* August 2, 2011.

40. Jason Bush et al., "When Putin Ordered Up New Hospitals, His Associates Botched the Operation," *Reuters,* May 22, 2014.

41. See, for instance, Svetlana Reyter, "Komu vygoden zapret na vvoz meditsinskoy tekhniki," *RosBiznesKonsalting,* June 23, 2014.

42. Slindile Khanyle, "New Breed of Traditional Healers Has Sharp Eye on Marketing," *Business Report,* May 15, 2008.

43. See, for instance, Nathan Geffen, *Echoes of Lysenko: State-Sponsored Pseudo-science in South Africa* (CSSR Working Paper No. 149, March 2006).

44. Maurizio Lazzarato, "Neoliberalism in Action Inequality, Insecurity and the Reconstitution of the Social," *Theory, Culture & Society* 26, no. 6 (2009): 109.

45. See, for instance, Coleen O'Manique, *Neoliberalism and AIDS Crisis in Sub-Saharan Africa: Globalization's Pandemic* (Basingstoke: Palgrave Macmillan, 2004), 6–10, 52–55, 78–96.

46. See, for instance, Rick Rowden, *The Deadly Ideas of Neoliberalism: How the IMF has Undermined Public Health and the Fight against AIDS* (New York: Zed Books, 2009).

47. Roberts, *Global Governance,* 101.

48. Michael J. Bosia, "Assassin! AIDS and Neoliberal Reform in France," *New Political Science* 27, no. 3 (2005): 291–308; Bosia, "Written in Blood: AIDS Prevention and the Politics of Failure in France," *Perspectives on Politics* 4, no. 4 (2006): 647–53.

49. On the evidence that the professional health community in fact influenced the health security agenda and successfully challenged neoliberalism, see Roberts, *Global Governance,* 52–62.

Chapter 2. Assembling the Purpose

1. Liliya Shevtsova, *Rezhim Borisa Yeltsina* (Moscow: Rosspen, 1999), 41–44.

2. Kathleen E. Smith, *Mythmaking in the New Russia: Politics and Memory during the Yeltsin Era* (Ithaca, NY: Cornell University Press, 2002).

3. Georgiy Satarov, *Rossiya v poiskah idei: Analiz pressy* (Moscow, 1997).

4. For a theoretical and empirical discussion of this concept, see Brian Taylor, *State Building in Putin's Russia: Policing and Coercion after Communism* (Cambridge: Cambridge University Press, 2011), 36–70.

5. "Spetssluzhba personala," *Kommersant*, October 3, 2012.

6. Viktor Cherkesov, "Nel'zya dopustit', chtoby voiny prevratilis' v torgovtsev," *Kommersant*, October 9, 2007.

7. Boris Gryzlov, *Politicheskiy doklad pered delegatami III s'ezda partii Edinaya Rossiya*, September 22, 2003.

8. *Put' natsional'nogo uspeha: Manifest vserossiyskoy politicheskoy partii Edinstvo i Otechestvo—Edinaya Rossiya*, April 23, 2003.

9. Detailed information about these clubs is available on their websites: http://cscp .ru/; http://gpclub.ru/; and http://www.inop.ru.

10. Vladimir Gel'man, "Party Politics in Russia: From Competition to Hierarchy," *Europe-Asia Studies* 60, no. 6 (2008): 913–30.

11. See, for instance, Vyacheslav Nikonov, "Strategiya Putina," *Rossiyskaya gazeta*, December 22, 2004; Vladislav Surkov, "Putin ukreplyaet gosudarstvo, a ne sebya," *Komsomol'skaya pravda*, September 28, 2004.

12. Vladimir Putin, "Rossiya na rubezhe tysyacheletiy," *Nezavisimaya gazeta*, December 30, 1999.

13. Vladislav Surkov, "Suverennaya demokratiya i Edinaya Rossiya," *Strategiya Rossii* 3 (2006).

14. Vladislav Surkov, "Russkaya politicheskaya kul'tura," *Strategiya Rossii* 7 (2007).

15. Available at http://archive.kremlin.ru/text/appears/2004/05/71501.shtml.

16. Federal Law No. 18, "On Introducing Amendments to Certain Legislative Acts of the Russian Federation" (2006). For detailed analysis of the amendments, see *Challenge to Civil Society: Russia's Amended Law on Noncommercial Organizations* (Washington, DC: United States Commission on International Religious Freedom, 2007).

17. Il'ya Kriger, "Dura lex," *Novaya gazeta*, July 24, 2008.

18. James Richter, "Putin and the Public Chamber," *Post-Soviet Affairs* 25, no. 1 (2009): 39–65; James Richter, "The Ministry of Civil Society? The Public Chambers in the Regions," *Problems of Post-Communism* 56, no. 6 (2009): 7–20.

19. Irina Nevinnaya, "NKO poluchat polmilliarda rubley na programmy po profilaktike VICH-infektsii," *Rossiyskaya gazeta*, June 2, 2011; Natal'ya Korchenkova et al., "Agenty uzakoneny," *Kommersant*, July 14, 2012.

20. *Issledovaniye informatsionnoy otkrytosti sistemy raspredeleniya gosudarstvennoy podderzhki NKO: 2011–2012* (Moscow: Transparency International, 2014).

21. See http://bolshoepravitelstvo.rf.

22. Dimitriy Medvedev, "Sokhranit' effektivnoe gosudarstvo v sushchestvuyushchikh granitsakh," *Ekspert*, no. 13 (2005).

23. See, for instance, Michael Loriaux, "The French Developmental State as Myth and Moral Ambition," in *The Developmental State*, ed. Meredith Woo-Cumings (Ithaca, NY: Cornell University Press, 1999), 235.

24. Leon Aron, *The Button and the Bear* (Washington, DC: American Enterprise Institute, 2009).

25. Vladimir Putin, "Mineral'no-syr'evye resursy v strategii razvitiya rossiyskoy ekonomiki," *Zapiski gornogo instituta* 144, no. 1 (1999): 1–11.

26. Vladimir Putin, "Rossiya na rubezhe tysyacheletiy," *Nezavisimaya gazeta*, December 30, 1999.

27. Gryzlov, *Politicheskiy doklad*.

28. Stenogramma vystupleniya Vladislava Surkova, *Gensovet Delovoy Rossii*, May 17, 2005.

29. Yevgeniy Primakov, "Sovremennaya Rossiya i liberalism," *Rossiyskaya gazeta*, December 17, 2012; Yevgeniy Primakov, "Rossiya pered vyborom," *Rossiyskaya gazeta*, January 14, 2010.

30. Vystuplenie prezidenta Rossiyskoy federatsii V. Putina po povodu prioritetnykh natsional'nykh proektov, September 5, 2005.

31. Dimitriy Medvedev, "Natsional'nye proekty: Ot stabilizatsii—k razvitiyu," *Kommersant*, January 25, 2007.

32. For one of the clearest examples of this matured economic outlook, see Vladimir Putin, "Ne otkazhemsya ot sotsial'nyh obyazatel'stv," *Strategiya Rossii* 5 (2011).

33. For a historical overview of Russia's identity as a great power, see Andrei P. Tsygankov, "Vladimir Putin's Vision of Russia as a Normal Great Power," *Post-Soviet Affairs* 21, no. 2 (2005): 132–58; Iver B. Neumann, "Russia as a Great Power, 1815–2007," *Journal of International Relations and Development* 11 (2008): 128–51; Richard Sakwa, "Russia's Identity: Between the 'Domestic' and the 'International,'" *Europe-Asia Studies* 63, no. 6 (2011): 957–75.

34. Ted Hopf, *Social Construction of International Politics: Identities and Foreign Policies, Moscow, 1955 and 1999* (Ithaca, NY: Cornell University Press, 2002), 105.

35. Alexey Chadaev, *Putin: Ego ideologiya* (Moscow: Evropa, 2006), 39–47.

36. See, for instance, Putin's speech at the Forty-Third Munich Conference on Security Policy, October 2, 2007.

37. Vyacheslav Nikonov, "Chernaya magiya," *Izvestiya*, May 30, 2007.

38. Vladimir Zhirinovsky, "Strana zhivet po poniyatiyam," in *Russkaya politicheskaya kul'tura: Vzglyad iz utopii*, ed. Konstantin Remchukov (Moscow: Izdatel'stvo Nezavisimaya gazeta, 2007), 56.

39. Vitaliy Ivanov, *Antirevolyutsioner: Pochemu Rossii ne nuzhna oranzhevaya revolytsiya* (Moscow: Evropa, 2006); Nataliya Narochnickaya, ed. *Oranzhevye seti: Ot Belgrada do Bishkeka* (Saint Petersburg: Aleteyya, 2008).

40. Vitaliy Tret'yakov, "Beskhrebetnaya Rossiya," *Politicheskiy klass* 1, no. 2 (2005).

41. See, for instance, Vladimir Putin, "Novyy integratsionnyy proyekt dlya Yevrazii—budushcheye, kotoroye rozhdayetsya segodnya," *Izvestiya*, October 3, 2011.

42. Boris Gryzlov, "Partiya—ot latinskogo slova chast," *Tribuna*, September 20, 2005.

43. Vladislav Surkov, "Russkaya politicheskaya kul'tura," *Strategiya Rossii* 7 (2007).

44. Aleksandr Tsipko, "Pochvenniki i liberaly: Vozmozhno li primirenie mezhdu nimi?," *Strategiya Rossii* 8 (2006).

45. Vladimir Putin, "Nichego u nikh ne vyydet," *Rossiyskaya gazeta*, November 21, 2007.

46. Yuriy Luzhkov and Gavriil Popov, "Eshche odno slovo o Gaidare," *Moskovskiy komsomolets*, January 21, 2010.

47. Yuriy Afanas'yev, "Vozmozhna li segodnya v Rossii liberal'naya missiya?," *Liberal.ru*, February 16, 2011.

48. I thank Irina Chechel for drawing my attention to this concept. For the discussion, see "Podavlyayushchee bol'shinstvo," *Gefter.ru*, July 17, 2013.

49. Gleb Pavlovskiy, *Genial'naya vlast': Slovar' abstraktsiy Kremlya* (Moscow: Evropa, 2012).

50. Thabo Mbeki, "I Am an African," in *Africa: The Time Has Come, Selected Speeches* (Cape Town: Tafelberg; Johannesburg: Mafube, 1998), 31–36.

51. Moeletsi Mbeki, "Issues in South African Foreign Policy: The African Renaissance," *Souls: A Critical Journal of Black Politics, Culture, and Society* 2, no. 2 (2000): 77.

52. "Tasks of the African Renaissance," NEC *Bulletin*, July 12–14, 2002.

53. Ibid.

54. On the political role and functions of these policy units, see Richard Calland, *Anatomy of South Africa* (Cape Town: Zebra Press, 2006), 35–41, and on the expansion of the presidency, see 22–28.

55. Frank Chikane, "A New Type of Partnership: The African Renaissance and the Development of NEPAD," *Umrabulo* 27, no. 3 (2006).

56. On the background of these individuals and their political views and positions, see Calland, *Anatomy of South Africa*, 27–35, 49–53, 122–24.

57. "Statement of the National Executive Committee on the Occasion of the 88th Anniversary of the ANC," January 8, 2000, http://www.anc.org.za/show.php?id=60.

58. See, for instance, Kimberly Lanegran, "South Africa's 1999 Election: Consolidating a Dominant Party System," *Africa Today* 48, no. 2 (2001): 81–102.

59. See Thabo Mbeki, "The African Renaissance, South Africa and the World," in Mbeki, *Africa: The Time Has Come*, 239–50.

60. Pitika Ntuli, "The Missing Link between the Culture and Education: Are We Still Chasing Gods That Are Not Our Own?," in *African Renaissance: The New Struggle*, ed. Malegapuru William Makgoba (Johannesburg: Mafube and Tafelberg, 1999), 187.

61. Githae Mugo, "African Culture in Education for Sustainable Development," in Makgoba, *African Renaissance*, 225.

62. See the Fifty-First National Conference, Resolutions 52–59, December 20, 2002, http://www.anc.org.za/show.php?id=2495.

63. See the White Paper on Traditional Leadership and Governance and the Traditional Leadership and Governance, *Staatskoerant*, September 10, 2003; speaking notes for Deputy President Phumzile Mlambo-Ngcuka at the House of Traditional Leaders Social Development Day, October 19, 2007, http://dev.absol.co.za/Presidency/show.asp?type=sp&include=deputy/sp/2007/sp1019167.htm&ID=1686.

64. On the importance of heritage, see Thabo Mbeki, "We Are Children of a Rich Heritage," ANC *Today* 7, no. 38 (2007); Pallo Jordan, "Celebrate Our Dance, Celebrate Our Heritage," ANC *Today* 8, no. 36 (2008).

65. See, for instance, Stanley B. Greenberg, "Ideological Struggles within the South African State," in *The Politics of Race, Class, and Nationalism in Twentieth-Century South Africa*, ed. Shula Marks and Stanley Trapido (London: Longman, 1987).

66. Archie Brown, *The Rise and Fall of Communism* (New York: Ecco, 2009), 362–63.

67. Nicoli Nattrass, "Economic Restructuring in South Africa: The Debate Continues," *Journal of Southern African Studies* 2, no. 4 (1994): 517–31.

68. Hein Marais, *South Africa: Limits to Change: The Political Economy of Transition*, 2nd ed. (London: Zed Books; Cape Town: University of Cape Town, 2001).

69. John Weeks, "Stuck in Low GEAR? Macroeconomic Policy in South Africa 1996–98," *Cambridge Journal of Economics* 23, no. 6 (1999): 795–812. Coined by John Williamson and endorsed by major international financial institutions, the term "Washington Consensus" refers to ten specific economic ideas that stipulate a free-market way to development.

70. William Gumede, *Thabo Mbeki and the Battle for the Soul of the ANC* (London: Zed Books, 2007), 132.

71. Thabo Mbeki, "A New Patriotism: What Have I Contributed?," in Mbeki, *Africa: The Time Has Come*, 156.

72. Ibid.

73. Speech at the launch of the Global Business Unusual Tourism Campaign, Amsterdam, the Netherlands, November 1, 2005.

74. Eddy T. Maloka, "The South African 'African Renaissance' Debate: A Critique," paper written for the African Institute of South Africa, Pretoria, 2000.

75. David A. McDonald, "Ubuntu Bashing: The Marketisation of 'African Values' in South Africa," *Review of African Political Economy* 37, no. 124 (2010): 140.

76. See, for instance, Nickolaus Bauer, "ANCYL Warns of Zim-Style Land Invasions in South Africa," *Mail and Guardian*, June 6, 2012.

77. For a convincing explanation of this fundamental shift, see Jeremy Youde, "The Generational Shift in South African Foreign Policy," in *Theory and Application of the "Generation" in International Relations and Politics*, ed. Brent J. Steele and Jonathan M. Acuff (Basingstoke: Palgrave Macmillan, 2011), 97–122. See also Tristan Anne Borer and Kurt Mills, "Explaining Postapartheid South African Human Rights Foreign Policy: Unsettled Identity and Unclear Interests," *Journal of Human Rights* 10, no. 1 (2011): 76–98.

78. Peter Vale and Sipho Maseko, "Thabo Mbeki, South Africa, and the Idea of an African Renaissance," in *Thabo Mbeki's World: The Politics and Ideology of the South African President*, ed. S. Jacobs and R. Calland (Scottsville: University of Natal Press, Zed Books, 2002), 125.

79. See, for instance, Budget Vote 3: Speech Delivered by Minister Dlamini-Zuma, May 8, 2001; Foreign Affairs Budget Vote 11—Address by Minister Dlamini-Zuma to the National Assembly, March 14, 2000.

80. Sydney Mafumadi, "Challenges Facing Intellectuals in the African Renaissance," *Umrabulo* 15, no. 2 (2002).

81. Frank Chikane, "A New Type of Partnership: The African Renaissance and the Development of NEPAD," *Umrabulo* 27, no. 3 (2006).

82. See, for instance, Ian Phimister and Brian Raftopoulos, "Mugabe, Mbeki & the Politics of Anti-imperialism," *Review of African Political Economy* 31, no. 101 (2004): 385–400.

83. Mukoni Ratshitanga, "The African Cultural Milieu and Our Common Humanity," *ANC Today* 7, no. 40 (2007).

84. Semou Pathe Gueye, "African Renaissance as an Historical Challenge," in Makgoba, *African Renaissance*, 247.

85. Address of Deputy President Thabo Mbeki at the Unitra fund-raising dinner, April 30, 1998.

86. Thabo Mbeki, "Stop the Laughter," in Mbeki, *Africa: The Time Has Come*, 289–95.

87. Thabo Mbeki, "The African Renaissance, South Africa and the World," in Mbeki, *Africa: The Time Has Come*, 239–51.

88. Archives of *Umrabulo* are available at http://www.anc.org.za.

89. For the political context of the Native Club and a scholarly examination of its ideas, see Sabelo J. Ndlovu-Gatsheni, "Africa for Africans or Africa for 'Natives' Only? 'New Nationalism' and Nativism in Zimbabwe and South Africa," *Africa Spectrum* 44, no. 1 (2009): 61–78; Paul Tiyambe Zeleza, "What Happened to the African Renaissance? The Challenges of Development in the Twenty-First Century," *Comparative Studies of South Asia, Africa and the Middle East* 29, no. 2 (2009): 158.

90. Titus Mafolo, "The Third Pillar of Transformation," *Umrabulo* 26, no. 2 (2006).

91. Ibbo Mandaza, "Southern African Identity: A Critical Assessment," in *Shifting African Identities*, ed. S. Bekker, M. Dodds, and M. M. Khosa (Pretoria: HSRC, 2001), 137.

Chapter 3. Facing the Contagion

1. Christer Jöhnsson and Peter Söderholm, "IGO-NGO Relations and HIV/AIDS: Innovation or Stalemate?," *Third World Quarterly* 16, no. 3 (1995): 461–63.

2. Greg Behrman, *The Invisible People: How the U.S. Has Slept Through the Global AIDS Pandemic, the Greatest Humanitarian Catastrophe of Our Time* (New York: Free Press, 2004), 59–116.

3. http://www.who.int/trade/glossary/story034/en/.

4. Behrman, *The Invisible People*, 17–21.

5. United Nations General Assembly, "Political Declaration on HIV/AIDS," June 15, 2006; United Nations General Assembly, "Political Declaration on HIV and AIDS: Intensifying Our Efforts to Eliminate HIV and AIDS," June 10, 2011. For further details, see Amy Patterson, "The UN and the Fight against HIV/AIDS," in *The Global Politics of AIDS*, ed. Paul G. Harris and Patricia D. Siplon (Boulder, Colo.: Lynne Reiner Publishers, 2007), 210–12.

6. Jaime Sepúlveda et al., eds., PEPFAR *Implementation: Progress and Promise* (Washington, D.C.: National Academies Press, 2007).

7. Charles F. Gilks et al., "The WHO Public-Health Approach to Antiretroviral Treatment against HIV in Resource-Limited Settings," *Lancet* 368, no. 9,534 (2006): 509.

8. For the political contestation around AZT and the process of drug approval, see Daniel Carpenter, *Reputation and Power: Organizational Image and Pharmaceutical Regulation at the FDA* (Princeton, N.J.: Princeton University Press, 2010), chap. 6.

9. Bernhard Schwartländer, Ian Grubb, and Jon Perriens, "The 10-Year Struggle to Provide Antiretroviral Treatment to People with HIV in the Developing World," *Lancet* 368, no. 9,534 (2006): 541.

10. *Guidance for Industry: Fixed Dose Combinations, Co-packaged Drug Products, and Single-Entity Versions of Previously Approved Antiretrovirals for the Treatment of HIV* (Washington, D.C.: U.S. Department of Health and Human Services, Food and Drug Administration, 2006), 4.

11. *Scaling Up Antiretroviral Therapy in Resource-Limited Settings: Treatment Guidelines for a Public Health Approach: 2003 Revision* (Geneva: World Health Organization, 2003), 60 (Annex D).

12. For updates, see *Consolidated Guidelines on General HIV Care and the Use of Antiretroviral Drugs for Treating and Preventing HIV Infection: Recommendations for a Public Health Approach* (Geneva: World Health Organization, 2013).

13. *Approved and Tentatively Approved Antiretrovirals in Association with the President's Emergency Plan*, FDA, last updated March 18, 2014.

14. For detailed information on the prices and availability of different ARVs over the past thirteen years, see the numerous Access Campaign reports entitled *Accessing ARVs: Untangling the Web of Price Reductions for Developing Countries*. The latest one was published by Médecins sans frontières in 2013.

15. Available at http://www.duesberg.com/subject/africa2.html.

16. See Steven Epstein, *Impure Science: AIDS, Activism, and the Politics of Knowledge* (Berkeley: University of California Press, 1998), 105–13; Peter H. Duesberg, *Inventing the AIDS Virus* (Washington, D.C.: Regnery Publishing, 1996).

17. See Jad Adams, "Virus Hunters," in *AIDS: The HIV Myth* (New York: St. Martin's Press, 1989).

18. Peter Duesberg, Claus Koehnlein, and David Rasnick, "The Chemical Bases of the Various AIDS Epidemics: Recreational Drugs, Anti-viral Chemotherapy and Malnutrition," *Journal of Biosciences* 28 (2003): 383.

19. John Lauritsen, "Petrushka Was Poisoned? Did AZT Contribute to Nureyev's Untimely Death?," *New York Native*, February 1, 1993.

20. For the authoritative clarifications, refer to the definitions supplied by the National Center for Complementary and Alternative Medicine of the National Institutes of Health, http://nccam.nih.gov/health/whatiscam.

21. *WHO Traditional Medicine Strategy, 2002–2005* (Geneva, Switzerland: World Health Organization, 2002), 1.

22. See, for instance, Intellectual Property and Traditional Medical Knowledge, Background Brief No. 6; *http://www.wipo.int/tk/en/resources/pdf/tk_brief6.pdf*.

23. K. Peltzer et al., "HIV/AIDS/STI/TB Knowledge, Beliefs and Practices of Traditional Healers in KwaZulu-Natal, South Africa," *AIDS Care* 18, no. 6 (2006): 608–13; V. G. Chipfakacha, "STD/HIV/AIDS Knowledge, Beliefs and Practices of Traditional Healers in Botswana," *AIDS Care* 9, no. 4 (1997): 417–25; Jane Mufamadi, "Cross-Cultural Dilemmas in the Management of HIV/AIDS: The Role of African Traditional Healers: Indigenous African Healing Practices," *Indilinga* 8, no. 1 (2009): 24–35.

24. World Health Assembly, "Revised Drug Strategy," May 24, 1999 (WHA 52.19).

25. For useful overviews of TRIPS, see Ellen 't Hoen, *The Global Politics of Pharmaceutical Monopoly Power: Drug Patents, Access, Innovation and the Application of the WTO Doha Declaration on TRIPS and Public Health* (Diemen, the Netherlands: AMB Publishers, 2009).

26. Draft Ministerial Declaration: Proposal from a Group of Developed Countries, October 4, 2001, http://www.wto.org/english/tratop_e/trips_e/mindecdraft_w313_e.htm.

27. Declaration on the TRIPS Agreement and Public Health, Adopted on November 14, 2001, http://www.wto.org/english/thewto_e/minist_e/min01_e/mindecl_trips_e.htm.

28. Ellen't Hoen, "TRIPS, Pharmaceutical Patents and Access to Essential Medicines: Seattle, Doha and Beyond," in *Economics of AIDS and Access to HIV/AIDS Care in Developing Countries: Issues and Challenges*, ed. Jean-Paul Moatti et al. (Paris: ANRS, 2003), 46–47.

29. Smith and Siplon, *Drugs into Bodies*, 125, 130–37.

30. *Accelerating Access Initiative: Widening Access to Care and Support for People Living with HIV/AIDS: Progress Report, June 2002* (Geneva, Switzerland: WHO and UNAIDS, 2002).

31. Brenda Waning, Ellen Diedrichsen, and Suerie Moon, "A Lifeline to Treatment: The Role of Indian Generic Manufacturers in Supplying Antiretroviral Medicines to Developing Countries," *Journal of the International AIDS Society* 13, no. 35 (2010).

32. Colleen V. Chien, "HIV/AIDS Drugs for Sub-Saharan Africa: How Do Brand and Generic Supply Compare?," *PLoS ONE* 2, no. 3 (2007): e278.

33. "PEPFAR Secures Cost Savings and Low Prices on Lifesaving Medicines for Developing Countries," Press Release no. 83,466, http://2006-2009.pepfar.gov/press/83466 .htm.

34. Charles B. Holmes et al., "PEPFAR's Past and Future Efforts to Cut Costs, Improve Efficiency, and Increase the Impact of Global HIV Programs," *Health Affairs* 31, no. 7 (2012): 1555.

35. http://www.medicinespatentpool.org.

36. See, for instance, "UNITAID Welcomes Bristol Myers Squibb's Agreement with the Medicines Patent Pool," *UNITAID Press Release*, December 12, 2013.

37. Elizabeth Whitman, "Rich Nations Step Up Assault on Generic AIDS Drugs," *Guardian*, June 10, 2011.

38. See, for instance, Kenneth C. Shadlen, "Is AIDS Treatment Sustainable?," in *The Global Governance of HIV/AIDS: Intellectual Property and Access to Essential Medicines*, ed. Obijiofor Aginam, John Harrington, and Peter K. Yu (Cheltenham: Edward Elgar, 2013), 29–56.

39. For an overview of public health in post-Communist Russia, see Patricio Marquez et al., "Adult Health in the Russian Federation: More than Just a Health Problem," *Health Affairs* 26, no. 4 (2007): 1040–51.

40. UNAIDS *World AIDS Day Report* (Geneva: Joint United Nations Programme on HIV/AIDS, 2011), 8.

41. "Prezident razrabotal mery po bor'be so SPIDom," *Kommersant*, April 22, 2006.

42. Robert Coalson, "Media's AIDS Awareness Campaign Off to Slow Start," *Radio Free Europe / Radio Liberty*, April 11, 2005.

43. Mikhail Khodorkovskiy, "Levyy povorot-2," *Kommersant*, November 11, 2005.

44. Vladimir Yakunin et al., *Novyye tekhnologii bor'by s rossiyskoy gosudarstvennost'yu* (Moscow: Nauchnyy Ekspert, 2009), 150–73.

45. http://www.pravoslavie.ru/analit/global/demograf.htm

46. Gennadiy Onishchenko, "vich-politizirovannyy," *Rossiyskaya gazeta*, March 15, 2005.

47. Ellen Mickiewicz, *Television, Power, and the Public in Russia* (Cambridge: Cambridge University Press, 2008), 45–47.

48. "Bor'ba so spidom, a ne s opponentami," *Press-sluzhba Obshchestvennoy palaty RF*, March 31, 2012.

49. Elena Gorlanova, "vich vernetsya na staroe mesto," *Gazeta.ru*, December 20, 2006.

50. Elena Gorlanova, "Zurabov oshibsya na $37 milliona," *Gazeta.ru*, January 18, 2007.

51. Vladimir Starodubov, "vich-infitsirovannye patsienty ne ostanutsya bez lekarstv," *Ria-novosti*, December 21, 2006.

52. Yuliya Taratuta and Dmitriy Kryazhev, "Minzdrav ne nashel u sebya simptomov korruptsii," *Kommersant*, December 22, 2006.

53. "who Statement on Roche's Viracept Recall," June 14, 2007.

54. Anastasiya Makryashina, "vich ostalsya bez lekarstva," *Gazeta.ru*, June 16, 2007.

55. Anastasiya Makryashina, "vich krepchal," *Gazeta.ru*, June 20, 2006.

56. Vyacheslav Kozlov, "vich-infektsiya ne vpisalas' v kontrakt," *Kommersant*, March 23, 2014.

57. http://www.rost.ru/themes/2006/07/251825_4422.shtml.

58. Elena Gorlanova, "spid vmesto organa pravitel'stva," *Gazeta.ru*, May 17, 2008.

59. Sasha Volgina, "Pereboi v boyah s vich," *Grani.ru*, August 16, 2011; Polina Nikol'skaya, "U minzdrava snova problemy s vich," *Gazeta.ru*, May 27, 2011.

60. Rustem Falyahov, Gleb Kliment'ev, and Ekaterina Gerashchenko, "Eksklyuzivnyy zavoz sohranitsya," *Gazeta.ru*, August 17, 2011.

61. *Strategiya razvitiya meditsinskoy promyshlennosti Rossiyskoy federatsii na period do 2020 goda* (Moscow: Minpromtorg 2009), esp. sec. 1.

62. Ekaterina Karpenko, "Rabotat' na tabletki," *Gazeta.ru*, October 18, 2012.

63. Anna Stepko, "Importnym lekarstvam pridetsya potesnit'sya?," *Meditsinskaya gazeta*, June 20, 2007.

64. Tat'yana Yakovleva, "Chem bolen farmatsevticheskiy rynok," *Strategiya rossii* 12 (2009).

65. Vladimir Putin, "O nashikh ekonomicheskikh zadachakh," *Vedomosti*, January 30, 2012.

66. Tat'yana Batenova, "Import popadet pod zapret," *Rossiyskaya biznes-gazeta*, April 1, 2014.

67. Rustem Falyahov and Gleb Kliment'ev, "Chemezovu vypishut vse tabletki," *Gazeta.ru*, August 13, 2009.

68. Interview with Tatiyana Nikolenko, Andrey Ivashchenko, and Tat'yana Gremyakova, *Itogi* 3, no. 657, January 12, 2009.

69. Vadim Volkov, "Russia's New 'State Corporations': Locomotives of Modernization or Covert Privatization Schemes?," *PONARS Eurasia Policy Memo*, no. 25 (2008).

70. Mikhail Grishankov, "Rasprostranenie SPIDa v Rossii: Sposobno li gosudarstvo ego sderzhivat'," *Ekho Moskvy*, January 12, 2005.

71. Pieter Fourie, *The Political Management of HIV and AIDS in South Africa: One Burden Too Many?* (Basingstoke: Palgrave Macmillan, 2006), 141.

72. Michael Cherry, "Letter Fuels South Africa's AIDS Furore," *Nature* 404 (2000); Tony Karon, "Why South Africa Questions the Link between HIV and AIDS," *Time*, April 21, 2000.

73. Alec Russell, *Bring Me My Machine Gun: The Battle for the Soul of South Africa, from Mandela to Zuma* (New York: Public Affairs, 2009), 222.

74. The text is available at http://www.virusmyth.com/aids/hiv/ancdoc.htm.

75. Andrew Feinstein, *After the Party: A Personal and Political Journey inside the ANC* (Johannesburg: Jonathan Ball, 2007), 112.

76. Joan Shenton, "Interview with Professor Sam Mhlongo," *New African*, July–August 2000.

77. For a similar interpretation, see Joy Wang, "AIDS Denialism and the Humanisation of the African," *Race and Class* 49, no. 3 (2008): 1–18.

78. Quotes taken from Tim Butcher, "West Blames 'Lustful' Blacks for AIDS, Says Mbeki," *Telegraph*, October 27, 2001.

79. Ronald Suresh Roberts, *Fit to Govern: The Native Intelligence of Thabo Mbeki* (Johannesburg: Ste Publishers, 2007), 186–91.

80. Ibid., 181.

81. See Helen Epstein's interview with Nxesi in Epstein, *The Invisible Cure*, 170–71.

82. For NAPWA's official website, see http://www.napwa.org.za.

83. See NAPWA Resolutions at First NAPWA Congress, May 25–27, 2001.

84. "Zuma 'Committed and Serious' on HIV and AIDS," *SA Government News Agency*, December 2, 2009.

85. Virginia van der Vliet, "South Africa Divided against AIDS: A Crisis of Leadership," in *AIDS and South Africa: The Social Expression of a Pandemic*, ed. Kyle D. Kaufman and David L. Lindauer (Basingstoke: Palgrave Macmillan, 2004), 73, 85.

86. Virginia van der Vliet, "AIDS: Losing 'the New Struggle'?," *Daedalus* 130 (2001): 151–84.

87. Anne-Christine d'Adesky, *Moving Mountains: The Race to Treat Global AIDS* (London: Verso, 2004), 183.

88. This book manuscript can be found online on Brink's home page, http://www.tig.org.za/.

89. Kerry Cullinan, "Health Minister Promotes Nutritional Alternative to ARV Roll-Out," *Health-e News*, May 30, 2005.

90. Kanya Ndaki, "Traditional Alternatives?," in *The Virus, Vitamins & Vegetables: The South African HIV/AIDS Mystery*, ed. Kerry Cullinan and Anso Thom (Johannesburg: Jacana Media, 2009), 146.

91. "TAC Refuses to Back Down from Qunta Attack," *Health-e News*, October 5, 2007.

92. *Operational Plan for Comprehensive HIV and AIDS Care, Management and Treatment for South Africa* (Pretoria: Ministry of Health, 2003), 86.

93. Staff Reporter, "UCT Acts against Academic Associated with Aids Tonic," *Mail & Guardian*, July 3, 2006.

94. "Traditional Health Practitioners Act (No. 35 of 2004)," *Government Gazette*, February 11, 2005.

95. "The Presidential Task Team on African Traditional Medicine in South Africa (No. 1030 of 2006)," *Staatskoerant*, October 11, 2006.

96. Kerry Cullinan, "KZN Health Minister Mimics Manto and Punts Herbal Remedies for AIDS," *Health-e News*, November 23, 2006; "MEC Wants Traditional Medicine in Hospice," *Health-e News*, November 11, 2008.

97. Kerry Cullinan, "Health Officials Promote Untested uBhejane," *Health-e News*, March 22, 2006.

98. Jo-Anne Smetherham, "Natural Cures to Get the All-Clear from Manto," *Independent Online*, January 17, 2005.

99. Robert J. Thornton, *Unimagined Community: Sex, Networks, and Aids in Uganda and South Africa* (Berkeley: University of California Press, 2008), 176.

100. Tamar Kahn, "Alternative Medicines to Be Scrutinized," *Business Day*, August 26, 2011; Tamar Kahn, "Council Set to Regulate Alternative Medicines," *Business Day*, August 6, 2011.

101. Tamar Kahn, "Alternative Medicine Deadline Missed," *Business Day*, February 17, 2014.

102. Lesley Cowling, "AIDS 'Breakthrough' Broke All the Rules," *Mail & Guardian*, January 23, 1997.

103. For further details, see James Myburgh, "In the Beginning There Was Virodene," in Cullinan and Thom, *The Virus, Vitamins & Vegetables*, 1–15.

104. For further discussion, see David Barnard, "In the High Court of South Africa, Case No. 4138/98: The Global Politics Of Access to Low-Cost AIDS Drugs in Poor Countries," *Kennedy Institute of Ethics Journal* 12, no. 2 (2002): 159–74.

105. Kerry Cullinan, "Free AIDS Drug Still Not Available," *Health-e News*, August 24, 2001.

106. Anso Thom, "Registration of Critical ARV Drug Delayed," *Health-e News*, February 9, 2006.

107. Theo Smart, "South Africa Completes Negotiations for Large-Scale Antiretroviral Procurement," *Aidsmap.com*, February 22, 2005.

108. Kerry Cullinan, "Aspen's Generics Ensure Affordable AIDS Treatment," *Health-e News*, January 18, 2006.

109. Carlos Correa, "Pharmaceutical Innovation, Incremental Patenting and Compulsory Licensing," Research Paper 41, South Centre, 2011, 7–8.

110. Marcus Low, "Patent Plot to Deceive," *Financial Mail*, January 23, 2014.

111. For a detailed discussion of controversies arising around intellectual property issues, see Andy Gray, Yousuf Vawda, and Caron Jack, "Health Policy and Legislation," in *South African Health Review 2012/13*, ed. Ashnie Padarath and René English (Durban: Health Systems Trust, 2013), 11–13.

112. Catherine Tomlinson, "People before Patents," *NSP Review* 4 (October–November 2012); Lotti Rutter, "Patents: Reform or Lose," *NSP Review* 9, December, 2013.

113. Parks Mankahlana, "Buying Anti-AIDS Drugs Benefits the Rich," *Business Day*, March 20, 2000.

114. William Gumede, *Thabo Mbeki and the Battle for the Soul of the ANC* (London: Zed Books, 2007), 196.

115. *End AIDS! Break the Chains of Pharmaceutical Colonialism* (Dr. Rath Foundation, South African National Civil Organization, 2007), 33.

116. Ibid., 236.

117. Roberts, *Fit to Govern*, 185, 198–99, 201.

118. Sarah Wild, "ARV Plan Bounces Back," *Mail & Guardian*, May 24, 2013.

119. Matt Price, "Now's the Time to Think Smart about ARVs," *Mail & Guardian*, June 25, 2010.

Chapter 4. Expanding Access

1. United Nations General Assembly, "Declaration of Commitment on HIV/AIDS: 'Global Crisis—Global Action,'" June 27, 2001.

2. Michel Sidibé, Sonja Tanaka, and Kent Buse, "People, Passion & Politics: Looking Back and Moving Forward in the Governance of the AIDS Response," *Global Health Governance* 4, no. 1 (2010).

3. For further discussion, see Tony Evans, "A Human Right to Health?," *Third World Quarterly* 23, no. 2 (2002): 197–215.

4. United Nations General Assembly, "Political Declaration on HIV/AIDS," June 2, 2006; United Nations General Assembly, "Political Declaration on HIV and AIDS: 'Intensifying Our Efforts to Eliminate HIV and AIDS,'" June 10, 2011.

5. See, for instance, "The Global HIV/AIDS Epidemic," Kaiser Family Foundation, October 10, 2013.

6. "FDA Panel Recommends Approval of Truvada as HIV Prevention Tool," *Kaiser Daily Global Health Policy Report*, May 11, 2012.

7. Jon Cohen, "Breakthrough of the Year: HIV Treatment as Prevention," *Science* 34 (2011): 1628–29.

8. Holly Burkhalter, "The Politics of AIDS: Engaging Conservative Activists," *Foreign Policy* 83, no. 1 (2004): 8–14.

9. On the evolution of the scientific understanding of the disease from the "gay disease" and lifestyle argument overturned by retrovirology, see Steven Epstein, *Impure Science: AIDS, Activism, and the Politics of Knowledge* (Berkeley: University of California Press, 1998), 45–79.

10. On quarantine as a discussed solution to the AIDS crisis, see David F. Musto, "Quarantine and the Problem of AIDS," in *AIDS: The Burdens of History*, ed. Elizabeth Fee and Daniel M. Fox (Berkeley: University of California Press, 1988), 67–85.

11. Timothy F. Murphy, *Ethics in an Epidemic: AIDS, Morality, and Culture* (Berkeley: University of California Press, 1994), 129–43.

12. See B. H. Shepard, "Shifting Priorities in U.S. AIDS Policy," in *The Global Politics of AIDS*, edited by Paul G. Harris and Patricia D. Siplon (Boulder, Colo.: Lynne Reiner, 2007), 182–89.

13. Jonathan M. Mann et al., "Health and Human Rights," *Health and Human Rights: An International Journal* 1, no. 1 (1994).

14. The text is available at http://www.unicef.org/ceecis/The_Dublin_Declaration .pdf.

15. *Implementing the Dublin Declaration on Partnership to Fight HIV/AIDS in Europe and Central Asia: 2010 Progress Report* (Stockholm: European Centre for Disease Prevention and Control, 2010).

16. Methadone hydrochloride (Dolophine), Food and Drug Administration, safety information, November 11, 2006. For the list of other opioids, see "FDA Works to Reduce Risk of Opioid Pain Relievers," *FDA Consumer Health Information*, July 9, 2012; "List of Extended-Release and Long-Acting Opioid Products Required to Have an Opioid Risk Evaluation and Mitigation Strategy (REMS)," FDA, last updated, September 7, 2012.

17. Simon Lenton and Eric Single, "The Definition of Harm Reduction," *Drug and Alcohol Review* 17, no. 2 (1998): 216.

18. Claudia Stoicescu, ed., *The Global State of Harm Reduction 2012: Towards an Integrated Response* (London: Harm Reduction International, 2012), 14–15.

19. See Rifat Atun and Michel Kazatchkine, "The Global Fund's Leadership on Harm Reduction: 2002–2009," *International Journal of Drug Policy* 21, no. 2 (2010): 103–6.

20. http://www.ihra.net/what-we-do.

21. Catherine Cook, ed., *The Global State of Harm Reduction 2010: Key Issues for Broadening the Response* (London: International Harm Reduction Association, 2010), 73.

22. *Global Report: UNAIDS Report on the Global AIDS Epidemic 2013* (Geneva: Joint United Nations Programme on HIV/AIDS, 2013), 30.

23. Paul A. Wilson et al., "Combating HIV/AIDS in the Developing World: The Interim Report Task Force 5 Working Group on HIV/AIDS," Millennium Project, February 1, 2004, 42.

24. *Scaling Up Antiretroviral Therapy in Resource-Limited Settings: Treatment Guidelines for a Public Health Approach, 2003 Revision* (Geneva: WHO, 2004), 7, 11.

25. United Nations General Assembly, "United Nations Millennium Declaration," September 8, 2000.

26. "Goal 6: Combat HIV/AIDS, Malaria and Other Diseases," http://www.un.org/millenniumgoals/aids.shtml.

27. More information is available at http://www.who.int/3by5/en/.

28. The archived information on the initiative is available at *http://www.who.int/3by5/en/*.

29. On the former, see Stefaan van der Borght et al., "The Accelerating Access Initiative: Experience with a Multinational Workplace Programme in Africa," *Bulletin of the World Health Organization* 87 (2009): 794–98.

30. *Confronting AIDS: Public Priorities in a Global Epidemic*, a World Bank Policy Research Report (New York: Published for the World Bank, Oxford University Press, 1993), 10.

31. Martha Ainsworth and Waranya Teokul, "Breaking the Silence: Setting Realistic Priorities for AIDS Control in Less-Developed Countries," *Lancet* 356, no. 9,223 (2000): 57.

32. For the discussion of a broader historical context and the process that led to the success of the norm of universal antiretroviral access, see Jeremy Youde, "Is Universal Access to Antiretroviral Drugs an Emerging International Norm?," *Journal of International Relations and Development* 11, no. 4 (2008): 415–40. For further discussion, see Ethan B. Kapstein and Josh Busby, "Making Markets for Merit Goods: The Political Economy of Antiretrovirals," CGD Working Paper 179 (Washington, D.C.: Center for Global Development, 2009).

33. For an earlier discussion on the cost-effectiveness of treatment, see Lilani Kumaranayake and Damian Walker, "Cost-Effectiveness Analysis and Priority Setting: Global Approach without Local Meaning?," in *Health Policy in a Globalising World*, ed. Kelley Lee, Kent Buse, and Suzanne Fustukian (Cambridge: Cambridge University Press, 2002), 140–58.

34. Mead Over, "Prevention Failure: The Ballooning Entitlement Burden of U.S. Global AIDS Treatment Spending and What to Do about It," CGD Working Paper 144 (Washington, D.C.: Center for Global Development, 2008).

35. "High Drug Costs Could Jeopardize Brazil's No-Cost Antiretroviral Program," Kaiser Family Foundation, January 3, 2007.

36. Kenneth C. Shadlen, "Is AIDS Treatment Sustainable?," in *The Global Governance of HIV/AIDS: Intellectual Property and Access to Essential Medicines*, ed. Obijiofor Aginam, John Harrington, and Peter K. Yu (Cheltenham: Edward Elgar, 2013).

37. Julie Steenhuysen, "Insight: AIDS Science Leaping Ahead, but Will the Money Follow?," *Reuters*, September 6, 2012.

38. Dimitriy Medvedev, interview with Sergey Brilyov, Rossiya TV Channel, aired May 16, 2009.

39. Tat'yana Batenyeva, "Modernizatsiya rossiyskogo zdravoohraneniya nachalas' s sozdaniya novogo sovremennogo zakonodatel'stva," *Rossiyskaya gazeta*, December 12, 2011.

40. See, for instance, Tom Parfitt, "Russia's Health Promotion Efforts Blossom," *Lancet* 373, no. 9,682 (2009): 2186–87.

41. Vladimir D. Mendelevich, "Bioethical Differences between Drug Addiction Treatment Professionals Inside and Outside the Russian Federation," *Harm Reduction Journal* 8, no. 15 (2011).

42. See, for instance, Vladimir Putin, "Rossiya i menyayushchiysya mir," *Moskovskie novosti*, February 27, 2012.

43. Valeri Panyuskin et al., "V Kreml' zaneslo infektsiyu," *Kommersant*, April 20, 2006.

44. Nikolay Kaklyugin, "Strategiya snizheniya vreda v bor'be s VICH/SPIDOM kak faktor destabilizatsii demograficheskoy situatsii na territorii Rossiyskoy Federatsii: Etiologiya i patogenez," *Net—Narkotikam*, 2007, full text available at http://www.narkotiki.ru/mir_6514.html.

45. See, for instance, the interview with Aleksandr Mikhailov for the radio station Ekho Moskvy, March 23, 2005.

46. Ivanov's speeches are collected at http://gak.gov.ru/pages/gak/4601/4733/index.shtml.

47. See Yuriy Luzhkov, speech of the mayor of Moscow at the opening of the Second International Conference "HIV/AIDS in Developed Countries," February 4, 2008.

48. Interview with Alexey Nadezhdin available at http://www.narkotiki.ru/expert_5900.html.

49. Natal'ya Frolova and Georgiy Zazulin, *Aktual'nye voprosy antinarkoticheskoy politiki: Otechestvennyy i zarubezhnyy opyt* (Moscow: Orbita-M, 2003).

50. V. N. Krasnov et al., "Net metadonovym programmam v Rossiyskoy federatsii," *Meditsinskaya gazeta*, March 31, 2005.

51. Viktor Cherkesov, "Kak pobedit' legalizatsiyu narkodohodov," *Rossiyskaya gazeta*, March 12, 2008.

52. Viktor Ivanov, speech at the State Duma hearings, February 19, 2009.

53. Gennadiy Onishchenko, "Zamestitel'naya terapiya," *Rossiyskaya gazeta*, March 17, 2009.

54. Alla Shaboltas et al., "The Feasibility of an Intensive Case Management Program for Injection Drug Users on Antiretroviral Therapy in St. Petersburg, Russia," *Harm Reduction Journal* 10, no. 15 (2013).

55. For details on the inefficiency of the Russian practice of treating PLWA in narcological clinics and on continuing discrimination, see *Rehabilitation Required: Russia's Human Rights Obligation to Provide Evidence-Based Drug Dependence Treatment* (New York: Human Rights Watch, 2007).

56. Galina Papernaya, "Prinuditel'noe lechenie sprovotsirovalo gosnarkoraskol," *Moskovskie novosti*, December 26, 2011.

57. See, for instance, Maria Fikhte, "Shprits obmenu ne podlezhit," *Gazeta.ru*, August 25, 2008.

58. Daniel Wolfe, "Paradoxes in Antiretroviral Treatment for Injecting Drug Users: Access, Adherence and Structural Barriers in Asia and the Former Soviet Union," *International Journal of Drug Policy* 18 (2007): 246.

59. Federal Law 38-03 of 1995.

60. Valery Panyushkin, "SPID usmiren," *Kommersant*, December 1, 2005.

61. See *Country Progress Reports of the Russian Federation on the Implementation of the Declaration of Commitment on HIV/AIDS*, reporting periods: January 2006–December 2007 (March 30, 2008), p. 27; January 2008–December 2009 (June 8, 2010), p. 10.

62. Dimitriy Medvedev, "Natsional'nye proekty: Ot stabilizatsii—k razvitiyu," *Kommersant*, January 25, 2007.

63. See Putin's speech at the NPP Council meeting on February 28, 2008.

64. Kaiser Family Foundation daily updates, January 11, 2008.

65. See, for instance, Pavel Vorob'ev, ed., *Zdravoohranenie v Rossii 2010* (Moscow: Formulyarnyy Komitet, 2011).

66. "Meditsinskaya reforma skoroy ne vykhodit," *Kommersant*, April 15, 2010.

67. Knowledge for Action in HIV/AIDS in the Russian Federation, "Report of Findings," working document, October 2006, 14.

68. Charles D. H. Parry et al., "Rapid Assessment of HIV Risk Behavior in Drug Using Sex Workers in Three Cities in South Africa," *AIDS and Behavior* 13, no. 5 (2009): 849–59.

69. *HIV/AIDS and STDs: Strategic Plan for South Africa, 2000–2005*, 21; see also *HIV/AIDS and STI: Strategic Plan for South Africa, 2007–2011*, 14–15, 31–32.

70. Linda Ensor, "SA's HIV Plan to Focus on Health of Sex Workers," *Business Day*, December 11, 2013.

71. See, for instance, Catherine Campbell, "Political Will, Traditional Leaders and the Fight against HIV/AIDS: A South African Case Study," *AIDS Care: Psychological and Sociomedical Aspects of AIDS/HIV* 22, supplement 2 (2010): 1637–43.

72. On the virginity testing movement in South Africa, see Suzanne Leclerc-Madlala, "Popular Responses to HIV/AIDS and Policy," *Journal of Southern African Studies* 31, no. 4 (2005): 852–53.

73. For descriptive statistics, see *South African National HIV Prevalence, Incidence, Be-*

haviour and Communication Survey, 2008: A Turning Tide among Teenagers? (Cape Town: HSRC Press, 2009), 58–62; on loveLife, see http://kff.org/other/lovelife/.

74. "Sex Education—the Ugly Stepchild in Teacher Training," *IRIN/Plus News*, May 22, 2008. For a detailed discussion about sex education as a compulsory part of the Life Orientation curriculum, see Dennis A. Francis, "Sexuality Education in South Africa: Wedged within a Triad of Contradictory Values," *Journal of Psychology in Africa* 21, no. 2 (2011): 317–22.

75. Kerry Cullinan, "Bitter Court Battle Ahead over HIV Babies," *Health-e News*, November 23, 2001.

76. Alec Russell, *Bring Me My Machine Gun: The Battle for the Soul of South Africa, from Mandela to Zuma* (New York: PublicAffairs, 2009), 224.

77. Khopotso Bodibe, "Where Is the ARV Roll-Out?," *Health-e News*, February 9, 2004.

78. Nicoli Nattrass, *The Moral Economy of AIDS in South Africa* (Cambridge: Cambridge University Press, 2004), 71.

79. Kerry Cullinan, "HIV Babies May Grow Up Unaware of Their Infection," *Health-E News*, March 13, 2007.

80. Anso Thom, "New PMTCT Protocol in Two Weeks," *Health-e News*, November 30, 2007.

81. Nattrass, *The Moral Economy*, 47–48.

82. Patrick Furlong and Karen Ball, "The More Things Change: AIDS and the State in South Africa, 1987–2005," in *The African State and the AIDS Crisis*, ed. Amy S. Patterson (Aldershot: Ashgate, 2005), 142.

83. Information taken from http://www.pepfar.gov/countries/southafrica/index.htm.

84. Tanya Doherty et al., "Implications of the New WHO Guidelines on HIV and Infant Feeding for Child Survival in South Africa," *Bulletin of the World Health Organization* 89 (2001): 62–67.

85. http://www.avert.org/hiv-aids-south-africa.htm.

86. See Krista Johnson, "The Politics of AIDS Policy Development and Implementation in Postapartheid South Africa," *Africa Today* 51, no. 2 (2004): 110–12, 124–25.

87. Petrida Ijumba et al., "Access to Antiretroviral Therapy," in *South African Health Review, 2003/2004* (Durban: Health Systems Trust, 2003), 323–36.

88. See, for instance, Rob Stewart and Marian Loveday, *Public HAART Projects in South Africa: Progress to November 2004* (Durban: Health Systems Trust, 2005), 224–46.

89. Fatima Hassan, "Country Report: South Africa," in *Missing the Target: Report on HIV/AIDS Treatment Access from the Frontlines* (New York: International Treatment Preparedness Coalition, 2005), 73.

90. For detailed analysis of resource allocation and expenditure, see Alison Hickey and Nhlanhla Ndlovu, "Budgeting for HIV/AIDS in South Africa: An Analysis of Provincial Health Budgets," *South African Journal of Economics* 73 (2005): 627–40; Nhlanhla

Ndlovu and Rabelani Daswa, "Review of Progress and Expenditure on the Comprehensive Plan for HIV and AIDS for South Africa," *South African Journal of Economics* 76 (2008): S34–S51.

91. Anso Thom, "'Tyrant' Manana Made to Pay Doctor," *Health-e News*, October 22, 2008.

92. See, for instance, "Antiretroviral Treatment Moratorium in the Free State November 2008–February," *AIDS Law Project*, February 11, 2009.

93. Kira E. Foster, "Clinics, Communities, and Cost Recovery: Primary Health Care and Neoliberalism in Postapartheid South Africa," *Cultural Dynamics* 17 (2005): 239–66.

94. Anso Thom, "866 000 Waiting on ARV Treatment in SA," *Health-e News*, July 29, 2005.

95. Zwelinzima Vavi, input to TAC Congress, September 2005.

96. "Activists Welcome Ambitious New AIDS Plan," *IRIN PlusNews*, March 15, 2007.

97. For the general review of drug policies in sub-Saharan Africa and the continuing practice of reusing syringes in clinical settings in South Africa, see Savanna R. Reid, "Injection Drug Use, Unsafe Medical Injections, and HIV in Africa: A Systematic Review," *Harm Reduction Journal* 6, no. 24 (2009). See also Bruce Trathen, Charles D. H. Parry, and Neo K. Morojele, "Harm Reduction in Sub-Saharan Africa," in *Harm Reduction in Substance Use and High-Risk Behaviour*, ed. Richard Pates and Diane Riley (Hoboken, N.J.: Wiley-Blackwell, 2012), 425–43.

98. Cook, *Harm Reduction 2010*, 22.

Chapter 5. Selecting Partners

1. For some conceptual clarifications of the vast literature exploring "governance without government," see Thomas Risse, "Transnational Actor and World Politics," in *Handbook of International Relations*, ed. Walter Carlsnaes, Tom Risse, and Beth Simmons (London: Sage, 2012), 255–74; James N. Rosenau, "Governance in the Twenty-First Century," *Global Governance* 1, no. 1 (1995): 13–43. This vast literature sometimes overstated the weakness of the traditional structures of authority, such as states, but made an important point about the spread and effectiveness of nonstate governance.

2. For a detailed conceptualization, see Stephen H. Linder and Pauline Vaillancourt Rosenau, "Mapping the Terrain of the Public-Private Policy Partnership," in *Public/Private Policy Partnerships*, ed. Pauline Vaillancourt Rosenau (Cambridge: MIT University Press, 2000), 1–10; Marco Schäferhoff, Sabine Campe, and Christopher Kaan, "Transnational Public-Private Partnerships in International Relations: Making Sense of Concepts, Research Frameworks, and Results," *International Studies Review* 11, no. 3 (2009): 451–74.

3. The definition is available at http://www.ncppp.org/howpart/index.shtml#define.

4. Christer Jönsson, "Coordinating Actors in the Fight against HIV/AIDS: From 'Lead

Agency' to Public-Private Partnerships," in *Democracy and Public-Private Partnerships in Global Governance*, ed. Magdalena Bexell and Ulrika Mörth (Basingstoke: Macmillan, 2010), 167–89.

5. For an analysis of public-private partnerships in the context of global health issues and the right to health, see Kent Buse and Gill Walt, "Global Public-Private Partnerships: Part I—a New Development in Health?," *Bulletin of the World Health Organization* 78, no. 4 (2000); Kent Buse and Gill Walt, "Global Public-Private Partnerships: Part II—What Are the Health Issues for Global Governance?," *Bulletin of the World Health Organization* 78, no. 5 (2000).

6. The list of Merk's HIV and AIDS Partnerships and Programs is available at http://www.merck.com/corporate-responsibility/access/access-hiv-aids/access-hiv-aids-partnerships/global.html.

7. Bill Rau, "The Politics of Civil Society in Confronting HIV/AIDS," *International Affairs* 82, no. 2 (2006): 285–95. See also Kasia Malinowska-Sempruch, Roxana Bonnell, and Jeff Hoover, "Civil Society—a Leader in HIV Prevention and Tobacco Control," *Drug and Alcohol Review* 25 (2006): 625–32.

8. See Leon Gordenker, Roger Coate, Christer Jönsson, and Peter Söderholm, *International Cooperation in Response to AIDS* (London: Frances Pinter, 1994), 74–77, 128–29; Peter Söderholm, *Global Governance of AIDS: Partnerships with Civil Society* (Lund, Sweden: Lund University Press, 1997), 125–30; Behrman, *Invisible People*, 40–57.

9. The document is available at http://www.theglobalfund.org/documents/TGF_Framework.pdf.

10. See the series by the Center for Strategic and International Studies (CSIS).

11. For a detailed account of the global health architecture, consult Jeremy Youde, *Global Health Governance* (Cambridge: Polity Press, 2012).

12. Princeton N. Lyman and Stephen B. Wittels, "No Good Deed Goes Unpunished," *Foreign Affairs* 89, no. 4 (2010): 75–77.

13. A special issue of *Health Affairs* 31, no. 7 (2012) is dedicated to the President's Emergency Plan for AIDS Relief.

14. *The President's Emergency Plan for AIDS Relief: U.S. Five Year Global HIV/AIDS Strategy* (Washington, D.C.: Office of the United States Global AIDS Coordinator, 2004). For the relevant updates, see PEPFAR's annual reports.

15. See http://www.pepfar.gov/countries/southafrica/; http://www.pepfar.gov/press/docs/c22228.htm; Ingrid T. Katz et al., "PEPFAR in Transition—Implications for HIV Care in South Africa," *New England Journal of Medicine*, no. 369 (2013): 1385–87.

16. http://89.rospotrebnadzor.ru/documents/postanovlenia/609/.

17. Dar'ya Nikolaeva, "Farmatsevty vyzvali konkurentam doktora," *Kommersant*, October 7, 2009.

18. Anatoliy Berestov, Yuliya Shevtsova, and Nikolay Kaklyugin, *Ostorozhno—*

metadon! (Moscow: Tsentr Ioanna Kronshtadtskogo, Tsentr sotsial'noy i sudebnoy psikhiatrii Imeni V. P. Serbskogo, 2006).

19. Viktor Ivanov, "O konsolidirovannoy antinarkoticheskoy politike gosudarstva, obshhestva i tserkvi," *Narkologiya* 2 (2010): 13–16.

20. Vyacheslav Kozlov, "FSKN poluchila dozu obshchestvennogo poritsaniya," *Kommersant*, December 12, 2013.

21. See Nataliya Mustafina, "Rossiyskuyu ekonomiku pogubit SPID," *Kommersant*, March 31, 2004.

22. "Na modernizatsiyu zdravoohraneniya planiruetsya vydelit' 460 milliardov rubley," *Kommersant*, April 23, 2010.

23. *O finansirovanii mer po profilaktike i bor'be s VICH/SPIDom v Rossii* (Moscow: Transatlanticheskie partnery protiv SPIDa, 2006).

24. See, for instance, the report by Anatoliy Vishnevsky et al., "Rossiyskoe zdravoohranenie: Kak vyyti iz krizisa: Modernizatsiya ekonomiki i gosudarstvo," *Otechestvennye zapiski* 2 (2006).

25. Vadim Visloguzov et al., "Bol'she gippokratii, bol'she sotsializma," *Kommersant*, April 21, 2010.

26. Dar'ya Nikolaeva, "Minzdrav zateyal dvukhprotsentnyy remont," *Kommersant*, April 22, 2010.

27. Francesca Perlman and Dina Balabanova, "Prescription for Change: Accessing Medication in Transitional Russia," *Health Policy and Planning* 26, no. 6 (2011): 453–63.

28. Irina Stepanova, "Bolezni rosta," *Meditsinskaya gazeta*, June 18, 2008.

29. Anastasiya Bashkatova, "Snizhenie tsen na lekarstva okazalos' illyuziey," *Nezavisimaya gazeta*, September 9, 2010; Anastasiya Bashkatova, "V Rossii ischezayut vazhneyshie lekarstva," *Nezavisimaya gazeta*, October 2, 2011.

30. *On the Frontline of an Epidemic: The Need for Urgency in Russia's Fight against AIDS* (New York: Transatlantic Partners against AIDS, 2003), 23.

31. Elena Dmitrieva, "Use of Mobile Technologies to Promote Reproductive Health in the Russian Federation," presentation at Brown University, March 6, 2012.

32. For a detailed description of the Russian nongovernmental health landscape, see Ulla Pape, *The Politics of HIV/AIDS in Russia* (Abington: Routledge, 2013).

33. Galina Papernaya, "Izlishki profilaktiki," *Moskovskie novosti*, December 9, 2011.

34. Oksana Petrovskaya and Vladislava Filyanova, eds., *Zarubezhnye nepravitel'stvennye nekommercheskie i religioznye organizatsii v Rossii* (Moscow: RISS, 2011), 132.

35. Galina Papernaya, "Nasledstvo pionerii," *Moskovskie novosti*, March 3, 2012.

36. *An Uncivil Approach to Civil Society: Continuing State Curbs on Independent NGOs and Activists in Russia* (New York: Human Rights Watch, 2009), 10–21.

37. See, for instance, "Russia: USG World Health Assembly Objectives Delivered," Cable 07MOSCOW2199, created May 11, 2007, released August 30, 2011; "Russia's Chief

Medical Officer Wants to Expand Cooperation," Cable 09MOSCOW3072, created December 21, 2009, released August 30, 2011.

38. For a brief overview, see Judyth Twigg, *U.S.-Russia Collaboration on Health: Moving toward Engagement* (Washington, D.C.: CSIS, 2009); William H. Frist, "Improving Russian-U.S. Collaboration on Health," *Washington Quarterly* 30, no. 4 (2007): 7–17.

39. See the *Kaiser Family Foundation Daily Report*, May 5, 2008.

40. "YuNISEF lobbiruet interesy zapadnyh farmatsevticheskikh kompaniy v ushcherb interesam Rossii," *Gazeta.ru*, August 29, 2011.

41. Kommentariy ofitsial'nogo predstavitelya MID Rossii A. K. Lukashevicha o prekrashchenii deyatel'nosti v Rossiyskoy federatsii Agentstva SSHA po mezhdunarodnomu razvitiyu (USAID), September 19, 2012.

42. The text of the Moscow Declaration is available at http://www.unodc.org/pdf/event_2005-03-31_declaration.pdf.

43. Available at http://en.g8russia.ru/agenda/.

44. *Summary Statement from the Conference Organizing Committee with Input from the Conference Delegates* (2006), 2–3.

45. Diana McConachy, *Evaluation Report: Eastern Europe and Central Asia AIDS Conference* (Moscow, 2006); Diana McConachy, *Evaluation Report: Second Eastern Europe and Central Asia AIDS Conference* (Moscow, 2008).

46. Laetitia Lienart, *Third Eastern Europe and Central Asia AIDS Conference-Evaluation Report* (International AIDS Society, 2010).

47. Anya Sarang et al., open letter to UNAIDS regarding EECAAC 2014, April 24, 2014.

48. The Federal Agency for the Commonwealth of Independent States, Expatriates and International Humanitarian Cooperation, commonly referred to as Rossotrudnichestvo (http://www.rs.gov.ru/).

49. See, for instance, Judyth Twigg, "Russia's Global Health Outlook: Building Capacity to Match Aspirations," in *Key Players in Global Health: How Brazil, Russia, India, China, and South Africa Are Influencing the Game*, ed. Katherine Bliss (Washington, D.C.: CSIS, 2010), 34–41.

50. For a detailed analysis of the Russian Orthodox views on HIV, human rights, and the responsibilities of the individual, see Jarrett Zigon, *"HIV Is God's Blessing": Rehabilitating Morality in Neoliberal Russia* (Berkeley: University of California Press, 2010).

51. For a detailed history of the South African organizational response to HIV/AIDS, see Ann Strode and Kitty Barrett Grant, eds., *Understanding the Institutional Dynamics of South Africa's Response to the HIV/AIDS Pandemic* (Pretoria: IDASA, 2004), 10–17.

52. See, for instance, the opening speech by President Thabo Mbeki at the First Meeting of the Presidential Advisory Panel on AIDS, May 6, 2000.

53. *A Synthesis Report of the Deliberations by the Panel of Experts Invited by the President of the Republic of South Africa, the Honourable Mr. Thabo Mbeki* (Pretoria: Presidential Aids Advisory Panel, 2001), 59.

54. Ronald Suresh Roberts, *Fit to Govern: The Native Intelligence of Thabo Mbeki* (Johannesburg: Ste Publishers, 2007), 181, 192, 195, 202.

55. Mandy Rossouw, "Move to Manto-ise Aids Council Fails," *Mail & Guardian*, September 14, 2007.

56. "Building Consensus on HIV Prevention, Treatment and Care," summary of the conference available at http://www.info.gov.za/issues/hiv/consensus.htm.

57. Adele Baleta, "No Clinical Trials Sanctioned for South Africa's Controversial HIV drug," *Lancet* 353, no. 9,147 (1999): 125.

58. The quote is taken from http://www.dr-rath-foundation.org.za/open_letters /open_letter_2004_10_07.html.

59. Clare Kapp, "New Hope for Health in South Africa," *Lancet* 372, no. 9,645 (2008): 1207–8.

60. Nicoli Nattrass, "AIDS and the Scientific Governance of Medicine in Post-Apartheid South Africa," *African Affairs* 107, no. 427 (2008): 167–72.

61. Hoosen Coovadia et al., "The Health and Health System of South Africa: Historical Roots of Current Public Health Challenges," *Lancet* 374, no. 9,692 (2009): 817–34; Mickey Chopra et al., "Achieving the Health Millennium Development Goals for South Africa: Challenges and Priorities," *Lancet* 374, no. 9,694 (2009): 1023–31.

62. Craig Timberg, "S. Africans with AIDS See Ray of Hope: Drugs Begin to Help the Few Poor Patients Who Can Get Them," *Washington Post Foreign Service*, November 30, 2004.

63. *South African Health Review 2007* (Durban: Health Systems Trust, 2007), 223–36.

64. Natalie Leon and Ray Mabope, "Private Health Sector," in *South African Health Review 2005*, ed. Petrida Ijumba and Peter Barron (Durban: Health Systems Trust, 2005), 33.

65. Petrida Ijumba et al., "Access to Antiretroviral Therapy," in *South African Health Review, 2003/2004* (Durban: Health Systems Trust, 2003), 334.

66. Julian Meldrum and Theo Smart, "South African HIV Treatment to Depend on Generic Drugs," *Aidsmap.com*, July 8, 2003.

67. Viviane Brunne, "Public-Private Partnerships as a Strategy against HIV/AIDS in South Africa: The Influence of Historical Legacies," *African Journal of AIDS Research* 8, no. 3 (2009): 339–48.

68. On the discussion of the corporate response to AIDS in South Africa, see David Dickinson, "Corporate South Africa's Response to HIV/AIDS: Why So Slow?," *Journal of Southern African Studies* 30, no. 3 (2004): 627–50; Jeremy Seekings and Nicoli Nattrass, "State-Business Relations and Pro-poor Growth in South Africa," *Journal of International Development* 23, no. 3 (2011): 338–57.

69. *Stop Stockouts: Stock Outs in South Africa—a National Crisis* (2013).

70. Nathan Geffen, *Debunking Delusions: The Inside Story of the Treatment Action Campaign* (Johannesburg: Jacana Media, 2010), 135–36.

71. See Kerry Cullinan and Anso Thom, eds., *The Virus, Vitamins & Vegetables: The South African HIV/AIDS Mystery* (Johannesburg: Jacana Media, 2009), 104–6.

72. *Operational Plan for Comprehensive* HIV *and* AIDS *Care, Management and Treatment for South Africa* (Pretoria: Ministry of Health, 2003), 79–86.

73. Lucky Mazibuko, "AIDS Body in Deep Financial Trouble," *Sowetan*, October 12, 2004; Lucky Mazibuko, "Scandalous Shenanigans," *Sowetan*, October 12, 2004.

74. See, for instance, Namhla Tshisela, "12 Years with HIV, Getting Married," *Sowetan*, November 30, 2010; Ayanda Mkhwanazi, "Concern over Theft of ARVs," *Health-e News*, April 4, 2011.

75. Kanya Ndaki, "Traditional Alternatives?," in Cullinan and Thom, *The Virus*, 145.

76. "Activists Launch Pan-African Drive to Demand Treatment," *U.N. Wire*, August 23, 2002.

77. Jo-Anne Richards, "The Agitator: Zackie Achmat," *Vanity Fair*, July 2007.

78. For the history of TAC's activism and its strategy of using the human rights approach and litigation as a principal strategy, see, for instance, Gaffen, *Debunking Delusions*.

79. Andrew Feinstein, *After the Party: A Personal and Political Journey inside the ANC* (Johannesburg: Jonathan Ball, 2007), 113.

80. Sue Valentine, "TAC Appeals to AIDS Conference," *Health-e News*, July 14, 2004.

81. Roberts, *Fit to Govern*, 213–14.

82. Anthony Brink, *In the International Criminal Court at The Hague Criminal Complaint against Abdulrazack "Zackie" Achmat* (Cape Town: Treatment Information Group, 2007).

83. Kerry Cullinan, "Government's Strange Bedfellows," in Cullinan and Thom, *The Virus*, 96.

84. Janine Stephen, "Saints and Sinners: The Treatment Action Campaign," in Cullinan and Thom, *The Virus*, 164.

85. Krista Johnson, "Framing AIDS Mobilization and Human Rights in Post-apartheid South Africa," *Perspectives on Politics* 4, no. 4 (2006): 663–70.

86. Pieter Fourie, *The Political Management of* HIV *and* AIDS *in South Africa: One Burden Too Many?* (Basingstoke: Palgrave Macmillan, 2006), 119.

87. See, for instance, Steven Robins, "Long Live Zackie, Long Live: AIDS Activism, Science and Citizenship after Apartheid," *Journal of Southern African Studies* 30, no. 3 (2004): 651–72; Steven Friedman and Shauna Mottiar, "A Rewarding Engagement? The Treatment Action Campaign and the Politics of HIV/AIDS," *Politics & Society* 33, no. 4 (2005): 511–65.

88. Mark Heywood, "Civil Society and Uncivil Government: The Treatment Action Campaign (TAC) versus Thabo Mbeki, 1998–2008," in *Mbeki and After: Reflections on the Legacy of Thabo Mbeki*, ed. Daryl Glaser (Johannesburg: Wits University Press, 2010), 128–62.

89. Fourie, *The Political Management*, 109.

90. For a general discussion, see Nhlanhla Ndlovu and Daswa Rabelani, "Review of Progress and Expenditure on the Comprehensive Plan for HIV and AIDS for South Africa," *South African Journal of Economics* 76, supplement 1 (2008): 34–51.

91. *The HIV & AIDS and STI Strategic Plan for South Africa, 2007–2011* (Pretoria: Department of Health, 2007).

92. "South African President Mbeki Criticizes UN AIDS Fund Grant," available at http://www.thebody.com/content/policy/art20730.html.

93. Virginia van der Vliet, "South Africa Divided against AIDS," in *AIDS and South Africa: The Social Expression of a Pandemic*, ed. Kyle D. Kauffman and David L. Lindauer (New York: Palgrave Macmillan, 2004), 79.

94. Fatima Hassan, "Country Report: South Africa," in *Missing the Target: A Report on HIV/AIDS Treatment Access from the Frontlines* (Cape Town: International Treatment Preparedness Coalition, 2005), 80–81.

95. Fatima Hassan, "South Africa: Update on Treatment Delivery," in *Missing the Target: Off Target for 2010: How to Avoid Breaking the Promise of Universal Access* (Cape Town: International Treatment Preparedness Coalition, 2006), 38.

96. See Theo Smart, "PEPFAR Working Closely with South African Government to Support HIV Treatment and Care," *Aidsmap.com*, June 13, 2005.

97. Kerry Cullinan, "SA Minister Wants More Control over U.S. Funds," *Health-e News*, June 12, 2006.

98. See, for instance, speech by Zwelinzima Vavi, COSATU general secretary, at the International Day of Action against Pharmaceutical Company Profiteering.

99. *The Status of Traditional Medicine in Africa and Review of Progress Made on the Implementation of the Plan of Action on the African Union Decade of Traditional Medicine (2001–2010)*, Third Ordinary Session of the African Union Conference of Ministers of Health, April 9–13, 2007; *Plan of Action on the AU Decade of Traditional Medicine: Implementation of the Decision of the Lusaka Summit of the Heads of State and Government*, Second Ordinary Session of the Conference of African Ministers of Health, Gaborone, Botswana, October 10–14, 2005.

100. See Amy S. Patterson and David Ciemenis, "Weak and Ineffective? African States and Recent International AIDS Policies," in *The African State and the AIDS Crisis*, ed. Amy Patterson (Aldershot: Ashgate Publishing, 2005), 182.

101. See, for instance, Jennifer G. Cooke, "South Africa and Global Health: Minding the Home Front First," in *Key Players in Global Health: How Brazil, Russia, India, China, and South Africa Are Influencing the Game*, ed. Katherine Bliss (Washington, D.C.: CSIS, 2010), 41–49.

Conclusion

1. This definition of conceptual power is borrowed from Daniel Carpenter, *Reputation and Power: Organizational Image and Pharmaceutical Regulation at the FDA* (Princeton, NJ: Princeton University Press, 2010), 17.

2. See the models discussed in chapter 1.

3. For such an assertion, see, for instance, Achille Mbembe, *On the Postcolony* (Berkeley: University of California Press, 2001), 75–76.

4. For a discussion about different types of ideas, see Nina Tannenwald, "Ideas and Explanation: Advancing the Theoretical Agenda," *Journal of Cold War Studies* 7, no. 2 (2005): 14–17. For the rationalist tradition, see Judith Goldstein and Robert O. Keohane, eds., *Ideas and Foreign Policy: Beliefs, Institutions, and Political Change* (Ithaca, NY: Cornell University Press, 1993), 13, 16. For a succinct contrast between rationalist and constructivist accounts of ideas, see John Gerard Ruggie, "What Makes the World Hang Together? Neo-utilitarianism and the Social Constructivist Challenge," *International Organization* 52, no. 4 (1998): 865–69.

5. For an explicitly constructivist approach to ideas, see Mark Laffey and Jutta Weldes, "Beyond Belief: Ideas and Symbolic Technologies in the Study of International Relations," *European Journal of International Relations* 3, no. 2 (1997): 193–237.

6. Brian D. Taylor, *Russia's Power Ministries: Coercion and Commerce* (Syracuse, NY: Institute for National Security and Counterterrorism, 2007), 41.

7. An insightful elaboration on the nature of the ideational argument and the formulation of the criteria to which such an argument must conform is in Craig Parsons, *How to Map Arguments in Political Science* (New York: Oxford University Press, 2007), 94–132.

8. For a notable exception, see Vincent Navarro, "Politics and Health: A Neglected Area of Research," *European Journal of Public Health* 18, no. 4 (2008): 354–55.

9. See, for instance, Paul G. Harris and Patricia D. Siplon, eds., *The Global Politics of AIDS* (Boulder, CO: Lynne Reiner, 2007).

10. For an example, see Simon Rushton and Owain David Williams, "Frames, Paradigms and Power: Global Health Policy-Making under Neoliberalism," *Global Society* 26, no. 2 (2012): 147–67.

11. Emanuel Adler and Vincent Pouliot, eds., *International Practices* (Cambridge: Cambridge University Press, 2011), 6–10.

12. For an excellent edited volume that examines African HIV/AIDS politics from the perspective of the African states' efficiency and capacity and documents various crucial aspects of how the absence of capacity and efficiency debilitated responses to the epidemic at a state level, see Amy Patterson, ed., *The African State and the AIDS Crisis* (Aldershot: Ashgate Publishing, 2005).

13. On the key characteristics of harm reduction versus a punitive approach, see Tuukka Tammi and Toivo Hurme, "How the Harm Reduction Movement Contrasts Itself against Punitive Prohibition," *International Journal of Drug Policy* 18, no. 2 (2007): 86.

14. For the ongoing debate, see Saul Takahashi, "Drug Control, Human Rights, and the Right to the Highest Attainable Standard of Health: By No Means Straightforward Issues," *Human Rights Quarterly* 31, no. 3 (2009): 748–76; Craig Reinarman, "Public Health

and Human Rights: The Virtues of Ambiguity," *International Journal of Drug Policy* 15, no. 4 (2004): 239–41; Neil Hunt, "Public Health or Human Rights: What Comes First?," *International Journal of Drug Policy* 15, no. 4 (2004): 231–37.

15. Kanya Ndaki, "Traditional Alternatives?," in *The Virus, Vitamins & Vegetables: The South African HIV/AIDS Mystery*, ed. Kerry Cullinan and Anso Thom (Johannesburg: Jacana Media, 2009), 143–45.

INDEX